AF807030

# Shoulder Instability Across the Life Span

Andreas B. Imhoff • Felix H. Savoie III
Editors

# Shoulder Instability Across the Life Span

Springer

INTERNATIONAL SOCIETY OF ARTHROSCOPY, KNEE SURGERY & ORTHOPAEDIC SPORTS MEDICINE • 1995 •

*Editors*
Andreas B. Imhoff
Department of Orthopaedic
Sports Medicine
Technical University of Munich (TUM)
Munich
Germany

Felix H. Savoie III
Department of Orthopaedics
Tulane University School of Medicine
Department of Orthopaedics
New Orleans
Louisiana
USA

ISBN 978-3-662-54076-3 ISBN 978-3-662-54077-0 (eBook)
DOI 10.1007/978-3-662-54077-0

Library of Congress Control Number: 2017938119

© ISAKOS 2017
This work is subject to copyright. All rights are reserved by the Publisher, whether the whole or part of the material is concerned, specifically the rights of translation, reprinting, reuse of illustrations, recitation, broadcasting, reproduction on microfilms or in any other physical way, and transmission or information storage and retrieval, electronic adaptation, computer software, or by similar or dissimilar methodology now known or hereafter developed.
The use of general descriptive names, registered names, trademarks, service marks, etc. in this publication does not imply, even in the absence of a specific statement, that such names are exempt from the relevant protective laws and regulations and therefore free for general use.
The publisher, the authors and the editors are safe to assume that the advice and information in this book are believed to be true and accurate at the date of publication. Neither the publisher nor the authors or the editors give a warranty, express or implied, with respect to the material contained herein or for any errors or omissions that may have been made. The publisher remains neutral with regard to jurisdictional claims in published maps and institutional affiliations.

Printed on acid-free paper

This Springer imprint is published by Springer Nature
The registered company is Springer-Verlag GmbH Germany
The registered company address is: Heidelberger Platz 3, 14197 Berlin, Germany

# Contents


**Part I The Young Patient with Shoulder Instability (Age <20)**

1 **Overview of the Spectrum of Instability in the Very Young: Evolving Concepts** . . . . . . . . . . . . . . . . . . . . . . 3
A.B. Imhoff, K. Beitzel, and A. Voss

2 **Classification of Glenohumeral Instability: A Proposed Modification of the FEDS System** . . . . . . . . . . . . . . . 7
Kevin P. Shea

3 **Genetics of the Unstable Shoulder** . . . . . . . . . . . . . . . . . . . . . . . . 15
Carina Cohen, Paulo S. Belangero, Benno Ejnisman, and Mariana F. Leal

4 **Multidirectional Instability/Hyperlaxity of the Glenohumeral Joint** . . . . . . . . . . . . . . . . . . . . . . . . . . . . . . . . 21
Felix H. Savoie, Enrique Salas, and Michael O'Brien

5 **Posterior Shoulder Instability in the Young Patient** . . . . . . . . . . 35
Diana C. Patterson and Leesa M. Galatz

6 **Management of Acute Shoulder Instability: Conservative Treatment** . . . . . . . . . . . . . . . . . . . . . . . . . . . . . . . . 49
Rebecca A. Carr and Geoffrey D. Abrams

7 **Arthroscopic Repair for Initial Anterior Dislocation** . . . . . . . . . 57
Robert A. Arciero and Andreas Voss

8 **Management of Acute Shoulder Instability: The Combined Lax Shoulder with Added Acute Trauma** . . . . . 65
S.C. Petterson, A.M. Green, and Kevin D. Plancher

9 **Stabilization Options in the Adolescent: Open Bankart Repair** . . . . . . . . . . . . . . . . . . . . . . . . . . . . . . . . . . 73
Stephen C. Weber

**Part II The Young Athletic High Risk Patient with Shoulder Instability (Age 18–30)**

10 **Spectrum of Instability in the Athletic Young Adult** . . . . . . . . . . 81
K. Beitzel, A.B. Imhoff, and A. Voss

**11 Overview of Evaluation and Management of the Unstable Shoulder With and Without Bone Loss: Definition, Measurement, and Guidelines on Treatment** ..... 83
Eiji Itoi, Nobuyuki Yamamoto, Taku Hatta, and Jun Kawakami

**12 Arthroscopic Soft Tissue Repair: Bankart Repair and Remplissage Procedure** ..... 93
Jiwu Chen

**13 Modified Open Bankart Repair and Capsular Shift for Recurrent Traumatic Anterior Shoulder Instability** ..... 103
Robert A. Arciero and Felix Dyrna

**14 Humeral Avulsion of the Glenohumeral Ligaments (HAGL) in Shoulder Instability** ..... 109
Mark Ferguson

**15 Open Coracoid Transfer: Indications, Technique, and Results** ..... 115
Giovanni Di Giacomo and Mark Ferguson

**16 Arthroscopic Latarjet: Technique and Results** ..... 127
Emilio Calvo and María Valencia-Mora

**17 Prevention of Complications of Bone Block Procedures: Latarjet** ..... 137
Kevin D. Plancher, Allison M. Green, Margaret A. Harvey, and Stephanie C. Petterson

**18 Posterior Instability of the Shoulder** ..... 143
Blandine Marion, André Thès, and Philippe Hardy

**19 Arthroscopic Repair of Extended Labral Tears After a Traumatic Shoulder Dislocation** ..... 169
Felix Dyrna, Jessica DiVenere, and Augustus D. Mazzocca

**Part III Instability in the Middle Ages (Age 25–50)**

**20 Spectrum of Instability in the Middle-Age Range** ..... 179
A.B. Imhoff, K. Beitzel, and A. Voss

**21 The Association of Bankart and Rotator Cuff Tear in Patients Aged 25–50** ..... 183
Francesco Franceschi, Edoardo Franceschetti, and Enrique Alberto Salas

**22 SLAP** ..... 187
Carina Cohen, Bernardo Terra, Benno Ejnisman, Dan Guttmann, and Andreas Voss

**23 Biceps Injuries: What to Do and Where?** ..... 203
Stephen C. Weber

**24 The Unstable and Painful Long Head of the Biceps** . . . . . . . . . 211
Juan P. Previgliano and Guillermo Arce

**25 Subscapularis Tears and Instability** . . . . . . . . . . . . . . . . . . . . . . 217
Geoffrey D. Abrams

**26 Cartilage Defects** . . . . . . . . . . . . . . . . . . . . . . . . . . . . . . . . . . . . 227
Julian Mehl and Knut Beitzel

**Part IV Instability in the "Older" Patient (Age >50)**

**27 Spectrum of Instability in the Older Patient** . . . . . . . . . . . . . . . 239
A.B. Imhoff, K. Beitzel, and A. Voss

**28 Acute RCT as a Part of Dislocation** . . . . . . . . . . . . . . . . . . . . . . . 243
Francesco Franceschi, Edoardo Franceschetti, and Enrique Alberto Salas

**29 Acute Dislocation Superimposed on Chronic RCT** . . . . . . . . . . 247
Mike H. Baums

**30 Dislocation Arthropathy of the Shoulder** . . . . . . . . . . . . . . . . . . 251
María Valencia and Emilio Calvo

**Part V Miscellaneous Instability Topics in the Various Ages**

**31 Glenoid Fracture** . . . . . . . . . . . . . . . . . . . . . . . . . . . . . . . . . . . . . 261
Jean Michel Hovsepian, Felix Dyrna, and Knut Beitzel

**32 Locked Posterior Shoulder Dislocation (LPSD)** . . . . . . . . . . . . . 269
J. Pogorzelski and A.B. Imhoff

**33 Chronic Locked Anterior and Posterior Dislocations** . . . . . . . . 277
Felix H. Savoie and Michael O'Brien

**34 Brachial Plexus Injuries and Rotator Cuff Tears with Dislocations** . . . . . . . . . . . . . . . . . . . . . . . . . . . . . . . . . . . . 283
Kevin D. Plancher, Joseph Ajdinovich, and Stephanie C. Petterson

**Part VI Complications**

**35 Complications After Instability Surgery** . . . . . . . . . . . . . . . . . . 291
Andrew J. Sheean and Stephen S. Burkhart

**Index** . . . . . . . . . . . . . . . . . . . . . . . . . . . . . . . . . . . . . . . . . . . . . . 299

# Part I

# The Young Patient with Shoulder Instability (Age <20)

# 1 Overview of the Spectrum of Instability in the Very Young: Evolving Concepts

A.B. Imhoff, K. Beitzel, and A. Voss

## Content

References .................................................................. 4

To encounter the challenges of shoulder instability in a population younger than 20 years old, it is important to distinguish between the skeletally mature and immature population. It has been shown that because of the growing skeletally immature patient with open physes, traumatic shoulder events resulting in a shoulder dislocation are relatively rare. One of the first studies by Rowe investigating 500 shoulder dislocations found that 20% of these dislocations occurred to patients at the age between 10 and 20 but only about 2% to patients younger than 10 years [15]. Therefore, these pediatric traumas more often result in humeral physeal or metaphyseal fractures. In addition the younger patient population is showing a higher recurrence rate after first-time traumatic shoulder dislocation with a rate up to 100% in patients younger than 10 [15] and 60–94% between 10 and 20 years of age [5, 7, 15]. Children between 14 and 18 years of age are 24 times more likely to experience recurrent instability compared to infants aged 13 years and less, with a 14 times more likelihood of recurrent instability with a closed physis compared with those with an open physis [12]. There are several factors reported which may explain the high recurrence rate in this collective: (1) structural age-related factors such as a higher composition of collagen type III fibers in the glenohumeral capsule [18], (2) anatomical-related factors like a more lateral insertion of the capsules on the glenoid [14], or (3) the severity of impact during

A.B. Imhoff (✉) • K. Beitzel • A. Voss
Department of Orthopaedic Sports Medicine, Technical University of Munich (TUM), Munich, Germany
e-mail: Imhoff@tum.de

© ISAKOS 2017
A.B. Imhoff, F.H. Savoie III (eds.), *Shoulder Instability Across the Life Span*, DOI 10.1007/978-3-662-54077-0_1

first-time traumatic shoulder dislocation with and without bony deficiency [9]. For these patients, treatment options are still debatable. Whether a conservative or an operative treatment is the best option has not finally been shown, due to the lack of differentiation between skeletally mature and immature patients. Most of the studies refer to an adolescent population, and some propose a surgical procedure due to the mentioned high recurrence rate. But each of these cases has to be considered individually, and factors like activity level, sports, and general conditions have to be taken into account before proposing a treatment option.

Another aspect that has to be considered in these young patients is the occurrence of hyperlaxity with joint hypermobility. The incidence in the skeletal immature population is estimated to be between 4% and 13% and not associated with soft tissue disease like the Ehlers-Danlos or Marfan syndrome [2, 19]. Among these individuals, the condition of shoulder hyperlaxity is somewhat higher in women with poor muscular development and adolescent overhead athletes, due to the activity demanding with increased flexibility and range of motion [8, 13]. These patients are able to maintain their stability by a balancing act of dynamic muscular compensation. However, these patients can suffer from a traumatic shoulder event interrupting this balancing act with a consequently structural damage, resulting in unidirectional shoulder instability [17]. Most of the time though, this young population with an increased laxity experiences several subluxations resulting in an elongation of the static shoulder stabilizing structures [16]. This pathological change between static bony and capsulo-labral anatomy and dynamic muscular stabilizers leads to a symptomatic multidirectional instability (MDI), an atraumatic instability in two or more directions [1, 17]. The recent literature reveals a variation of definitions of MDI, which makes the classification difficult, leading to a high variation of MDI diagnoses [10]. Even though there is limited data particularly regarding children and adolescents, the incidence of MDI is estimated to be approximately 10% because of increased capsular laxity associated with youth and seems to be even higher in overhead athletes [6]. Most of the recent literature proposed a conservative treatment in these atraumatic hyperlax shoulder instabilities, expecting a decline of symptoms through aging and maturation. The treatment consists of a specific program for muscular control [3]. If conservative treatment fails, these patients may benefit from surgical stabilization. The arthroscopic techniques nowadays provide similar results to the traditional used open capsular shift procedures [4, 11].

There is still a high demand for clinical studies to investigate the differences among this young population, especially the differences in skeletal mature and immature patients. The subsequent chapters should help and provide further information on how to treat these patients in the context of traumatic and atraumatic instability as well as hyperlaxity.

## References


1. Alpert JM, Verma N, Wysocki R, Yanke AB, Romeo AA. Arthroscopic treatment of multidirectional shoulder instability with minimum 270 degrees labral repair: minimum 2-year follow-up. Arthroscopy. 2008;24(6):704–11. doi:10.1016/j.arthro.2008.01.008.
2. Biro F, Gewanter HL, Baum J. The hypermobility syndrome. Pediatrics. 1983;72(5):701–6.
3. Burkhead Jr WZ, Rockwood Jr CA. Treatment of instability of the shoulder with an exercise program. J Bone Joint Surg Am. 1992;74(6):890–6.
4. Chalmers PN, Mascarenhas R, Leroux T, Sayegh ET, Verma NN, Cole BJ, Romeo AA. Do arthroscopic and open stabilization techniques restore equivalent stability to the shoulder in the setting of anterior glenohumeral instability? a systematic review of overlapping meta-analyses. Arthroscopy. 2015;31(2):355–63. doi:10.1016/j.arthro.2014.07.008.
5. Deitch J, Mehlman CT, Foad SL, Obbehat A, Mallory M. Traumatic anterior shoulder dislocation in adolescents. Am J Sports Med. 2003;31(5):758–63.
6. Good CR, MacGillivray JD. Traumatic shoulder dislocation in the adolescent athlete: advances in surgical treatment. Curr Opin Pediatr. 2005;17(1):25–9.
7. Hovelius L, Olofsson A, Sandstrom B, Augustini BG, Krantz L, Fredin H, Tillander B, Skoglund U, Salomonsson B, Nowak J, Sennerby U. Nonoperative treatment of primary anterior shoulder dislocation in patients forty years of age and younger. a prospective twenty-five-year follow-up. J Bone Joint Surg Am. 2008;90(5):945–52. doi:10.2106/JBJS.G.00070.

8. Jansson A, Saartok T, Werner S, Renstrom P. Evaluation of general joint laxity, shoulder laxity and mobility in competitive swimmers during growth and in normal controls. Scand J Med Sci Sports. 2005;15(3):169–76. doi:10.1111/j.1600-0838.2004.00417.x.
9. Lee TQ, Dettling J, Sandusky MD, McMahon PJ. Age related biomechanical properties of the glenoid-anterior band of the inferior glenohumeral ligament-humerus complex. Clin Biomech (Bristol, Avon). 1999;14(7):471–6.
10. Longo UG, Rizzello G, Loppini M, Locher J, Buchmann S, Maffulli N, Denaro V. Multidirectional instability of the shoulder: a systematic review. Arthroscopy. 2015;31(12):2431–43. doi:10.1016/j.arthro.2015.06.006.
11. Milewski MD, Nissen CW. Pediatric and adolescent shoulder instability. Clin Sports Med. 2013;32(4):761–79. doi:10.1016/j.csm.2013.07.010.
12. Olds M, Donaldson K, Ellis R, Kersten P. In children 18 years and under, what promotes recurrent shoulder instability after traumatic anterior shoulder dislocation? A systematic review and meta-analysis of risk factors. Br J Sports Med. 2015; doi:10.1136/bjsports-2015-095149.
13. Perry J. Anatomy and biomechanics of the shoulder in throwing, swimming, gymnastics, and tennis. Clin Sports Med. 1983;2(2):247–70.
14. Rockwood CA, Matsen FA. The shoulder. 4th ed. Philadelphia: Saunders/Elsevier; 2009.
15. Rowe CR. Prognosis in dislocations of the shoulder. J Bone Joint Surg Am. 1956;38-A(5):957–77.
16. Urayama M, Itoi E, Sashi R, Minagawa H, Sato K. Capsular elongation in shoulders with recurrent anterior dislocation. Quantitative assessment with magnetic resonance arthrography. Am J Sports Med. 2003;31(1):64–7.
17. Vavken P, Tepolt FA, Kocher MS. Open inferior capsular shift for multidirectional shoulder instability in adolescents with generalized ligamentous hyperlaxity or Ehlers-Danlos syndrome. J Shoulder Elb Surg. 2016;25(6):907–12. doi:10.1016/j.jse.2015.10.010.
18. Walton J, Paxinos A, Tzannes A, Callanan M, Hayes K, Murrell GA. The unstable shoulder in the adolescent athlete. Am J Sports Med. 2002;30(5):758–67.
19. Wichman M, Snyder S. Arthroscopic capsular plication for multidirectional instability of the shoulder. Oper Tech Sports Med. 1997;5:238–43.

# Classification of Glenohumeral Instability: A Proposed Modification of the FEDS System

2

Kevin P. Shea

## Contents

2.1 **Introduction** 7

2.2 **Previous Shoulder Instability Classification** 7

2.3 **The FEDS System** 9

2.4 **Deficiencies of the FEDS System** 9

2.5 **The Modified FEDS System** 11

2.6 **Future Directions** 12

**References** 13

K.P. Shea, MD
Division of Sports Medicine and Shoulder Surgery, University of Connecticut School of Medicine, 263 Avenue Farmington, Farmington, CT 06034-4038, USA
e-mail: Shea@uchc.edu

## 2.1 Introduction

Classification systems have been found to be very useful in many areas of medicine. Once a system is formulated and validated, it can guide the physician to select an appropriate treatment leading to better outcome based on the experience of others. In a research setting, using a classification system can be extremely helpful, in particular, for multicenter research, to ensure that investigators at different centers are looking at the same type of condition or injury. The AO systems of fracture classification are the most widely recognized examples in orthopedic surgery.

While shoulder instability is a very common orthopedic condition, a widely recognized classification system is not yet available. Developing comprehensive and easily used classification system for shoulder instability would be useful to guide research in surgical outcomes for the various types of shoulder instability. In this chapter, historical classifications of shoulder instability will be reviewed, and a new classification system will be proposed based upon these previous systems.

## 2.2 Previous Shoulder Instability Classification

Shoulder dislocations occur more frequently than any other joint in the human body. Shoulder dislocations appear in Egyptian murals as early as

© ISAKOS 2017
A.B. Imhoff, F.H. Savoie III (eds.), *Shoulder Instability Across the Life Span*,
DOI 10.1007/978-3-662-54077-0_2

3000 BC. Likely, other ancient people also suffered from recurrent shoulder instability as well. Hippocrates described two types of shoulder instability, those resulting from injuries and those that loose-jointed people could produce "at will," formulating the first classification of shoulder instability [1]. It is not known whether or not he used this classification system to determine who was treated with the hot irons in the axilla, the first known surgical treatment for instability. Very little progress was made in the treatment of shoulder instability until Lister published his work on aseptic surgical technique, leading to the beginnings of modern surgery [2].

Codman [3] recognized seven causes of recurrent shoulder instability (initially described by Speed [4]):

1. Defect in the humeral head acquired at the first dislocation
2. Defect in the glenoid-acquired fracture of the edge
3. Rupture of the insertions of the external rotators of the head of the humerus
4. Avulsion of the tuberosities with/without rupture of the rotators
5. Detachment of capsule from the anterior lip of the glenoid
6. Enlarged joint from relaxed capsule following tears which have been given insufficient time for strong cicatrization or repeated stretching without tears
7. Failure of neuromuscular cooperation

It was Codman's belief that the treatment of recurrent instability, almost always anterior, should address the pathologic lesion. This is likely the first classification system that provided some basis for guiding operative treatment of shoulder instability.

DePalma [5] confirmed Codman's various pathologic findings as anatomic causes of recurrent shoulder instability. He was one of the first to differentiate between anterior and posterior shoulder subluxations and dislocation. He also described anterior pouch redundancy and hypermobility of the shoulder as additional pathologies that resulted in recurrent shoulder instability.

Rowe published the next comprehensive classification of shoulder instability in which there were five categories of shoulder instability and six causative lesions [6].

| Type of shoulder instability | Causative lesion |
|---|---|
| Traumatic | Capsule avulsion (Bankart lesion) |
| Atraumatic | Capsule excessive laxity |
| Transient ("dead arm syndrome") | Bone Hill-Sachs lesion |
| Voluntary | Bone-fractured glenoid rim |
| Involuntary chronic laxity, (multidirectional) | Glenoid tilt |
| | Muscle rupture (rotator cuff) |

He reasoned that there was no one "essential lesion" of shoulder instability; the treatment of shoulder instability addresses the anatomic lesion.

Neer [7] classified anterior shoulder instability into three categories, based on the mechanism of the initial instability event: (1) atraumatic, including patients with generalized joint laxity; (2) traumatic, one major injury resulting in a dislocation; and (3) acquired, patients with repeated microtrauma including throwers, swimmers, etc. He advised exercise for groups 1 and 2, immobilization and surgery if recurrences continue, and inferior capsular shift for group 3. His classification did not specifically address specific anatomic lesions.

Gerber and Nyffeler [8] classified shoulder instability as static or dynamic. Superior static instability was attributed to massive rotator cuff tears. Static posterior instability was due to progressive static subluxation, usually associated with glenoid dysplasia or degenerative joint disease. Inferior subluxation was usually neurologic or luxatio erecta.

Dynamic instabilities were classified according to direction including multidirectional, presence or absence of hyperlaxity, and involuntary versus three types of voluntary dislocations. They included locked anterior and posterior dislocations in the dynamic group.

The treatment of the instability was directed at the type of pathology.

Despite the common occurrence of recurrent shoulder instability, no single classification system has been adopted by the orthopedic community.

## 2.3 The FEDS System

Kuhn [10, 11] introduced the FEDS classification of shoulder instability to address the inconsistencies in defining shoulder instability. He recognized that most systems were procedure based and not condition based. Additionally, the many terms used to describe instability, e.g., voluntary, multidirectional, traumatic, bidirectional, etc., were poorly defined and thus made it difficult to directly compare the results of many published studies. As an example, in one of the first reports on multidirectional instability, Neer and Foster included several different patterns of shoulder instability under the term "multidirectional": the common theme was that he treated every type with an anterior-inferior shift.

From the outset, he reasoned that the term "instability" needed to be defined. After a review of the literature, he concluded that instability required *both* discomfort and a feeling of looseness, slipping, or the shoulder "going out" of joint. He then performed a systematic review of the orthopedic literature to identify criteria used by previous authors to define types of shoulder instability. Etiology, direction, severity, and frequency (all define below) were the four most commonly used features. He then used this information to develop the FEDS system.

*Frequency* was felt to be an indirect measure of the severity of the pathology and was divided into three categories: *solitary,* one episode of instability; *occasional,* two to five episodes; and *frequent,* more than five episodes. The difference between occasional and frequent is somewhat arbitrary.

*Etiology* was divided between those with a *traumatic* etiology and those who did not have a specific event that led to their instability (*atraumatic*). Athletes with pain with overhead activities, but no feeling of slipping, were not included as the author felt that they did not have true instability by their definition.

*Direction* was defined as the direction of the patient's most severe symptoms (*anterior, inferior, posterior*). If the patient could not tell the physician which direction was most symptomatic, the physician was to use common provocative examination tests, i.e., apprehension test, sulcus sign, and jerk test, to determine the most symptomatic direction of instability. They purposely did not include the term "multidirectional" in the classification because of the confusing and often contradictory descriptions of this entity in the literature.

*Severity* was divided into *subluxations* and *dislocations* depending on whether the shoulder auto-reduced or required a maneuver to reduce it.

The advantages of the system are obvious. The FEDS system required data only from a history and physical examination to classify the patient's instability type. It has been shown to have content validity and is highly reliable for classifying glenohumeral instability [10, 11]. The classification of instability is immediately identified without additional imaging. For the most part, the classifications follow the outline as set forth in ICD-10, making the system also very useful for coding and billing purposes as well.

## 2.4 Deficiencies of the FEDS System

While extremely useful and easy to utilize, classifying a patient's shoulder instability in FEDS system does not classify instability sufficiently to direct appropriate treatment or to allow several researchers at multiple institutions assurance that their patients all have the same type of instability. Consider the three following cases of first-time shoulder dislocations that illustrate this point.

**Case #2.1**

A 17-year-old male suffered a first-time anterior shoulder dislocation when his dominant right arm was hit while shooting on goal in a water polo game. The shoulder did not relocate spontaneously but did relocate with gentle internal rotation once he got out of the pool. The MRI is seen in Fig. 2.1a.

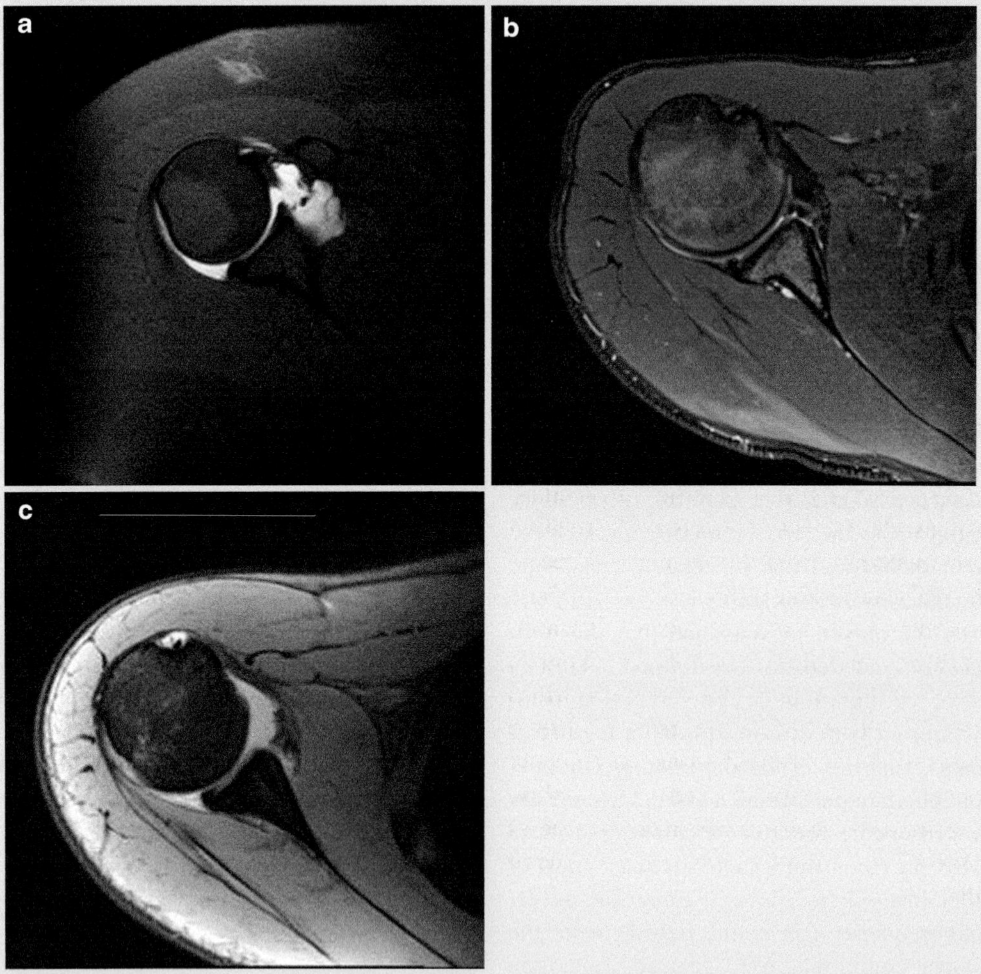


**Fig. 2.1** Selective axial MRI images for three patients with a first-time anterior shoulder dislocation. Image (**a**) does not show any structural lesion. Image (**b**) shows a labral avulsion off of the anterior-inferior glenoid (classic Bankart lesion). Image (**c**) shows a displaced fracture of the anterior inferior glenoid rim. Please see text for more details

**Case #2.2**

A 17-year-old male baseball player sustained a first-time anterior shoulder dislocation diving into second base. The on-site athletic trainer was able to reduce the dislocation on the field. The MRI is seen in Fig. 2.1b.

**Case #2.3**

A 17-year-old male American football player sustained a first-time anterior shoulder dislocation when he was attempting to make a tackle and was upended, landing on his outstretched right arm. He required a reduction in the emergency room. MRI is seen in Fig. 2.1c.

If one uses the FEDS system to classify the instability on these three cases, each would be classified as solitary, traumatic, anterior, and dislocation. However, most orthopedic surgeons who treat shoulder injuries would immediately recognize that the treatment for each case should be very different to achieve a satisfactory outcome. The first case will likely improve with therapy, the second likely requires surgical labral repair, and the third case requires glenoid reconstruction or bone grafting. Based on this type of example, it is the author's opinion that the anatomic lesion responsible for the instability is also very important in classifying shoulder instability similar to Codman and Gerber.

In 2013, we published the first modification of the FEDS system that was developed by Kuhn et al. [12]. In this first revision, we added a category for the anatomic lesion(s) that were identified on imaging that were thought to either be responsible for the instability or required specific treatment in order to prevent recurrence. We also included locked anterior and posterior dislocations as these forms of instability were not included in the FEDS system. While it could be argued that these conditions are not "recurrent," they are treated with a reduction with or without bone grafting or arthroplasty, as opposed to fixed static subluxation, especially posterior, that is recognized as a sequela of long-standing glenohumeral arthritis.

## 2.5 The Modified FEDS System

This chapter is intended to reflect further modification to the FEDS system to arrive at an all-inclusive, easy-to-use instability classification for all types of shoulder instability. We based the classification system on the FEDS with the following modifications (see Table 2.1):

*Frequency* – No changes. The category of two to five episodes of recurrence as compared to greater than five episodes of instability remains somewhat arbitrary, but there is no other literature that clearly demonstrates when the prognosis for recurrence changes.

*Etiology* – We strongly felt that a third category should be added for "acquired instability" to differentiate truly atraumatic onset from those patients who recurrently participate in an activity or sport known to be associated with the development of shoulder instability. "Repetitive microtrauma," another phase used to identify these patients, is frequently identified in patients with recurrent posterior instability and should be included as its own separate category.

*Direction* – Again, we did not feel that changes should be made. Many will argue that "multidirectional" instability should be included as a separate category in this section. We strongly agree with Kuhn that this term is used in a number of ways in the literature leading to confusion. By elimination, the term multidirectional, the system focuses on the direction

**Table 2.1** Modified FEDS classification of shoulder instability

| Frequency | Etiology | Direction | Severity | Anatomic Lesion |
|---|---|---|---|---|
| First time | Traumatic | Anterior | Subluxation | Capsule |
| 2–5 episodes | Atraumatic | Inferior | Dislocations | Labrum |
| >5 episodes | Acquired | Posterior | Locked | Bone-Glenoid |
| | | | Pain | Bone-Humerus |
| | | | | Rotator Cuff Muscle |

The components of the original FEDS system are shown in black. The additions made in the modified system are shown in red. Please see text for details in which the patient has the predominance of symptoms. As the system is further modified, it is likely that those patients with instability in more than one direction will be identified by both directions, with the direction of the preponderance of symptoms being first, i.e., anterior/inferior.

*Severity* – The original FEDS system included only subluxations and dislocations. We felt that two additional categories were needed to completely classify all types of shoulder instability. The recent literature shows that *pain*, and not subluxation/dislocation, is the predominant complaint of patients with recurrent posterior instability [13]. Failure to include pain in this category would eliminate many patients with posterior instability from the classification scheme. Similarly, those with inferior instability often complain of pain and not inferior subluxation [9].

As was noted above, we also included *locked dislocations* in this category to be complete as the dislocation occurs because of some type of instability.

*Anatomic lesion* – In our example above, we illustrated the value in directing treatment by understanding the anatomic injuries that are present in the shoulder instability. In this modification, we include injuries to the labrum, capsule, bone, rotator cuff tendon, and muscle. As most shoulder surgeons are aware, avulsion of the labrum was called the "essential lesion of shoulder instability" by Bankart, and repair of the "Bankart lesion" open, and more recently arthroscopically, was the standard anatomic repair. However, labral injury is not always present, necessitating capsulorrhaphy or other methods to compensate for capsular laxity. Capsular avulsions of the glenohumeral capsule (HAGL and reverse HAGL) are recognized as unique patterns of capsular injury requiring specialized treatment.

Burkhart and De Beers [14] renewed interest in glenoid bone loss and its contributions to recurrent instability. Understanding both the pattern and extent of glenoid bone loss is critical to understanding the appropriate treatment of recurrent shoulder instability. It is likely that this category will be subdivided in the future, and we will more thoroughly understand how much bone loss can still be treated arthroscopically, what can be directly repaired, and what needs to be augmented by either bone transfer or allograft reconstruction.

More recently, there has been a focus on humeral head bone loss, i.e., the Hill-Sachs lesion and the role that it can play in recurrent instability, primarily anterior instability [15]. Further research has discovered that the exact interplay between the humeral head and glenoid bone loss (the glenoid track) is also critical in understanding and correcting some types of shoulder instability.

Scapular dyskinesis (muscle) has been shown to be an important factor in treating posterior shoulder instability [13] and in our opinion should be included as either present or absent in any shoulder instability classification.

Recurrent instability in older patients has been shown to be more a function of rotator cuff tearing and insufficiency [3–8] and, of course, requires separate treatment.

## 2.6 Future Directions

The modified FEDS classification is another step in fully classifying shoulder instability. We recognize that further modifications will be required with time. However, with this latest version, we have included all of the various anatomic lesions that may singly or in combination be responsible for the shoulder instability pattern. It is fully expected that each of these categories will be further subdivided to direct more specific treatment as our understanding of shoulder instability advances, i.e., how much bone loss on the glenoid can present and still successfully treated arthroscopically versus bony repair and/or bone augmentation.

Once the system is completed, validation studies will need to be performed. Until then, we feel that this modified FEDS system can be used as an additional tool to understand, classify, and direct treatment of shoulder instability.

## References

1. Withington ET. Hippocrates. London: Hinemann; 1922.
2. Moseley HF. Recurrent dislocations of the shoulder. Montreal: McGill University Press; 1961.
3. Codman EA. The shoulder. Boston: Thomas Todd Company; 1934. p. 293.
4. Speed K. Recurrent anterior dislocation of the shoulder. Operative cure by bone graft. Surg Gynecol Obstet. 1927;44:468–77.
5. DePalma AF. Surgery of the shoulder. Philadelphia: JB Lippincott; 1950.
6. Rowe CR. The shoulder. New York: Churchill Livingstone, Inc; 1988.
7. Neer CS. Shoulder reconstruction. Philadelphia: WB Saunders Co.; 1990.
8. Gerber C, Nyffeler RW. Classification of glenohumeral joint instability. Clin Orthop Relat Res. 2002;400:65–76.
9. Neer II CS, Foster CR. Inferior capsular shift for involuntary inferior and multidirectional instability of the shoulder. A preliminary report. J Bone Joint Surg. 1980;62-A:897.
10. Kuhn JE. A new classification system for shoulder instability. Br J Sports Med. 2010;44:341–6. doi:10.1136/bjsm.2009.071183.
11. Kuhn JE, Helmer TT, Dunn WP, Throckmorton TW. Development and reliability testing of the frequency, etiology, direction, and severity (FEDS) system for classifying glenohumeral instability. J Shoulder Elb Surg. 2011;20:548–56. doi:10.1016/j.jse.2010.10.027.
12. Shea KP. ISAKOS consensus shoulder instability classification system. In: Arce G, Bak K, Shea KP, et al., editors. Shoulder concepts 2013: consensus and concerns. Berlin/New York: Springer; 2013.
13. DeLong JM, Jiang K, Bradley JP. Posterior instability of the shoulder: a systematic review and meta-analysis of clinical outcomes. Am J Sports Med. 2015;43(7):1805–17. doi:10.1177/0363546515577622.
14. Burkhart SS, De Beer JF. Traumatic glenohumeral bone defects and their relationship to failure of arthroscopic Bankart repairs. Significance of the inverted-pear glenoid and the humeral engaging Hill-Sachs lesion. Arthroscopy. 2000;16:667–94.
15. Provencher MT, Frank RM, LeClere LE, Metzger PD, Bernhardson A, Romeo AA. The Hill-Sachs lesion: diagnosis, classification, and management. JAAOS. 2012;20:242–52.

# Genetics of the Unstable Shoulder

# 3

Carina Cohen, Paulo S. Belangero,
Benno Ejnisman, and Mariana F. Leal

## Content

**References** ........ 18

Although the earliest description of a shoulder dislocation dates back to ancient Egyptian times with other early depictions from the Greeks and Romans, shoulder instability has received much attention and study over the years and has seen important advancements in the understanding and treatment [1]. The use of arthroscopic surgery has allowed the discovery of previously unrecognised pathologic entities, thus improving our understanding of aetiology, residual pain and treatment failures.

The term "instability" constitutes a spectrum of disorders which includes hyperlaxity, subluxation and dislocation. A multitude of classification systems have been suggested, which perhaps in itself reflects the complexity of the problem. Mainly, glenohumeral instability can be classified according to its aetiology, degree, frequency and direction. The classic classification of affected individuals into two groups with traumatic and atraumatic instability is the Thomas and Matsen classification [2] represented by the mnemonics TUBS and AMBRII (Table 3.1); that latter has been supplemented by a further grouping located between these two extremes defined as minor or microinstability that is mainly comprised of overhead athletes and that has been labelled with the acronym AIOS (acquired instability overstress surgery) [3]. However, it should be emphasised that congenital or acquired hyperlaxity, microinstability and traumatic instability can overlap particularly in athletes engaged in overhead sports [4].

C. Cohen (✉) • P.S. Belangero • B. Ejnisman
Universidade Federal de Sao Paulo, SP Brazil, Grupo de Ombro e Cotovelo do Centro de Traumatologia do Esporte- UNIFESP, Sao Paulo, SP, Brazil
e-mail: cacohen18@gmail.com

M.F. Leal
Universidade Federal de Sao Paulo, SP Brazil, Disciplina de Genetica- Depto. de Morfologia e Genetica- UNIFESP, Sao Paulo, SP, Brazil

© ISAKOS 2017
A.B. Imhoff, F.H. Savoie III (eds.), *Shoulder Instability Across the Life Span*,
DOI 10.1007/978-3-662-54077-0_3

**Table 3.1** Thomas and Matsen classification of instability in mnemonics (TUBS and AMBRII) supplemented by AIOS group

| | |
|---|---|
| TUBS | *T*raumatic<br>*U*nidirectional<br>*B*ankart lesion<br>*S*urgery |
| AMBRII | *A*traumatic<br>*M*ultidirectional<br>*B*ilateral<br>*R*ehabilitation<br>*I*nferior capsular shift<br>*I*nterval closure |
| AIOS | *A*cquired<br>*I*nstability<br>*O*verstress<br>*S*urgery |

Anterior shoulder dislocations contribute 96–98 % of all shoulder dislocations. The incidence of first-time anterior shoulder dislocation ranges from 8 to 8.2/100,000 population/year [5]. Shoulder instability is often observed after the initial episode of shoulder dislocation, with a recurrence rate of up to 100 % in young athletes. [6] The anterior glenohumeral joint capsule is affected in 90 % of shoulder dislocations after a traumatic shoulder dislocation [7], with patients presenting a plastic deformation of the capsule, which results in capsular laxity [8]. The anteroinferior (AI) region of the capsule is the site most often injured and was described as the real pathogenic pattern of the shoulder dislocation [8, 9]. Whether the AI capsule is previously a more fragile area propense to plastic deformation or it gets damaged after the traumatic episode is currently unknown.

A genetic propensity may give a contribution to it; therefore, genetic research is expanding increasingly within orthopaedics. There is a growing body of evidence that positive directional selection has a pervasive impact on genetic variation within and between species [10, 11]. A great deal of emphasis has therefore been placed on identifying the population genetic signatures of adaptation, in hopes of revealing the genetic basis of recent phenotypic innovations. Typically this is done by investigating genetic variation at a locus of interest using one or more summary statistics capturing information about allele frequencies [12–16], linkage disequilibrium [17, 18] or haplotypic diversity [19, 20] and asking whether the values of these statistics differ from the expectation under neutrality [21].

A "genetic" approach is now being given at shoulder instability, opening the first steps to genetic studies. Clinical association of recurrent dislocation of the shoulder and of the patella with familial joint laxity also suggests an inherited genetic predisposition [22]. Later, gene variants (COL1A1, COL5A1 and COL12A1 genes) previously associated with ACL injury risk were in large part also associated with joint laxity [23].

The healing process in damaged ligament/capsule is complex and requires deposition and accumulation of newly synthesised structural proteins as well as degradation of old or damaged structures composed mainly of the extracellular matrix (ECM) [24].

The capsule is composed of cellular and fibrous elements. Types 1, 3 and 5 fibrillar collagens are the most common types present in the shoulder capsule [25]. Mutations in genes encoding the collagens have been identified in osteogenesis imperfecta [26] and in most forms of Ehlers–Danlos syndrome (EDS) [27] which present frequent joint dislocations, including dislocations of the shoulder. Thus, alterations in these genes may also play a role in shoulder instability.

The anteroinferior (AI) portion of the glenohumeral capsule of shoulder instability patients commonly exhibits macroscopic alteration such as the capsular deformation that is observed during arthroscopic treatment [8]. Previously, a macroscopic analysis of the collagen fibre bundle architecture in the AI region of the glenohumeral capsule revealed that a system of bundles spirally crossing one another permits the entire capsule to resist tensile and shear loads [28]. Later, Wang et al. suggested there is a reciprocal load-sharing relationship in the capsule, whereby tensile load in either the anterior or superior structures is simultaneously accompanied by laxity in the posterior or inferior portion, respectively. So, the complex structure of the joint capsule would suggest that the capsular cylinder has to be regarded as a functional entity, and this biomechanical concept should be considered for the stabilising effect [8].

Corroborating to these findings, Belangero et al. [29] published the first study to detect collagen gene expression alterations in the glenohumeral capsule of shoulder instability patients compared to controls. The COL1A1 and COL3A1 expression were increased not only in AI portion but in all sites, including anterosuperior (AS) and posterior (P) portions of the capsule that may be indicative of a global biomechanic tissue disorders suggesting that anterior shoulder dislocation might lead to molecular alterations across all the capsule even in patients without multidirectional instability. Moreover, COL1A2 was also upregulated in the AS and P sites of the capsule of shoulder instability patients. Upregulation of these genes or their protein products has been reported in several joint injuries, including injured Achilles tendon [30], anterior cruciate ligament [31, 32] and rotator cuff tear [33, 34].

Collagen type 1 (COL1) is the most prominent protein of the capsule, as well as of ligaments and tendons, and the primary protein responsible for resisting physiological loads for different activities. In turn, collagen type 3 (COL3), with its ability to form extensive cross-links, seems to modulate the growth in the diameter of the collagen fibrils [35]. During joint healing, COL3 is postulated to form the architecture of an early repair construct, which is then infiltrated and replaced with COL1. In tendons, it has been suggested that the ratio of COL1/COL3 may be an indicator of total repair response, with the early increase of COL3 initiating the repair, the later increase of COL1 reflecting maturation and the return to baseline ratio level indicating conclusion of the repair process [36].

We detected an imbalance in the expression ratio of several collagen genes, suggesting that the repair process was still incomplete, particularly in the AI site [29]. These molecular alterations may lead to modifications of collagen fibril structure and of the tissue healing process, as well as to capsular deformation. Therefore, the expression of COL1A1, COL1A2, COL3A1 and COL5A1 may play a role in shoulder instability.

Later Belangero et al. [37] evaluated the expression of transforming growth factor b1 (TGFb1), transforming growth factor bR1 (TGFbR1), lysyl oxidase (LOX), PLOD1 and PLOD2 mRNA in these three sites of the glenohumeral capsule in patients with traumatic anterior shoulder instability and controls.

An increase of TGFb1 accompanies the acute inflammatory phase and appears to act as a signal that modulates the production of matrix macromolecules by fibrogenic cells at the injury site [38]. In the shoulder capsule of patients with adhesive capsulitis, TGFb1 was associated with fibrosis and accumulation of a dense matrix of type 1 and type 3 collagen within the capsule [39, 40]. TGFb1 regulates important collagen-modifying enzymes, such as the lysyl oxidase (LOX) that plays a key role in the maturation of the extracellular matrix and is also essential to maintain the tensile and elastic features of connective tissues [41] and lysyl hydroxylases 1 and 2 (encoded by PLOD1 and PLOD2) [42–44]. In many pathological fibrotic situations, the expression of the cross-linked enzyme LOX and its enzymatic activity are controlled by TGFb1. Additionally, differential variations of TGFb1 were able to induce the LOX activity in an in vitro model of mechanical injury in ligament cells [45].

We found increased PLOD2 expression in the macroscopically injured (anteroinferior) region of the glenohumeral capsule of shoulder instability patients [37]. PLOD2 is a lysyl hydroxylase that hydroxylates the telopeptides [46]. Therefore, the shoulder dislocation episode may lead to PLOD2 upregulation in an attempt to heal the capsule through the cross-linking of the new collagen fibrils by the hydroxyallysine route in the injured tissue. Upregulation of TGFb1, TGFbR1 and PLOD2 seemed to be related to patients with more than two episodes of shoulder dislocation and with longer duration of symptoms especially in the posterior region of the capsule [37]. TGFbR1 is a key element in the regulation of wound healing; therefore, the continuation of symptoms may contribute to activation of the TGFb pathway in the posterior region.

LOX upregulation seemed to occur only in an initial phase of the disease, and gene expression was inversely correlated to the duration of symptoms. It was significantly higher in patients with only one dislocation episode compared to controls and compared to patients with recurrent dislocations. [37] It is generally accepted that the total amount of enzymatic cross-linking is controlled by the expression of LOX. Several previous studies have demonstrated that collagen cross-link formation directly affects the strength of bones, tendons and ligaments [47, 48]. With concomitant collagen upregulation, we should expect LOX upregulation across the capsule. Therefore, the authors suggest that the lack of LOX upregulation in later phase suggests that the new collagen fibrils may have reduced resistance to mechanical stress.

On the other hand, capsule modifications may occur due to physical activity involving the superior member which can lead to biomechanical and structural capsule modifications, such as capsular tightness, especially in the posterior region [49]. Belangero et al. [37] found PLOD2 and TGFb1 were reduced in the posterior portion and PLOD1 was reduced in the anterosuperior portion of the capsule of patients who undertook physical activity involving the upper limbs compared to those who did not. Although additional investigations are still necessary, they hypothesise that these capsule modifications due to physical activity may explain the reduced PLOD2, TGFb1 and PLOD1 expression in the capsule of a subgroup of patients [37].

Therefore, genetics may play an important but still unclear role in shoulder instability represented by this moment by the expression of COL1A1, COL1A2 and COL3A1 and also TGFb1, TGFbR1, LOX and PLOD2 [29, 37]. Whether it corresponds to previously inherited characteristics or the consecutive shoulder dislocations are an adaptation to the traumatic process and sports activities is not clearly known.

Further we believe that in the future, knowing the gene expression profile of patients with shoulder instability can help to identify new risk factors, understand more about genetic inheritance and thus help to avoid mistakes of surgical indication, failure to recognise capsular laxity and underappreciation of technical decisions and missed associated pathology. More high-quality research is required to better understand and characterise this spectrum of conditions so that successful evidence-based information can clarify causal pathways and provide a clue for therapeutic targets.

## References

1. Randelli P, Cucchi D, Butt U. History of shoulder instability surgery. Knee Surg Sports Traumatol Arthrosc. 2016;2(24):305–29.doi:10.1007/s00167-015-3947-3.
2. Thomas SC, Matsen FA. An approach to the repair of avulsion of the glenohumeral ligaments in the management of traumatic anterior glenohumeral instability. J Bone Joint Surg Am. 1989;71:506–13.
3. Castagna A, Nordenson U, Garofalo R, Karlsson J. Minor shoulder instability. Arthroscopy. 2007;23(2):211–5.
4. Lewis A, Kitamura T, Bayley JIL. The classification of shoulder instability: new light through old windows! Curr Orthop. 2004;18:97–108.
5. Kirkley A, Werstine R, Ratjek A, et al. Prospective randomized clinical trial comparing the effectiveness of immediate arthroscopic stabilization versus immobilization and rehabilitation in first traumatic anterior dislocations of the shoulder: long-term evaluation. Arthroscopy. 2005;21:55–63.
6. te Slaa RL, Wijffels MP, Brand R, et al. The prognosis following acute primary glenohumeral dislocation. J Bone Joint Surg. 2004;86:58–64.
7. Goss TP. Anterior glenohumeral instability. Orthope Dics. 1988;11:87–95.
8. Wang VM, Flatow EL. Pathomechanics of acquired shoulder instability: a basic science perspective. J Shoulder Elb Surg. 2005;14:2S–11S.
9. Burkart AC, Debski RE. Anatomy and function of the glenohumeral ligaments in anterior shoulder instability. Clin Orthop. 2002:32.
10. reviewed in Hahn NW. Toward a selection theory of molecular evolution. Evolution. 2008;62(2):255–65.
11. Cutter AD, Payseur BA. Genomic signatures of selection at linked sites: unifying the disparity among species. Nat Rev Genet. 2013;14(4):262–74. doi:10.1038/nrg3425. Epub 2013 Mar 12
12. Tajima F. Statistical method for testing the neutral mutation hypothesis by DNA polymorphism. Genetics. 1989;123(3):585–95.
13. Fu YX, Li WH. Statistical tests of neutrality of mutations. Genetics. 1993;133(3):693–709.
14. Fay JC, Wu CI. Hitchhiking under positive Darwinian selection. Genetics. 2000;155(3):1405–13.
15. Kim Y, Stephan W. Detecting a local signature of genetic hitchhiking along a recombining chromosome. Genetics. 2002;160(2):765–77.
16. Achaz G. Frequency spectrum neutrality tests: one for all and all for one. Genetics. 2009;183(1):249–58.
17. Kelly JK. A test of neutrality based on interlocus associations. Genetics. 1997;146(3):1197–206.
18. Kim Y, Nielsen R. Linkage disequilibrium as a signature of selective sweeps. Genetics. 2004;167(3):1513–24.
19. Sabeti PC et al. Detecting recent positive selection in the human genome from haplotype structure. Nature. 2002;419:832–7. doi:10.1038/nature0114.

20. Voight BF, Kudaravalli S, Wen X, Pritchard JK. A map of recent positive selection in the human genome. PLoS Biol. 2006;4(3):e72. Epub 2006 Mar 7
21. Schrider DR, Mendes FK, Hahn MW, Kern AD. Soft shoulders ahead: spurious signatures of soft and partial selective sweeps result from linked hard sweeps. Genetics. 2015;200(1):267–84.
22. Carter C, Sweetnam R. Recurrent dislocation of the patella and of the shoulder. Their association with familial joint laxity. J Bone Joint Surg Br. 1960;42-R:721–7.
23. Bell RD, Schuktz SJ, WidemanWideman L, Henrich VC. Collagen gene variants previously associated with anterior cruciate ligament injury risk are also associated with joint laxity. Sports Health. 2012;4(4):312–8.
24. Zhou D, Lee HS, Villarreal F, et al. Differential MMP-2 activity of ligament cells under mechanical stretch injury: an in vitro study on human ACL and MCL fibroblasts. J Orthop Res. 2005;23:949–57.
25. Kaltsas DS. Comparative study of the properties of the shoulder joint capsule with those of other joint capsules. Clin Orthop. 1983;(173):20–6.
26. van Dijk FS, Cobben JM, Kariminejad A, et al. Osteogenesis imperfecta: a review with clinical examples. Mol Syndromol. 2011;2:1–20.
27. Pope FM, Burrows NP. Ehlers-Danlos syndrome has varied molecular mechanisms. J Med Genet. 1997;34:400–10.
28. Gohlke F, Essigkrug B, Schmitz F. The pattern of the collagen fiber bundles of the capsule of the glenohumeral joint. J Shoulder Elb Surg. 1994;3:111–28.
29. Belangero PS, Leal MF, Figueiredo EA, et al. Gene expression analysis in patients with traumatic anterior shoulder instability suggests deregulation of collagen genes. J Orthop Res. 2014;32:1311–6.
30. Xu Y, Murrell GA. The basic science of tendinopathy. Clin Orthop. 2008;466:1528–38.
31. Bramono DS, Richmond JC, Weitzel PP, et al. Characterization of transcript levels for matrix molecules and proteases in ruptured human anterior cruciate ligaments. Connect Tissue Res. 2005;46:53–65.
32. Lo IK, Marchuk L, Hart DA, et al. Messenger ribonucleic acid levels in disrupted human anterior cruciate ligaments. Clin Orthop. 2003;(407):249–58.
33. Lo IK, Boorman R, Marchuk L, et al. Matrix molecule mRNA levels in the bursa and rotator cuff of patients with full-thickness rotator cuff tears. Arthroscopy. 2005;21:645–51.
34. Shirachi I, Gotoh M, Mitsui Y, et al. Collagen production at the edge of ruptured rotator cuff tendon is correlated with postoperative cuff integrity. Arthroscopy. 2011;27:1173–9.
35. Birk DE, Mayne R. Localization of collagen types I, III and V during tendon development. Changes in collagen types I and III are correlated with changes in fibril diameter. Eur J Cell Biol. 1997;72:352–61.
36. Robertson CM, Chen CT, Shindle MK, et al. Failed healing of rotator cuff repair correlates with altered collagenase and gelatinase in supraspinatus and subscapularis tendons. Am J Sports Med. 2012;40:1993–2001.
37. Belangero PS, Leal MF, Cohen C, Figueiredo EA, Smith MC, Andreoli CV, de Castro PA, Ejnisman B, Cohen M. Expression analysis of genes involved in collagen cross-linking and its regulation in traumatic anterior shoulder instability. J Orthop Res. 2016;34(3):510–7.
38. Sakai T, Yasuda K, Tohyama H, et al. Effects of combined administration of transforming growth factor-beta1 and epidermal growth factor on properties of the in situ frozen anterior cruciate ligament in rabbits. J Orthop Res. 2002;20:1345–51.
39. Rodeo SA, Hannafin JA, Tom J, et al. Immunolocalization of cytokines and their receptors in adhesive capsulitis of the shoulder. J Orthop Res. 1997;15:427–36.
40. Nago M, Mitsui Y, Gotoh M, et al. Hyaluronan modulates cell proliferation and mRNA expression of adhesion-related procollagens and cytokines in glenohumeral synovial/capsular fibroblasts in adhesive capsulitis. J Orthop Res. 2010;28:726–31.
41. Kagan HM, Li W. Lysyl oxidase: properties, specificity, and biological roles inside and outside of the cell. J Cell Biochem. 2003;88:660–72.
42. Knippenberg M, Helder MN, Doulabi BZ, et al. Differential effects of bone morphogenetic protein-2 and transforming growth factor-beta1 on gene expression of collagen-modifying enzymes in human adipose tissue-derived mesenchymal stem cells. Tissue Eng Part A. 2009;15:2213–25.
43. Remst DF, Blaney Davidson EN, Vitters EL, et al. TGF-ss induces Lysyl hydroxylase 2b in human synovial osteoarthritic fibroblasts through ALK5 signaling. Cell Tissue Res. 2014;355:163–71.
44. Witsch TJ, Turowski P, Sakkas E, et al. Deregulation of the lysyl hydroxylase matrix cross-linking system in experimental and clinical bronchopulmonary dysplasia. Am J Physiol Lung Cell Mol Physiol 2014;306:L246–59.
45. Xie J, Wang C, Huang DY, et al. TGF-beta1 induces the different expressions of lysyl oxidases and matrix metalloproteinases in anterior cruciate ligament and medial collateral ligament fibroblasts after mechanical injury. J Biomech. 2013;46:890–8.
46. van der Slot AJ, Zuurmond AM, Bardoel AF, et al. Identification of PLOD2 as telopeptide lysyl hydroxylase, an important enzyme in fibrosis. J Biol Chem. 2003;278:40967–72.
47. Kato S, Saito M, Funasaki H, et al. Distinctive collagen maturation process in fibroblasts derived from rabbit anterior cruciate ligament, medial collateral ligament, and patellar tendon in vitro. Knee Surg Sports Traumatol Arthrosc. 2013;23:1384–92.
48. Saito M, Marumo K. Collagen cross-links as a determinant of bone quality: a possible explanation for bone fragility in aging, osteoporosis, and diabetes mellitus. Osteoporos Int. 2010;21:195–214.
49. Nakagawa S, Yoneda M, Mizuno N, et al. Influence of posterior capsular tightness on throwing shoulder injury. Knee Surg Sports Traumatol Arthrosc. 2013;21:1598–602.

# Multidirectional Instability/ Hyperlaxity of the Glenohumeral Joint

4

Felix H. Savoie, Enrique Salas, and Michael O'Brien

## Contents

4.1 **Introduction/Literature Review** ............. 22
4.2 **Patient History** ............. 23
4.3 **Physical Examination** ............. 23
4.4 **Radiographic Findings** ............. 24
4.5 **Description of Management Techniques** ............. 25
4.5.1 Nonoperative Technique ............. 25
4.5.2 Indications ............. 25
4.5.3 Contraindications ............. 26
4.6 **Operative Arthroscopic Techniques** ............. 26
4.6.1 Surgical Anatomy and Patho-anatomy ............. 26
4.6.2 Exposure/Setup ............. 26
4.6.3 Specific Instruments/Equipment/ Implants ............. 27
4.6.4 Procedure ............. 27
4.7 **Treatment of the Lax Capsule** ............. 28
4.8 **Treatment of the Torn Capsule and Special Techniques** ............. 31
4.9 **Postoperative Protocols** ............. 32
4.9.1 Wound Closure ............. 32
4.9.2 Postoperative Regimen ............. 32
4.9.3 Avoiding Pitfalls and Complications ............. 32
4.10 **Summary** ............. 33
**References** ............. 33

F.H. Savoie, MD (✉) • M. O'Brien, MD
Department of Orthopaedic Surgery,
Tulane University School of Medicine,
New Orleans, LA, USA
e-mail: fsavoie@tulane.edu

E. Salas
Orthopaedic Sports Medicine,
University of Munich (TUM) Orthopaedic
Sports Medicine, München, Bayern, Germany

**Key Concepts**

1. Laxity of the shoulder is individually specific, with a wide variation. Instability is the pathologic excessive translational movement of the humeral head on the glenoid producing symptoms.
2. The diagnosis of multidirectional instability (MDI) is made by physical examination showing symptomatic subluxation in an anterior and/or posterior direction with associated inferior laxity demonstrated by a positive sulcus sign in adduction, abduction, and external rotation. Hyperlaxity is demonstrated by a positive Gage test.
3. MDI and hyperlaxity should be managed by nonoperative treatment including scapular bracing, taping and rehabilitation, control of inflammation, biofeedback therapy, and integrated rehabilitation prior for at least 3 months prior to any consideration of surgical intervention.
4. Arthroscopy provides the best surgical option in most cases of MDI.

© ISAKOS 2017
A.B. Imhoff, F.H. Savoie III (eds.), *Shoulder Instability Across the Life Span*,
DOI 10.1007/978-3-662-54077-0_4

5. Surgical techniques should center on restoration of the humeral head into the center of the glenoid by decreasing capsular volume by vertical shift of the capsule in a superior direction in both the anterior and posterior shoulder. The goal is to reform the anterior and posterior bands of the inferior glenohumeral ligament complex.
6. The pathologically widened rotator interval should be closed with multiple sutures in order to restore the normal resting tension of the coracohumeral ligament and provide support for the shoulder in adduction.
7. In severe cases of hyperlaxity and MDI (Ehlers-Danlos syndrome patients), allograft reconstruction of the IGHL and CHL may be necessary to restore stability.

## 4.1 Introduction/Literature Review

Multidirectional instability (MDI) of the shoulder is a condition in which the shoulder demonstrates symptomatic laxity in more than one direction, with one of the directions always being inferior. MDI was first described in 1980 by Neer and Foster [1]. They reported on a group of patients that had pain and laxity in the anterior, posterior, and inferior directions. They successfully eliminated the symptoms in most patients using a humeral-based open inferior capsular shift procedure. Savoie described the first arthroscopic treatment of MDI in a pilot study using a modification of the Caspari transglenoid capsular shift technique, and many surgeons have expanded and improved on this original idea of the use of arthroscopy for MDI [2].

Several reports have been published showing excellent results with arthroscopic treatment of the patient with multidirectional instability. Duncan and Savoie [9] presented a 1–3-year postoperative follow-up of a pilot study revealing improvement in all patients treated by an arthroscopic version of the Neer capsular shift. The average postoperative Rowe score was 90 and all rated as "satisfactory" according to the Neer system.

Wichman and Snyder [4] reported results of arthroscopic capsular shift for MDI in 24 patients with an average age of 26 and a minimum follow-up of 2 years. Five patients (21 %) had an "unsatisfactory" rating according to the Neer system. Of the unsatisfactory cases, one patient was in litigation for an MVA, and there were three workers compensation cases.

Treacy and Savoie [3] reported on 25 patients with multidirectional instability of the shoulder who underwent an arthroscopic capsular shift. At a minimum 5-year follow-up, three patients had episodes of subluxation, but none had recurrent dislocation. According to the Neer system, 88 % of the patients had "satisfactory" results.

Gartsman et al. [5] reported on 47 patients who underwent arthroscopic capsular plication for MDI. Ninety-four percent had "good" to "excellent" results at an average follow-up of 35 months. Eighty-five percent of athletes returned to their desired level of participation.

Lyons et al. [8] showed favorable results with an arthroscopic laser-assisted technique in which the rotator interval was plicated with multiple sutures to improve the stability. Twenty-six of 27 shoulders remained stable at 2-year follow-up. Eighty-six percent of athletes returned to their sport at the same level.

McIntyre et al. [6] reported results of arthroscopic capsular shift in MDI patients using a multiple suture technique in both the anterior and posterior capsules with 32-month follow-up. Recurrent instability occurred in one patient (5 %), who was treated successfully with a repeat arthroscopic stabilization. Thirteen athletes (93 %) returned to their previous level of performance.

Hewitt et al. [10] demonstrated favorable techniques and results in a review article of multidirectional instability of the shoulder using a pancapsular plication suture technique.

Tauro and Carter [7] reported preliminary results of a modified arthroscopic capsular shift for anterior and anterior-inferior instability in four patients with a minimum follow-up of 6 months. No patients developed recurrent instability in this short-term follow-up period.

The main areas of controversy in the management of MDI include proper diagnosis, how long a period of preoperative rehabilitation is satisfactory, and choice of surgical technique (open shift vs arthroscopic shift, how to, and the necessity for rotator interval closure) [11].

## 4.2 Patient History

A detailed history is extremely important in evaluating all shoulder patients, but this is especially true for the patient with MDI. The usual patient will be in their teens or twenties. The most common complaint is pain with activities of daily living in the midrange of function. The patient will usually complain of the shoulder popping out of place with minimal activity. The examiner must focus the history on the first asymptomatic subluxation event and whether the patient has always had "loose joints." The second area of questioning is how the first symptomatic subluxation event occurred and the activity level surrounding that event. Athletes may present with pain that began during a specific sporting event that followed an increased training schedule, leading to fatigue of the stabilizing musculature. The level of pain, timing of pain, and chronicity of pain must be recorded. The activity level of the patient and the specific sport (if any) should be recorded as well. Questions should be directed at the patient to determine if there are symptoms of popping, clicking, subluxation, or dislocations. The number of such episodes needs to be determined, as well as the amount of trauma it took to produce the episode. One should note if there has been one or multiple traumatic events, or if the symptoms have developed insidiously. Some patients will also give a history of transient neurological events.

Finally, one should be cognizant that non-shoulder factors may be a part of the problem; the symptomatic patient with MDI presents with pain, especially at night and with overhead activity. The relatively stoic individual or the patient that demonstrates instability on command without hesitation or pain should not be considered surgical candidates.

## 4.3 Physical Examination

The physical exam starts with visual inspection of the patient. Unclothe the shoulder to be able to see the entire arm, upper chest, scapula, and trapezius. Note the position of the scapula at rest. Symptomatic MDI patients present with a protracted shoulder, held in for "support," and are hesitant to move it at all due to coexisting inflammation of the rotator cuff. The entire body should be carefully inspected for laxity. Hyperextension of the elbow, fingers, and knee joints is usually present. Most of these patients will exhibit all nine Beighton criteria for ligamentous laxity.

We usually begin from the ground up, evaluating the looseness of the knee and hip joints. Hip and core strengths are evaluated via the two- and one-legged squat, looking for good posture control and stability.

The next step is to determine the current tracking patterns of the entire shoulder girdle, with a focus on the scapula. The patient is asked to move the arm in flexion, extension, abduction, and adduction within their pain-free arc of motion, while the scapula is observed for maltracking and winging. Almost all of these patients will exhibit significant scapular instability during motion.

Palpate the shoulder for widening of the rotator interval and for swelling of the rotator cuff tendons. Feel for areas of discomfort and spasm. Often in patients with long-standing MDI that have not worked on postural correction, there may be tightness and tenderness in the insertion of the pec minor tendon near the coracoid – a tip to long-standing problems.

Assess shoulder range of motion with the patient supine. Check forward flexion, abduction, IR/ER with the arm at the side, and IR/ER with the shoulder in 90° of abduction. Compare the motion to the contralateral shoulder.

Evaluate the degree and direction of instability. This is often determined both with the patient sitting up and in the supine position. With the patient sitting up, place one hand on the proximal humerus and the other hand on the elbow. Apply a load in the anterior, posterior, and inferior directions. A circumduction maneuver can demonstrate subtle instability and is a good way to start the exam. Note the degree of shoulder movement in each direction. Check for a sulcus sign in neutral rotation and repeat with the arm in external rotation. Check for a sulcus sign with the shoulder in greater than 45° of abduction. Have the patient lay on his or her back. Perform a load and shift test in the anterior and posterior directions in varying degrees of shoulder abduction as in the normal patient the degree of laxity will decrease with increasing degrees of abduction (Cofield test). This can also be performed with the patient on his or her side if the scapula is stabilized. Compare the results to the contralateral side. The Gage test should be performed during these maneuvers to evaluate for hyperlaxity.

Next, evaluate the rotator cuff strength and any pain associated with rotator cuff testing. MDI patients will often develop a rotator cuff tendonitis and exhibit significant pain with manual muscle testing. Preferred tests of the rotator cuff include the Whipple test, supraspinatus stress test, supraspinatus isolation test, external rotation test, and belly press test. The Whipple test is performed in 90° of forward flexion and slight adduction. Have the patient resist a downward pressure. The supraspinatus stress and isolation tests are performed in the scapular plane in 90° of abduction. Have the patient resist a downward pressure with the thumb turned down (SS stress test) and with the thumb turned up (SS isolation test). The supraspinatus stress test will be more painful in patients with posterior superior rotator cuff pathology. The supraspinatus isolation test will be more painful with anterior superior rotator cuff pathology. If the rotator cuff is weak, check for scapular protraction. If there is scapular protraction present and the rotator is weak and painful, check for normalization of shoulder strength with manual scapular stabilization. Next, perform the external rotation test with the arm in slight abduction and 45° of external rotation. Have the patient resist an inward pressure on the hand. The belly press test is performed by placing the hand on the abdomen and maintaining the elbow in front of the body. Have the patient resist an attempt to pull the hand off of the abdomen. Rate the strength as according to the standard manual muscle testing system and determine the level of pain associated with the tests. Compare it to the contralateral side. We believe that most cases of MDI can be managed nonoperatively. The Whipple test will be quite positive for pain, weakness, and buckling in most patients in their normal resting position but will become negative with the scapula manually stabilized in retraction.

Evaluate the cervical spine for motion. Determine if there are any nerve root compression symptoms.

The vascular status of the arm should be evaluated by performing the Adson test, checking the pulse with the arm abducted to 90° and externally rotated to 90°. In many MDI patients this will produce transient vascular compromise and a diminished pulse. Manual scapular retraction will relieve pressure and restore a normal pulse. This is termed positional or postural thoracic outlet syndrome. This variation of the Adson or Leffort's test demonstrates to the patient the etiology of the numbness, tingling, and vascular changes that may occur in this condition due to poor scapular control.

Evaluate the range of motion of the other extremities and check for hyperelasticity of the knees, elbows, and metacarpophalangeal joints. Note any and all joints that exhibit hyperextension and/or hypermobility.

Key points of the physical exam to document are the position of the scapula, the direction and degree of laxity, and the comparative size of the sulcus in adduction, external rotation, and abduction.

## 4.4 Radiographic Findings

Imaging modalities that are most commonly used are plain radiographs and MRI. Plain radiographs are often normal, but should be evaluated for any bony deficiency of the glenoid or humeral head. MRI scans are often employed in the evaluation of the patient with MDI. An MRI with intra-articular contrast is most helpful. The choice of contrast agent depends on the radiologist. If one is able to do so, normal saline is the safest agent to use. A typical MRI finding is an essentially normal shoulder with a large capsular volume.There may be mild tendonitis or tendinosis of the supraspinatus tendon. There will be a large axillary fold. The appearance is that of an upside-down bubble extending inferiorly below the glenoid in the coronal sections. One pathognomonic hallmark of MDI as described by Neer in some of his original thoughts on MDI is bulging of the rotator interval on arthrogram. If there is significant rotator interval laxity, you may be able to see the entire intra-articular portion of the biceps tendon silhouette. The underside of the rotator cuff and rotator interval may have space between them and the biceps tendon in the coronal sections. The axial sections will show capsular laxity in the anterior and posterior sides of the joint usually in the lower sections of the glenoid. In addition we recommend that each treating physician view the scan themselves in order to evaluate for size of labrum, any mild labral degeneration, tears, or malformation. Always try to determine the integrity of the rotator cuff. Evaluate for any cysts within the spinoglenoid notch. While unusually aberrant, check the quality and integrity of the rotator cuff and appearance of the supporting muscles.

## 4.5 Description of Management Techniques

### 4.5.1 Nonoperative Technique

The hallmark of the management of MDI is nonoperative management. If the treating physician considers a surgical repair to be a temporary stabilization to allow the patient to pursue adequate rehabilitation, then the ground can be set for nonoperative management. The principles of an adequate therapy program are centered on the scapular stabilizers, utilizing bracing, taping, and isometric exercises. It is extremely important to stress to the patient, the family, and the therapist that stabilization of the scapula must precede any attempts at rotator cuff strengthening. Starting rotator cuff exercises without stabilizing the scapula through bracing, taping, or manual forces will result in increased irritation and magnification of the pain. The focus of rehabilitation then progresses to the rotator cuff, attempting first to correct abnormal muscle firing patterns, then to improve deficient proprioceptive mechanisms, and finally to restore functional ability. If a patient has been properly educated, has been diligent in the rehabilitation process, and still has persistent symptoms of pain and functional impairment, then he/she is a surgical candidate.

Nonsurgical management is the mainstay of treatment for MDI. This program must be no less than 6 months in duration and include an emphasis on proper scapular control at all times to allow the new motor skill and coordination to become permanent. If this extensive process fails and abnormal firing patterns of the shoulder girdle continue, the patient should decide to discontinue the aggravating activity or progress to surgical intervention.

### 4.5.2 Indications

The symptomatic pattern of the instability should be ascertained prior to surgical treatment. The shoulder may demonstrate laxity in many directions and have symptomatic primary instability in only one direction. One must constantly be aware that laxity does not mean instability. Asymptomatic, normal laxity does not usually need to be surgically addressed.

Indication pitfalls: The primary cause of concern is the decision for surgery: the proper diagnosis is essential, and each patient should have had extensive, proper therapy prior to any indication for surgery. This must include postural correction and integrated rehabilitation. In Neer's original work he recommended a full year of therapy prior to any indication for surgery in the patient with true MDI.

### 4.5.3 Contraindications

There are several contraindications to surgical intervention in the MDI patient. The first is a failure to have attempted an adequate rehabilitation program. Another is the psychiatrically impaired voluntary dislocator. These patients often have secondary gain issues associated with this type of dislocation and will often try to redislocate the shoulder after the surgical shift of the tissues, making any surgery usually fruitless.

Patients with known connective tissue disorders are also poor surgical candidates for standard capsular shift procedures. Ehlers-Danlos syndrome is one such condition. It is characterized by skin hyperextensibility, joint hypermobility and dislocation, bone/skin fragility, and soft-tissue calcifications. There are multiple causes for the different subtypes of Ehlers-Danlos syndrome, but they all interfere in some way with the formation of Type I and Type III procollagens. With abnormal Type I and Type III collagen, healing occurs normally, but the scar tissue is replaced by the patients' own normal, poor quality ligaments. Surgically shifting this abnormal tissue gives a variable success rate. Laxity and capsular redundancy can redevelop very quickly after surgical shift of the tissue. In these patients we recommend the use of allograft tissue to supplement the repair [17].

As can be seen there are no absolute indications or contraindications for surgical intervention. The surgeon uses his best judgment to provide a solution for the patient. However, if there is any doubt, the prudent choice is to continue nonoperative management rather than opt for early surgery in patients with this disorder.

## 4.6 Operative Arthroscopic Techniques

### 4.6.1 Surgical Anatomy and Patho-anatomy

The underlying pathomechanical derangement is an increase in glenohumeral translation leading to symptoms. Static shoulder stabilizers include the glenohumeral ligaments, bony architecture, labrum, and negative intra-articular pressure. The dynamic stabilizers include the rotator cuff, scapular stabilizers, deltoid, and possibly the biceps brachii.

In patients with multidirectional instability there is an increased laxity of the joint capsule. Some patients acquire the laxity with activity and other patients have congenitally lax tissues. The most common surgical finding is a lax inferior capsule. The deficiency of the anterior and posterior pouches will differ between patients. There will be poorly defined bands of the IGHL in either the anterior pouch, posterior pouch, or both. The rotator interval will exhibit significant laxity and present with a "bulged out" appearance. The rotator interval contains the coracohumeral ligament, superior glenohumeral ligament, and the joint capsule. A "drive-through sign" is the ability to easily move the camera under the humeral head into the axillary pouch and is produced by the ability to laterally distract the humerus. This is a common finding in patients with MDI. Viewing the shoulder from posterior, there will be the "sky box view sign" if there is significant laxity posteriorly. This sign is demonstrated by the ability to view the entire glenoid as a pedestal from the posterior portal with the glenoid appearing distantly removed from the camera compared to a normal shoulder.

It is important in performing the diagnostic arthroscopy for MDI to remember that the chronic subluxations will cause significant stress to the labrum, capsule, and rotator cuff tendons, leading to tears, perforations, or partial tears. These lesions will need to be addressed at the time of the operation.

### 4.6.2 Exposure/Setup

Although this procedure may be performed in either the beach chair or the lateral decubitus position, we prefer the lateral decubitus position due to the ease of access to the inferior capsule. The use of the beach chair position may require the use of additional inferior portals to access and shift the capsule.

In the lateral decubitus position, the arm should be suspended with 5–10 lbs of traction. The amount of abduction and forward flexion can be varied. A generally accepted starting position is 45–60° of abduction and 15–20° of forward flexion. In shifting the anterior capsule and closing the rotator interval, it is helpful to have the arm positioned in 90° of external rotation to avoid overtightening the shoulder and producing a loss of external rotation. Maintenance of the arm in this position is much more readily accomplished in the lateral decubitus position. An easy external guide is to point the thumb toward the ceiling.

### 4.6.3 Specific Instruments/Equipment/Implants

A standard 4.0 mm arthroscope with the 30° lens is most often used in these cases, but a 70° arthroscope should also be readily available. 3.5 and 4.5 full radius and whisker soft tissue shavers should be available to debride and freshen the capsule without excising significant portions. A set of cannulas for the arthroscope, shaver, and instruments are necessary to work through without injuring the surrounding tissues. The instrument cannula should be clear to allow visualization of the suture and the knots as they enter the joint. They must be of sufficient size to allow passage of all the instruments. Usually 5 and 7 mm cannulas will be required for instrument passage. This is something that should be tested prior to the case.

Either gravity or pump inflow may be used during the case, but flow and pressure levels should be kept low to prevent excessive tissue swelling. A series of free sutures are also necessary. Additionally, some small diameter glenoid anchors should be available due to the possibility of an unexpected labral tear or deficient labrum.

Lastly, an instrument that allows you to pass suture through the capsule and the labrum is going to be required. There are many suture passing devices on the market. It is a good idea to evaluate as many as you can to see which system feels comfortable to you.

### 4.6.4 Procedure

Arthroscopy offers several advantages over open surgery in the management of MDI. The ability to detect injuries and abnormalities under magnification extends our diagnostic capability and allows direct repair of abnormal or injured structures on all sides of the joint. Diagnostically, one can get an overview of the joint ascertaining the presence of labral tears, capsular tears, and capsular and rotator interval laxity. Although the surgeon will already know the direction of the instability by the history and physical examination both awake and under anesthesia, repeating the exam while visualizing the movement with the arthroscope in the joint is quite useful. The usual advantages of arthroscopy include preserving muscle attachment, better visualization of pathology, anatomic-specific repairs based on this visualization, and small incisions. The patients usually experience less pain postoperatively by virtue of the minimally invasive nature of the procedure.

Once the decision to operate is made and the patient consents, surgery can be initiated. An interscalene block and catheter are routinely used for intraoperative and postoperative pain relief. This should be placed by an anesthesiologist with experience in regional anesthesia. Several methods are used today. To avoid unnecessary complications, it is recommended that the block be placed while the patient is awake and with ultrasound guidance [15, 16]. Due to reported complication rates, avoid intra-articular pain pumps.

Once adequate anesthesia, positioning, prepping, and draping have occurred, the diagnostic arthroscopy can begin. The lateral decubitus position offers an ergonomic advantage when doing labral and capsular reconstructions of the shoulder; however, if one has no experience with this position, the beach chair position can certainly be used. The diagnostic arthroscopy should begin with the standard posterior portal at the horizon of the glenohumeral joint. Several areas need to be evaluated which include the anterior capsule, the inferior capsule or axillary pouch (Fig. 4.1), the posterior capsule, the rotator interval (Fig. 4.2), the

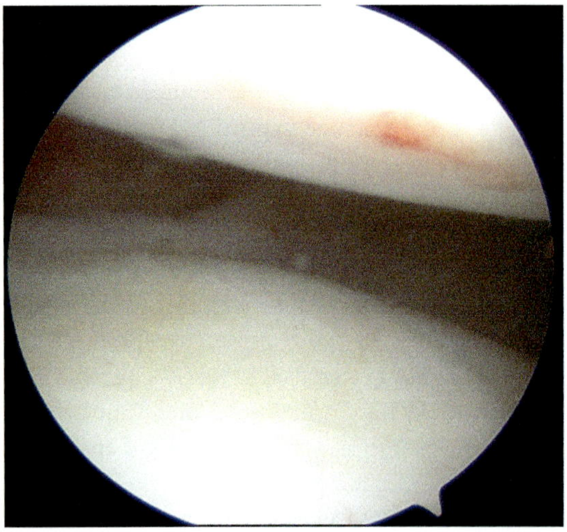

**Fig. 4.1** The view from posterior demonstrates the anterior shifting of the humeral head on the glenoid with minimal force in this right shoulder

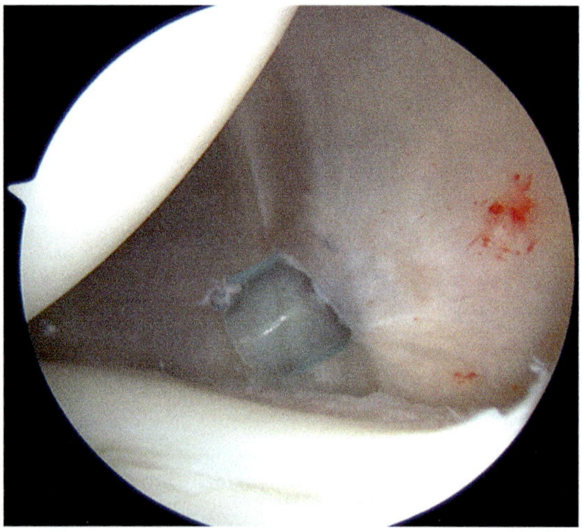

**Fig. 4.3** In many cases, the muscle fibers of the rotator cuff can be visualized through the very thin atrophic capsule

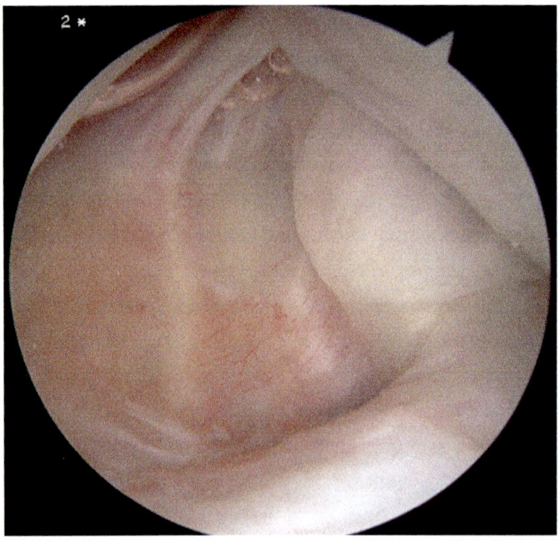

**Fig. 4.2** In this view from the posterior portal, the widening of the rotator interval can be visualized in this lax patient

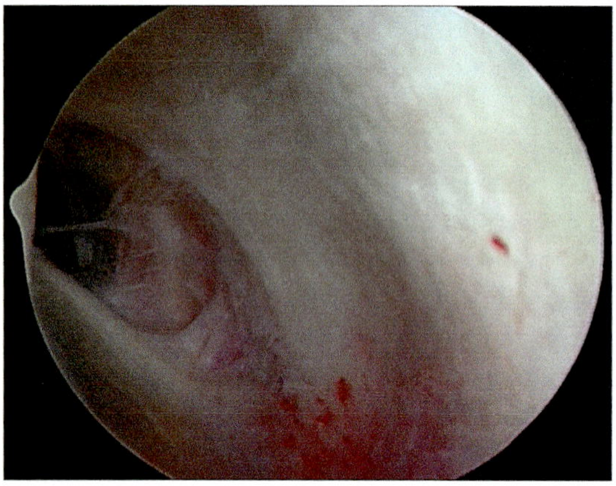

**Fig. 4.4** The capsule may also split or avulse from the humeral side in these patients as seen in this view from anterior

labrum, and the rotator cuff. In some patients with MDI, the posterior capsule may be so thin that the muscle of the infraspinatus can be visualized through it (Fig. 4.3).

The attachment of the anterior and posterior capsule to the humerus should be visualized looking for capsular splits, perforations, or HAGL lesions (Fig. 4.4).

## 4.7 Treatment of the Lax Capsule

The lax capsule is best managed by plication sutures. The basic principle is a superior shift of the capsule while also plicating the capsule to increase its strength. Absorbable or nonabsorbable sutures may be used. The choice of suture is up to the individual surgeon. Common choices include PDS or one of many permanent suture materials. The initial step involves abrading the capsule to stimulate a healing response. A full radius shaver without teeth, used with no suction, works well. Alternatively, a synovial rasp can be used to roughen up the capsule. The capsule can be left in situ or it can be cut at its attachment to the labrum. A suture hook is then used to perforate the capsule approximately 1 cm from the labrum. The area to be initially penetrated is determined by the amount of capsular laxity. A standard approach is to draw an imaginary line parallel to the horizon of the glenoid toward the capsule. This is the point of entry for the suture hook into the capsule. For a left shoulder, the anterior capsule is addressed as follows. The first suture hook is placed in the capsule at the 6 o'clock position at the point of the imaginary line and rotated until it pierces the capsule (Fig. 4.5a). The entire capsule is then advanced superiorly until the capsule appears taut (usually the 7 o'clock position-Fig. 4.5b). This is the point of advancement of the first suture. The same suture hook is then used to penetrate the labrum at the junction of the labrum and the articular margin at that point (Fig. 4.5c). A shuttle relay or some other monofilament suture is threaded through the suture hook. This suture is used to shuttle the final suture through both the capsule and the labrum, or, in some systems, the permanent suture can be passed. If a PDS has been passed, it can simply be tied (Fig. 4.5d). As the suture is tied, take care to ensure the post-limb of the suture is the limb that is through the capsule so that the knot is placed away from the articular surface. We prefer a sliding, self-locking (modified Roeder) knot. All knots have a tendency to migrate toward the articular margin as they are being tightened, so you must be cognizant to push the knot away as the suture and capsule are tightened. This advances the capsule superiorly and medially.

These steps are repeated up the face of the glenoid. The second capsular stitch is placed often at the 7 o'clock position and advanced until it is taut, which is usually near the 8 o'clock position on the glenoid. Additional sutures are placed in a similar manner up the glenoid face until the entire anterior capsular laxity is eliminated.

The posterior capsule is addressed in a similar way. For a left shoulder, start at the 6 o'clock position and shift the capsule superiorly until it is taut (usually around the 7 o'clock position) the same way as for the anterior procedure. Continue superiorly along the length of posterior glenoid until all capsular redundancy is eliminated.

In many cases of MDI, the posterior capsule is insufficient to hold a plication suture. In these cases, one may use a suture plication technique that includes the infraspinatus tendon. For this technique, the lateral capsule is pierced percutaneously with a large lumen 18 g spinal needle superiorly near the capsular insertion into the humerus. A suture is threaded through the needle into the joint. The initial stitch should be around the 7 o'clock position for a right shoulder and the 5 o'clock position for a left shoulder. The suture coming through the needle is grasped and the spinal needle is removed. A suture-retrieving device is then used to pierce the capsule adjacent to or just under the labrum, grasping the percutaneously placed suture. It is then removed out the posterior portal. The cannula is then retracted until it lies just outside the infraspinatus tendon. Using a switching stick, the cannula is placed into the subacromial space. A crochet hook is utilized to blindly grab the suture while watching from inside the joint. One should see the cannula indenting the infraspinatus during this retrieval. This suture is tied and the degree of capsular tightening is assessed. These steps are repeated until sufficient laxity has been eliminated. In most cases 2–4 sutures will be required (Fig. 4.6).

The arthroscope is then placed posteriorly above the level of the reconstruction and the rotator interval is assessed. In cases of MDI, true closure of the rotator interval is required to complete the stabilization of the shoulder (Fig. 4.7a, b). In order to tighten both the inner and outer layers of the rotator interval, a spinal needle is placed into the joint percutaneously approximately 1 cm from the articular margin just anterior to the edge of the supraspinatus tendon. A suture is threaded through the needle into the joint and placed anteriorly for retrieval. The anterior cannula is then retracted out of the joint until it is just anterior to the subscapularis tendon and the outer layer of the rotator interval. A suture-retrieving device is placed through the anterior layer of the rotator interval tissue and through the capsule entering the joint. The upper border of the subscapularis tendon may

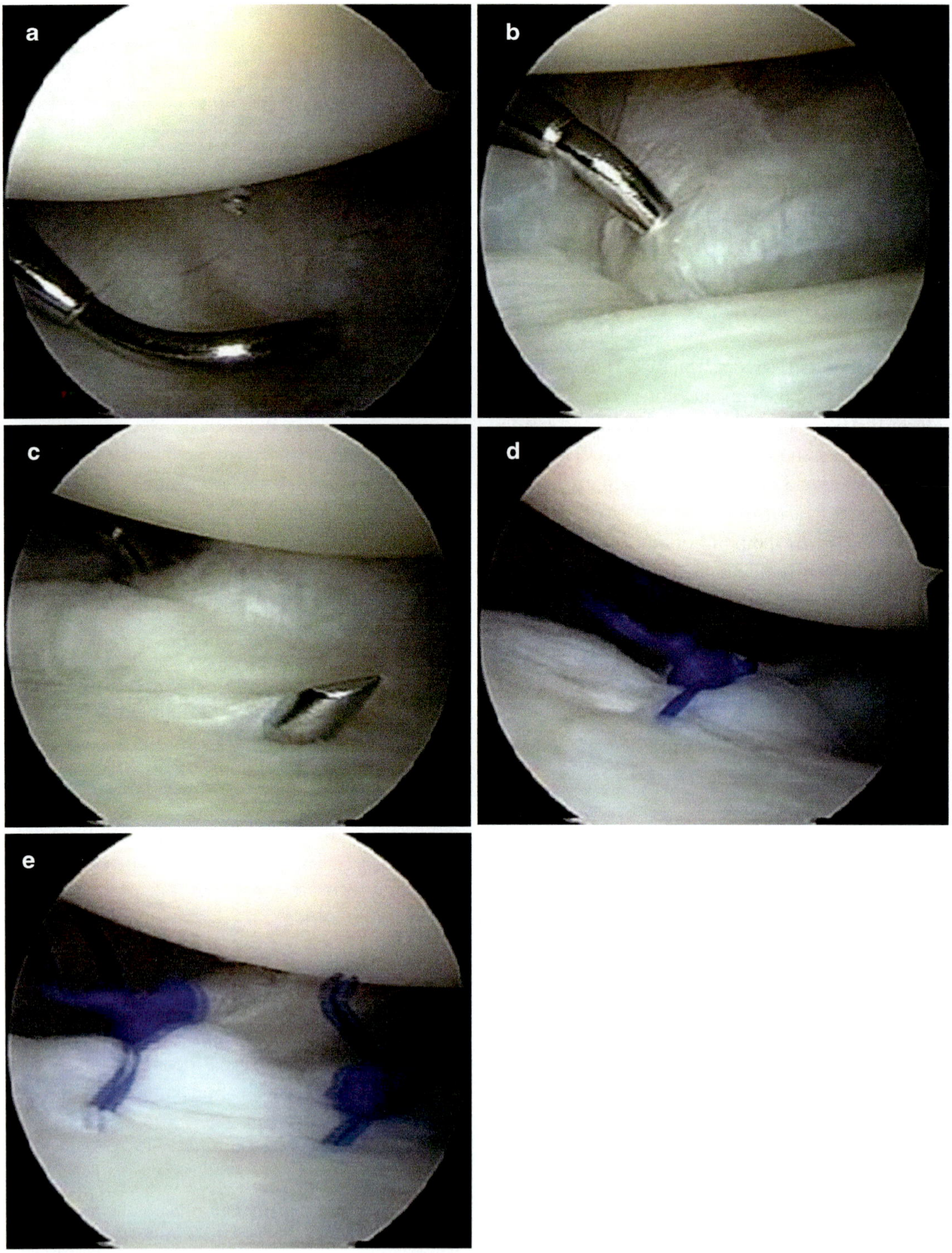

**Fig. 4.5** (**a**–**e**) In capsular plication, a suture hook is passed through the more inferior and lateral capsule (**a**). The hook is then advanced superiorly to take a second bite of the capsule, creating a plication of the capsule (**b**). The hook is then placed under the labrum, between the labrum and the bone to provide a solid anchor point for the suture (**c**). The suture, once the passage is completed, can then be tied to begin the process of capsular shift and repair (**d**). These steps can be repeated and the capsule plicated and shifted until the shoulder becomes stable (**e**)

be incorporated, or the device can simply grab the middle glenohumeral ligament. The suture passed percutaneously is then grabbed and pulled out the anterior cannula. A switching stick is then used to pass the cannula around the subscapularis tendon into the subacromial space. The cannula should be seen indenting the supraspinatus from inside the joint; it is then retracted until the indention is just anterior to the suture. A crochet hook is used to blindly grab the suture from the subacromial space and retrieve it out the anterior cannula as well. A sliding locking knot is used to close the interval. Additional sutures may be needed and are placed in the same manner. Work progressively more medially with each additional stitch. Alternatively, one may look in the subacromial space to retrieve and tie the suture. One must be careful not to incorporate the coracoacromial ligament into the rotator interval closure. When you see minor internal rotation of the arm, there has been adequate closure of the rotator interval.

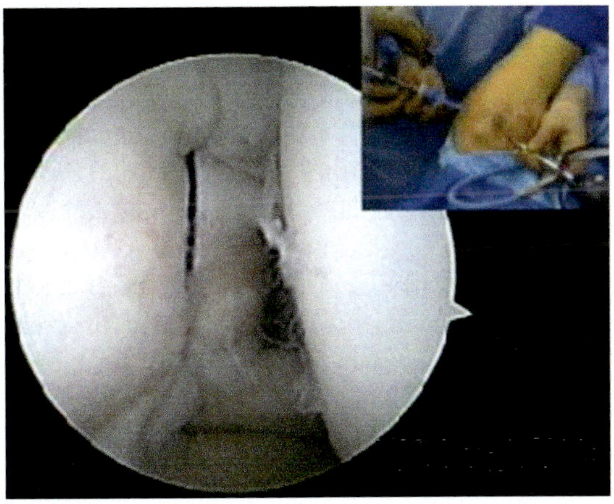

**Fig. 4.6** The capsule may be too thin posteriorly for plication, in which case sutures are placed through both the capsule and overlying infraspinatus tendon to provide stability to the posterior aspect of the shoulder

## 4.8 Treatment of the Torn Capsule and Special Techniques

Some patients with MDI may have associated labral or capsular tears, especially if they have had repeated subluxations or dislocations. In these patients it is important to remember to address the lax capsule in addition to the torn labrum. The labrum that is repaired using suture is placed through the capsule inferior to the tear and advanced superiorly under the free edge of the labral tear. This achieves a superior capsular shift and labral repair in one step. It is a good technique to mattress the sutures for greater tissue movement when possible. The second suture

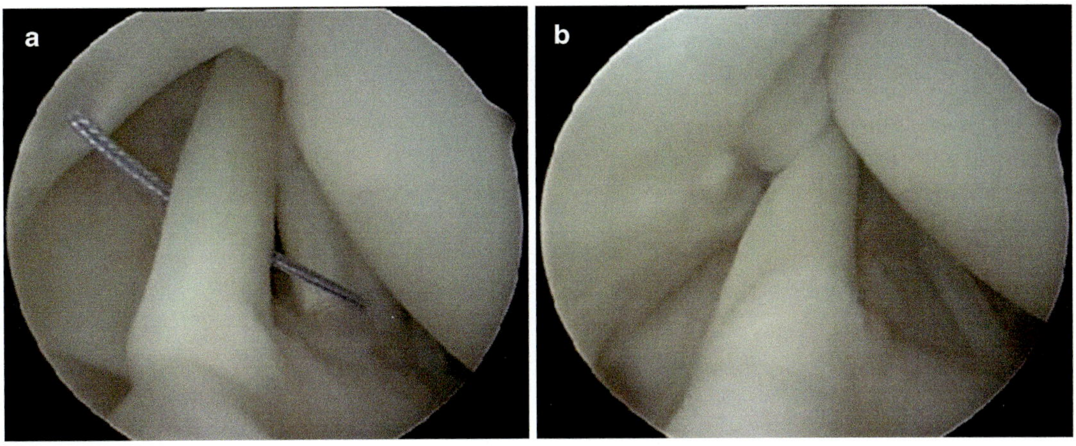

**Fig. 4.7** (**a**, **b**) In these individuals, the true rotator interval is closed by placing sutures between the supraspinatus and subscapularis to effectively shorten the coracohumeral and superior glenohumeral ligaments. The first suture is placed approximately 1 cm medial to the humeral head (**a**). The limbs of the suture are retrieved and tied, plicating the rotator interval and shortening the coracohumeral and superior glenohumeral ligaments

from the anchor can achieve more shift of the capsule when needed or simply be placed adjacent to the first stitch to hold the shifted tissue in place and help secure the labral tear. The placement of the anchor and suture depends on the location of the tear. Once the labrum has been reestablished and the capsule has been shifted superiorly, additional capsular plication stitches can be added to further shift the lax capsule in a manner similar to what has already been described. Once the labral repair and capsular shift are completed, the rotator interval can be addressed.

If there is no labral tear, but the labrum is hypoplastic, an anchor can be inserted on the glenoid and the capsule shifted toward it by passing sutures from the anchor through the capsule. In this instance, it is advisable to mattress the sutures to avoid suture irritation of the humeral head. This is also useful if there is a capsular split that needs to be addressed.

Lastly, in the ED-type patient with extremely poor connective tissue, we recommend allograft reconstruction of the IGHL and CHL to achieve stability for 5–7 years.

## 4.9 Postoperative Protocols

### 4.9.1 Wound Closure

The portals are closed with Steri-Strips only. If a larger cannula has to be used for labral repairs in addition to the capsular plication, we may use an absorbable subcutaneous stitch followed by a Steri-Strip. A sterile dressing is applied to the shoulder prior to the patient waking from anesthesia.

### 4.9.2 Postoperative Regimen

Depending on the procedure, the patient is placed in either an abduction brace or a gunslinger brace. The brace is maintained full-time, with the exception of showers, for 6 weeks. Initial rehab focuses on trying to maintain correct shoulder posture while in the brace.

Each patient has a unique response to healing after surgery. In those in whom the capsular shift is healing rapidly, passive motion and scapular stabilization exercises may begin when clinically indicated, but exercises for the majority of patients are delayed until 4–6 weeks postoperatively. Active exercise begins at 6–8 weeks, with careful attention to maintain correct scapular position during all exercises. In patients in whom the scapula remains protracted, early dynamic bracing is initiated to retrain the scapula to remain in its correct retracted position. This may include static bracing or taping for short periods of time. The need to reestablish proper shoulder positioning in space at all times is vital, especially during exercise. The patient and the therapist must both be aware of this. The more quickly normal shoulder posture is reestablished, the more likely a good recovery and a good result will occur.

Once the capsular reconstruction has healed, based on clinical endpoint exam and progressively decreasing pain, and the patient is able to maintain correct scapular position, the therapy is progressed to include rotator cuff strengthening exercises, proprioceptive neuromuscular facilitation exercises, and plyometrics. No passive stretching is allowed by the therapist for the first 3 months. Sometime in the 4–8 months postoperatively, integrated rehabilitation as described by Kibler [13] is initiated along with sport-specific conditioning in the athletic population. Sports are allowed between 6 and 12 months, depending primarily on shoulder position and tracking patterns.

### 4.9.3 Avoiding Pitfalls and Complications

One of the most common early pitfalls is placing incorrect or inadequate portals. Be sure to use the "outside in" technique to localize the placement of the portal. Take a spinal needle and insert it into the joint where you think your portal should be. Use that spinal needle to try to touch areas in the shoulder that need to be addressed. If the spinal needle is able to touch the areas of treatment, then likely this is a good portal. Remove the spinal needle and incise the skin there. Insert the cannula into the joint with the same angle as the spinal needle. Alternatively, there are newer cannula systems that allow penetration with a small needle device over which a cannulated switching stick is inserted into the joint. Again, it is important to try to touch the areas that need to be addressed surgically. The cannula is then advanced over the switching stick into the joint.

If you are using a pump system to inflow fluid, use the lowest setting that allows good distention to prevent much fluid extravasation. If the case takes more than 45 min, you may run into swelling that makes the rest of the case extremely difficult and taxing. Keeping the fluid flow and pressure as low as possible can help prolong your operating time.

The same risks apply to arthroscopic surgery as to open surgery. The axillary nerve is at risk in the axillary pouch. Be sure to grab separate bites of the capsule to shift it up to the labrum. One large enveloping suture could snare the axillary nerve.

If a knot is left adjacent to the articular surface, a patient may complain of clicking with shoulder range of motion. The long-term effect of this is unknown. Be sure to push the knots away from the articular surface when at all possible. The relatively recent development of high-tensile strength sutures, while excellent, presents a problem for the MDI patient. The normal tracking pattern in these patients is usually excessive, which would allow the cartilage of the humeral head to contact these more abrasive sutures and knots, creating damage to the articular surface. Thus, our recommendation is to use absorbable sutures in these patients.

The most devastating complication is chondrolysis. This has been associated with thermal devices and intra-articular pain pumps [12, 14]. Avoid the use of these to minimize your risk.

## 4.10 Summary

MDI and hyperlaxity should be managed nonoperatively. The arthroscopic management of multidirectional instability of the shoulder is successful in over 85 % of patients. The technique is minimally invasive and requires no detachment of the rotator cuff tendons. Experience is growing nationally and internationally and results of arthroscopic surgery are ever increasing. What one can accomplish arthroscopically is merely the extent of one's own imagination and technical skill.

## References

1. Neer CS, Foster CR. Inferior capsular shift for involuntary inferior and multidirectional instability of the shoulder. A preliminary report. J Bone Joint Surg Am. 1980;62(6):897–908.
2. Caspari RB, Savoie FH, Myers JF. Arthroscopic stabilization of traumatic anterior shoulder instability. In: Post M, Morrey B, Hawkins R, editors. Surgery of the shoulder. St. Louis: Yearbook Medical publishers; 1990.
3. Treacy SH, Savoie FH. Arthroscopic treatment of multidirectional instability. J Shoulder and Elbow Surg. 1999;8(4):345–50.
4. Wichman MT, Snyder SJ. Arthroscopic capsular plication for multidirectional instability of the shoulder. Oper Tech Sports Med. 1997;5:238–43.
5. Gartsman GM, Roddy TS, Hammerman SM. Arthroscopic treatment of multidirectional glenohumeral instability: 2 to 5 year follow-up. Arthroscopy. 2001;17(3):236–43.
6. McIntyre LF, Caspari RB, Savoie FH. The arthroscopic treatment of multidirectional shoulder instability: two year results of a multiple suture technique. Arthroscopy. 1997;13(4):418–25.
7. Tauro JC, Carter FM. Arthroscopic capsular advancement for anterior anterior-inferior shoulder instability. A preliminary report. Arthroscopy. 1994;10:513–7.
8. Lyons TR, Griffith PL, Savoie FH. Laser-assisted capsulorrhaphy for multidirectional instability of the shoulder. Arthroscopy. 2001;17(1):25–30.
9. Duncan R, Savoie FH. Arthroscopic inferior capsular shift for multidirectional instability of the shoulder: a preliminary report. Arthroscopy. 1993;9(1):24–7.
10. Hewitt M, Getelman MH, Snyder SJ. Arthroscopic management of multidirectional instability: Pancapsular plication. Orthop Clin North Am. 2003;34:549–57.
11. Wolf RS, Zheng N, Iero J, Weichel D. The effects of thermal capsulorrhaphy and rotator interval closure on multidirectional laxity in the glenohumeral joint: a cadaveric study. Arthroscopy. 2004;20(10):1044–9.
12. Levine WN, Clark AN, D'Allessandro DF, Yamaguchi K. Chondrolysis following arthroscopic thermal capsulorraphy to treat shoulder instability: a report of two cases. J Bone Joint Surg Am. 2005;87(3):616–21.

13. Kibler WB. Rehabilitation of the shoulder. In: Kibler WB, Herring SA, Press JM, editors. Functional rehabilitation of the Sports and Musculoskeletal injuries. Gaithersburg: Aspen Publishers; 1998.
14. Petty DH, Jazwari LM, Estrada LS, Andrews JR. Glenohumeral chondrolysis after shoulder arthroscopy: case reports and review of the literature. Am J Sports Med. 2004;32(2):509–15.
15. Soeding PA, Sha S, Royse CE, Marks P, Hoy G, Royse AG. A randomized trial of ultrasound-guided brachial plexus anesthesia in upper limb surgery. Anaesth Intensive Care. 2005;33(6):719–25.
16. Reuben SS. Interscalene block superior to general anesthesia. Anesthesiology. 2006;104(1):207.
17. Caspari RB, Savoie FH. Arthroscopic stabilization of traumatic anterior shoulder instability. In: Post M, Morreys B, Hawkins R, editors. Surgery of the shoulder. St. Louis: Yearbook Medical Publishers; 1990.

# Posterior Shoulder Instability in the Young Patient

# 5

Diana C. Patterson and Leesa M. Galatz

## Contents


5.1 **Introduction** ........ 35
5.2 **Anatomy** ........ 36
5.3 **Etiology** ........ 36
5.4 **Pathoanatomy** ........ 37
5.5 **Overhead Athletes (Thrower's Shoulder)** ........ 37
5.6 **Clinical Presentation** ........ 38
5.7 **Physical Exam** ........ 38
5.8 **Imaging** ........ 39
5.9 **Nonoperative Treatment** ........ 41
5.10 **Surgical Treatment** ........ 42
5.11 **Arthroscopic Treatment** ........ 42
5.12 **Open Procedures for Bone Deficiency** ........ 43
5.13 **Outcomes** ........ 44
**Conclusion** ........ 45
**References** ........ 45



D.C. Patterson
Department of Orthopaedic Surgery, Icahn School of Medicine at the Mount Sinai Health System, New York, NY, USA
e-mail: diana.patterson@mountsinai.org

L.M. Galatz, MD (✉)
Mount Sinai Professor and Chair, Leni and Peter May Department of Orthopedics, Icahn School of Medicine at Mount Sinai, Mount Sinai Health System, New York, NY, USA
e-mail: leesa.galatz@mountsinai.org


## 5.1 Introduction

Posterior shoulder instability is an increasingly recognized and treated shoulder problem. First described by McLaughlin in 1952 [1], posterior shoulder instability has historically been missed and more often treated nonoperatively compared to anterior instability. While it is far less common than anterior instability, only 2–10 % of all reported cases of instability [1–3], posterior shoulder instability is increasingly recognized as a problem in athletes and in posttraumatic settings. More comprehensive imaging modalities and expanded treatment options, especially with the development and application of arthroscopic techniques, have brought this problem into the forefront among athletic injuries of the shoulder. Posterior instability can occur after singular events or can be chronic in nature. For example, overhead athletes can develop pathologic progression of subtle instability that results in inability to participate. Traumatic dislocations can result in labral tears and glenoid fractures, mirroring those of anterior injuries. Posterior instability more commonly responds to nonoperative treatment with physical therapy, but surgical options are increasingly reported. Outcomes published in the literature are excellent, though most series contain small groups of patients. Return to play in athletes of all types is good, and many reach their prior level of performance.


© ISAKOS 2017


A.B. Imhoff, F.H. Savoie III (eds.), *Shoulder Instability Across the Life Span*,
DOI 10.1007/978-3-662-54077-0_5

## 5.2 Anatomy

The shoulder is intrinsically the least stable and most mobile joint in the body. Less than one-third of the articular surface of the humerus contacts the glenoid at any point during arc of motion and provides an enormous range of motion in all planes, including 360° of circumduction. The shoulder is stabilized by static and dynamic stabilizers. Static stabilizers include the glenoid labrum, capsular ligaments, and negative intra-articular pressure. Variations in the bony geometry, such as humeral or glenoid version and inclination, size, and width, can contribute to instability. The labrum, a fibrocartilaginous ring, is attached to the glenoid rim, adding stability to the articulation and functioning as a stable anchor for the glenohumeral ligaments. The four glenohumeral ligaments (anterior, middle, anterior band of inferior, and posterior band of inferior) each stabilize the shoulder with contributions varying according to the position of the shoulder [4]. The rotator interval, located between the subscapularis and supraspinatus tendons in the anterior shoulder, is viewed by some as important to overall and posterior stability of the shoulder, but its role remains controversial [5, 6].

The inferior glenohumeral ligament and posteroinferior capsule are the primary stabilizers against posterior translation of the humeral head between 45° and 90° of abduction [7, 8]. The posterior aspect of the joint capsule is the area between the intra-articular portion of the biceps tendon and the posterior band of the inferior glenohumeral ligament. However, it is also the thinnest portion of the shoulder capsule and is under the most stress with abduction, forward flexion, and internal rotation [4].

The rotator cuff muscles, anterior and middle deltoid, and pectoralis major are all dynamic stabilizers of the shoulder. Stability of the shoulder is closely dependent on scapular positioning, so scapular stabilizers indirectly contribute to shoulder stability. The subscapularis is the most important rotator cuff muscle to prevent posterior subluxation [9]. Co-contraction of shoulder girdle muscles forces the humeral head into the glenoid to create a unique concavity-compression force [10, 11].

## 5.3 Etiology

Historically, posterior instability was recognized following acute traumatic posterior dislocations. Acute dislocations occur with convulsive seizure and electrocution. Sports-related dislocations result from a posteriorly directed force applied to an adducted, internally rotated, and forward-flexed arm. Examples include a wrestler thrown onto his shoulder or the force applied to a football lineman's shoulder with his elbows locked out to block [12]. Mclaughlin described a boxer in the moment of punching with an internal twist and a wrestler who fell while in a "hammerlock," among other etiologies [1]. Athletes' shoulders can become more unstable during activity and competition as the muscular dynamic stabilizers fatigue and cease to function efficiently.

Posterior shoulder instability occurs in the absence of discrete trauma through a repetitive microtrauma model. These athletes may experience recurrent subclinical subluxation events, weakening and frequently tearing the weak posterior capsule [8, 13]. This more common etiology of progressive posterior shoulder instability has been diagnosed in baseball, golf, paddling sports, swimming, rugby, American football, and weight lifting [7, 8, 13]. Butterfly and freestyle athletes are at particularly high risk within the realm of swimming. In one case report, posterior instability developed after rifle shooting [14].

Overhead throwing sports, such as baseball pitching, volleyball, and the tennis serve, result in a clinical variant of posterior instability. The baseball swing applies tremendous force to the posterior complex of the shoulder, particularly the lead hand. Rotational velocities in the shoulder reach 937° per second and allow the bat to rotate at 1588° per second and reach a linear velocity of 31 m/s [15]. Reaching for an outside pitch increases the abduction angle to the shoulder, resulting in increased glenohumeral shear forces, particularly on missed outside pitches [16]. Without a ball strike on those pitches, there is nothing to offset the posterior pulling force of approximately 500 N, and the stabilizing muscles are not recruited, placing the shoulder at further risk [15, 16].

## 5.4 Pathoanatomy

Posterior instability can be predicated on alterations to the underlying anatomic variations in the bony morphology of the glenoid or humeral head. Glenoid hypoplasia, dysplasia of the posterior scapular neck, posterior glenoid rim deficiency, and increased glenoid retroversion can lead to posterior instability [17]. If the patient has had at least one specific traumatic posterior subluxation or dislocation, they may have a reverse Bankart; a reverse Hill-Sachs lesion on the anterior humerus, also coined a McLaughlin lesion; or an acute posterior humeral avulsion of the glenohumeral ligament (PHAGL) [13, 17, 18].

The repetitive microtrauma model of posterior instability results in attenuation and tearing of the posterior capsule posterosuperior labrum. In some individuals, it can also occur with insidious development laxity of the posterior capsule and its stabilizers. In both of these situations, but particularly the latter, patients should be questioned about a family history of congenital bone or connective tissue disorders [7, 13, 17].

## 5.5 Overhead Athletes (Thrower's Shoulder)

Overhead athletes often experience a "dead arm" which is a sensation experienced in association with instability. The shoulder is unable to throw with pre-injury velocity and/or control secondary to pain and a sensation of loss of control in the shoulder. Throwers report a sudden sharp pain and feeling the "arm going dead" when attempting to initiate early acceleration from the late cocking phase of the windup. Several theories were proposed to explain this. In various reports, it has been attributed to acromial osteophytes, coracoacromial impingement, posterior glenoid calcification, rotator cuff injury, biceps tendinitis, or internal impingement [19–22].

Jobe et al. initially described the overlap between instability and impingement [23]. Repetitive throwing gradually attenuates the anterior capsule and glenohumeral ligament complex. Loss of an anterior support results in anterosuperior migration of the humeral head during the throwing motion. Subacromial impingement syndrome symptoms develop and, eventually, the ability to throw is compromised. Since the process was thought to originate from an anterior lesion, surgical procedures to correct anterior instability were performed with regularity. Surgical results following acromioplasty [19] or open anterior capsulolabral reconstruction [24, 25] reported only 50 %, and 77 % of pitchers returned to pitching for at least one season following surgery, and in one study, only 68 % of pitchers reported excellent results.

In retrospect, posterior capsular contracture contributed to the imbalance, and some theorize the good outcomes were obtained due to tightening of the anterior capsule in shoulders with a preexisting contracted posterior capsule, thus creating an equalized shoulder which stretched out symmetrically during post-op rehabilitation [22].

Andrews was the first to describe a correlation between anterosuperior glenoid labrum tears and overhead throwing; he recommended treatment with arthroscopic debridement [26]. Walch et al. described an "internal impingement" that occurs in all shoulders in abduction and external rotation. The articular surface of the posterosuperior rotator cuff can become pinched between the labrum and the greater tuberosity in the abduction external rotation (ABER) position [27].

Contracture of the posterior shoulder capsule leads to glenohumeral internal rotation deficit (GIRD) [7, 22, 28, 29]. Posterior contracture is nearly universal in patients with painful throwing arms and can be subclinical. Eventually, the thickening of posterior capsule extends to the posterior band of the IGHL (PIGHL). As a result, when the arm is abducted and externally rotated, the tight PIGHL forces the humeral head posteriorly and superiorly. This translates the normal arc of motion of the humeral head on the glenoid in a posterior-superior direction. The greater tuberosity does not contact the glenoid at its normal point in external rotation, but is pulled superior, allowing the shoulder greater external rotation. With this, the humeral head "cam" effect on the anterior capsule ligaments, and the glenohumeral ligament sling over the lesser tuberosity, is reduced, which consequently allows further hyper-external rotation of the humerus [22, 30]. The hyperextension abduction of the arm leads to abnormal contact between the rotator cuff and the posterosuperior glenoid, particularly the articular side, leading to failure secondary from torsion and shear overload.

With the arm in excessive external rotation, the vector of the intra-articular biceps tendon shifts to a more posterior and vertical angle. This redirection twists the base of the biceps at its attachment to the superior labrum. The torsional force is then passed on to the labrum, which then rotates medially over the posterosuperior neck of the scapular neck. This pattern of injury, the "peel-back" mechanism, is seen in posterior and posterosuperior labrum tears, but is absent in normal controls and tears of the anterior labrum [22].

## 5.6 Clinical Presentation

Patients with posterior instability may present after a posterior shoulder dislocation or with seemingly atraumatic nonspecific, vague pain or fatigue in the shoulder. Types of sport activities should be elucidated, as well as any history of dislocation or subluxation events. The pain may worsen with activity or may only occur during certain activities. They may have mechanical symptoms or crepitus with range of motion or complain of instability symptoms ranging from subjective instability to true intermittent subluxation events. In one study, 90 % of patients with posterior instability noted mechanical symptoms (clicking or crepitation) with motion [31]. Pollock and Bigliani showed that two-thirds of athletes who eventually chose surgery presented with difficulty in using the shoulder outside of sports, particularly with the arm above the horizontal [32]. Overhead athletes can complain of "dead arm," significant fatigue, or an inability to reach usual velocity or pitch control. They may be unable to warm up or loosen the shoulder when warming up. The shoulder can be acutely painful at a specific moment during late cocking or early acceleration and subsequently lose velocity [7, 22, 28]. They may also notice a difference in the possible range of motion between the arms due to posterior capsular contracture.

## 5.7 Physical Exam

On inspection, patients with posterior instability may have muscle asymmetry or atrophy or scapular dysrhythmia on a range of motion. Winging of the medial border of the scapula is a compensatory mechanism for posterior instability. Tenderness can be elicited on the posterior joint line, greater tuberosity, and biceps tendon. This posterior tenderness can be due to inflammation or posterior rotator cuff synovitis. A posterior dimple, seen on posterior shoulder, 1 cm medial and 1 cm below to the posterior angle of the acromion has a sensitivity of 67 % and a specificity of 92 % for diagnosing posterior instability [33].

Range of motion of both shoulders should be assessed in all planes. Measurements for forward elevation, abduction in the scapular plane, external rotation with the arm at the side, and internal rotation to vertebral level are taken while standing. Internal and external rotation while supine, with the scapula stabilized and the arm abducted to 90°, is measured and compared to the contralateral side to assess for GIRD. Strength of the rotator cuff is assessed with standard commonly performed maneuvers. Tests for the subscapularis include the belly press (abdominal compression test), lift-off, and bear hug tests [7, 34, 35].

Testing for capsule or labral injuries can be performed via the jerk test, the Kim test, the circumduction test, and O'Brien's active compression test. The jerk test, a posteriorly directed force to the seated patient with the medial scapula stabilized and the arm in flexion, adduction, and internal rotation, is positive if it provokes posterior subluxation or dislocation, along with pain and apprehension. Variable sensitivities of this test have been reported [7, 36].

The Kim test has been shown to be 97 % sensitive in detecting a posteroinferior labral lesion when in combination with a positive jerk test [37]. While seated, the arm starts in 90° of abduction in the scapular plane while axially loaded and then is elevated 45° further with a posteroinferior vector for force. A positive test is sudden posterior subluxation with pain. Kim et al. found that patients with positive, painful Kim tests were more likely to require surgical intervention for symptom relief than those who did not [37].

The circumduction test, similar to the jerk test, is performed on a seated patient with the arm, elbow extended, brought into 90° of forward elevation and slight adduction. A posteriorly directed load is applied, subluxing or dislocating the humeral head, and then the arm is circumducted (abduction/extension rotation) until the head is felt to reduce into the glenoid. A positive test is a palpable and audible "clunk" as the humeral head reduces. This test is usually more useful in high grades of chronic instability, as it can often be performed without pain or guarding in these patients [7].

Posterosuperior labral tears, particularly in overhead athletes, can be suspected based on the O'Brien's compression test. While seated, a downward force is applied on the arm in 90° forward elevation, 10° adduction, and internal rotation. If there is deep pain in the shoulder with this motion that improves with the same position but externally rotated, the test is positive. Pain deep in the shoulder is indicative of labral pathology, but AC joint pain is a false positive. In a retrospective study of exam and arthroscopy findings, the O'Brien test had a sensitivity of 83 % and a positive predictive value of 90 % for the diagnosis of posterior labral tears [38].

In patients with atraumatic posterior instability, particularly those who show evidence of multidirectional instability, generalized ligamentous laxity conditions should be ruled out using the Beighton scale. The nine-point scale assesses hyperextension at elbows and knees beyond 10°: passively touch the thumb to the forearm with wrist flexion, hyperextend the small finger metacarpophalangeal joint greater than 90°, and touch the floor with palms (feet together). A score greater than 5 indicates generalized laxity.

## 5.8 Imaging

Orthogonal radiographs of the glenohumeral joint, anteroposterior (AP), scapular Y lateral, and axillary views assess bony anatomic anatomy of the shoulder. In the majority of cases, X-rays will be negative. Lesser tuberosity fractures may indicate a posterior shoulder dislocation. In some cases, the axillary view can reveal posterior glenoid lesions, Hill-Sachs lesions on anterior humeral head, and alterations in glenoid version (Fig. 5.1). CT scan is excellent for more detailed views of osseous structures and measurements of glenoid or humeral version (Fig. 5.2).

Magnetic resonance arthrogram (MRA) is more sensitive for diagnosis of chondrolabral pathology than standard MRI without contrast

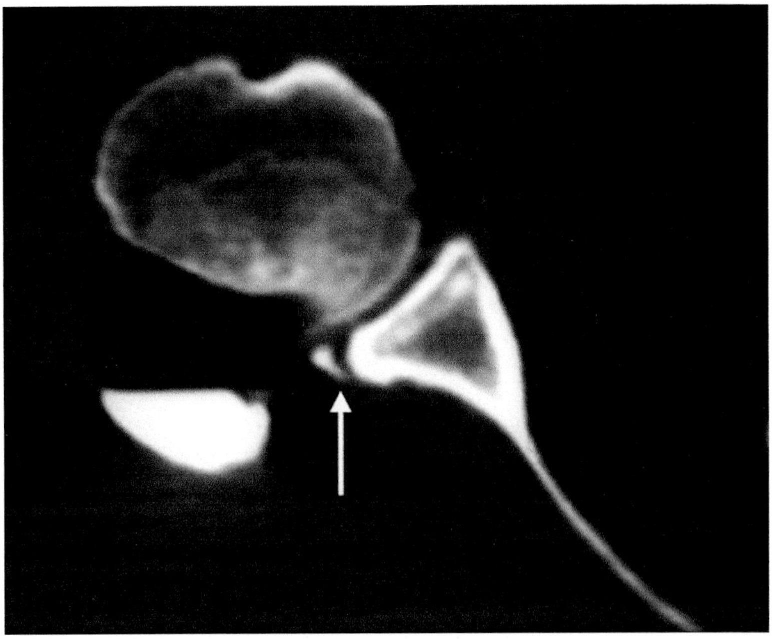

**Fig. 5.1** Axial CT view of patient with posterior boy Bankart lesion following traumatic posterior instability event (*arrow*). Hemarthrosis secondary to trauma is also visible intra-articularly

administration [39]. Pathology consistent with posterior instability injury, particularly when caused by internal impingement, seen on MRA includes posterior undersurface rotator cuff abnormalities, abnormal labral signal, and cystic changes at the posterosuperior humeral head [40–42]. Additionally, MRA reveals static posterior translation of humeral head on the glenoid, discrete tears in the posterior capsule (Fig. 5.3), labral tears/splits or labrocapsular lesions, posterior HAGL lesions, posterior labral periosteal sleeve avulsion (PLPSA), and subscapularis tendon avulsions (Fig. 5.4) [42, 43]. A Bennet lesion, enthesopathy, or heterotopic ossification at the origin of the posterior IGHL is also commonly seen in overhead throwers [44]. In a radiographic study of overhead athletes with GIRD and internal impingement symptoms, throwers tended to have a thicker labrum (6.4 vs. 2.9 mm), longer capsule-labrum length (8.8 mm vs. 5.4 mm), and shallower capsular recess in the posterior inferior shoulder (94° vs. 65°) than non-throwing controls [42].

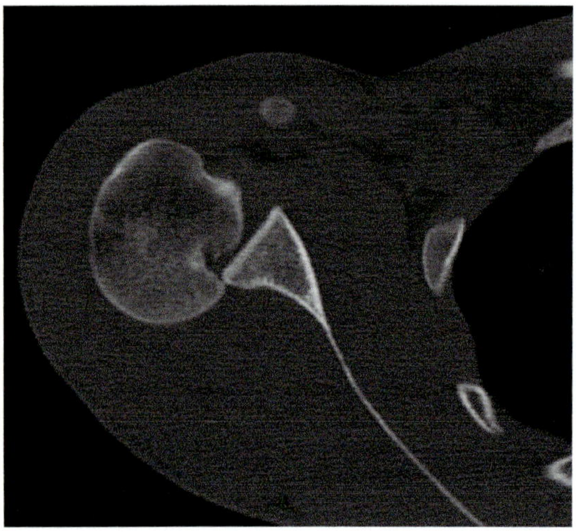

**Fig. 5.2** Axial view of CT scan with engaging reverse Hill-Sachs lesion on the anterior humeral head due to recurrent posterior instability

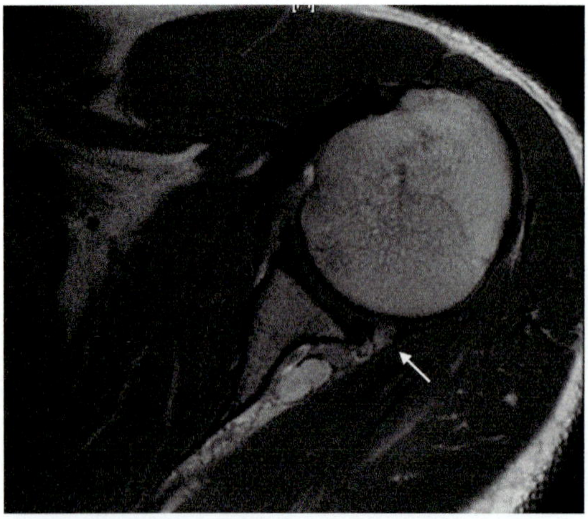

**Fig. 5.3** Axial MRI imaging showing posterior capsulolabral injury with capsular separation (*arrow*)

In a review of 28 shoulders with previously diagnosed posterior HAGL lesions, Rebolledo et al. found that the most common concurrent injuries were reverse Hill-Sachs lesions (36 %), anterior Bankart lesions (29 %) and posterosuperior rotator cuff tears (25 %), and bony HAGL avulsion (7 %). The posterior HAGL pathology was a complete tear in 71 %, a partial tear in 25 %, and a floating lesion in 4 % of patients [18].

The posterior labrum has a number of anatomic variants. Using CT arthrogram, Nourissat et al. defined four varieties of posterior labrum insertion: Type 1, the most common, was a posterior labrum fully inserted flush with cartilage, Type 2 was a medialized insertion of superior segment, Type 3 was a medialization of superior and medial segment, and Type 4 was a medialized insertion of the entire posterior labrum [45].

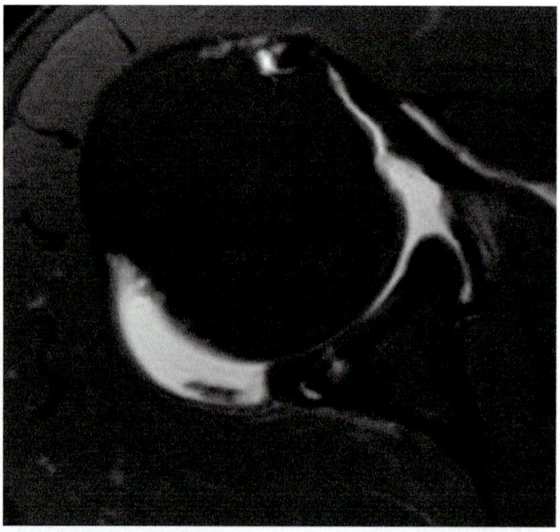

**Fig. 5.4** Axial cut of an MRA revealing a glenolabral articular disruption (GLAD) lesion. The displaced flap of articular cartilage is seen in the posteroinferior capsule

Kim et al. defined a classification for tears of the posterior labrum. Type I is an incomplete detachment, Type II the nominal "Kim lesion," Type III a chondrolabral erosion, and Type IV a flap tear of the posteroinferior labrum (Fig. 5.5) [46]. A "Kim lesion" is a concealed but complete detachment that can masquerade on arthroscopy as a superficial crack in the junction of the posteroinferior chondrolabral junction, but hides a complete detachment of the labrum from the glenoid rim.

Radiographic studies have consistently shown that shoulders with atraumatic posterior instability have alterations in the glenoid and chondrolabral version than age-matched controlled shoulders. Excessive retroversion of the glenoid has been defined as greater than −7° in the sagittal plane [47]. The increased retroversion is most frequently seen at the inferior aspect of the glenoid [48]. Kim et al. [49] examined 33 shoulders with atraumatic posterior instability and observed that the glenoid was more shallow and there was increased retroversion of the bony glenoid and chondrolabral complex at the middle and inferior glenoid in the unstable patients. Hurley et al. reported an average glenoid retroversion of −10° in patients with posterior instability as compared to −4° in uninjured controls [50]. In a series by Bradley et al., mean chondrolabral retroversion was 10.7° (controls 5.5°) and mean glenoid version 7.1° vs. 3.5°.

Rarely performed, but potentially useful in diagnosis, is an MRA performed with the shoulder in the abduction external rotation position. This arm position can reveal a "peel-back" lesion of posterosuperior labrum which may reduce to anatomic position in neutral arm position. This position can also help expose a Kim lesion, with the arm movement and position forcing intra-articular contrast to track into the Kim lesion under the labrum and reveal the extent of the damage. In a retrospective series of 34 MR in both the ABER and standard position with known labral peel-back seen on the ensuring arthroscopic repairs, this MR technique was 73 % sensitive and 100 % specific for the diagnosis; positive predictive value was 100 %, and negative predictive value was 78 %. Of these 34 patients, five had labral tears that would not be visible and went undiagnosed in MR in the standard neutral position [51].

MRA is also useful in the postoperative setting at a mean of just 6 months following surgery; 40 patients with recurrent instability underwent repeat MRA prior to undergoing revision shoulder stabilization. Finding was compared with pathology observed at revision arthroscopy. MRA was 91.9 % accurate for diagnosis of labral tears with a 96.2 % sensitivity. Accuracy for detecting rotator cuff lesions was 87.2 % (sensitivity 94.1 %) and for biceps injury was 95.7 % (sensitivity 85.7 %) [52].

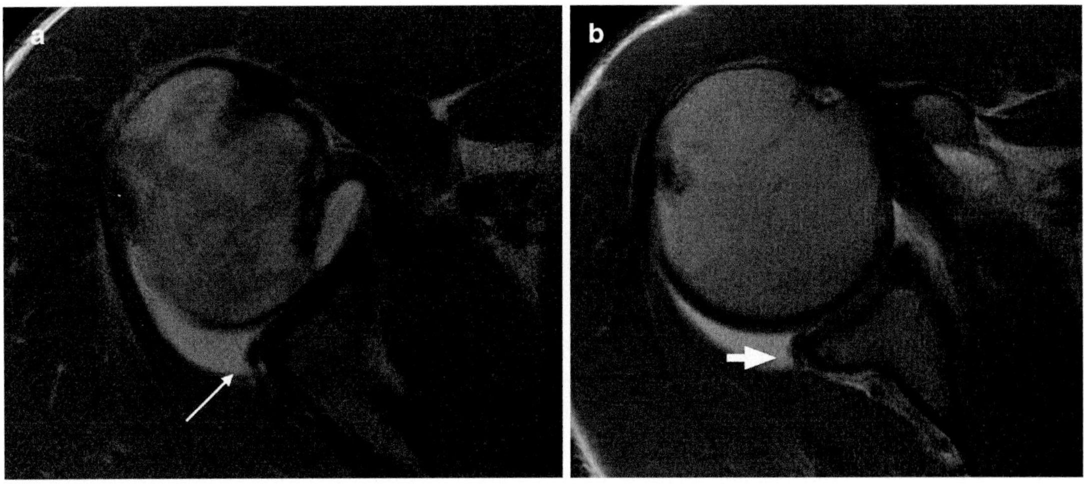


**Fig. 5.5** (**a**) Axial cut, proton density MRI images showing posteroinferior labrum degeneration and tearing (*arrow*), and (**b**) inferior blunting of the posteroinferior margin of the labrum (*arrowhead*)

## 5.9 Nonoperative Treatment

Conservative treatment for a minimum of 6 months is almost universally recommended. Activity modification and physical therapy, with particular focus on dynamic muscular stabilizers of the shoulder, have been shown to result in significant improvement in many patients [12, 32, 53, 54]. Elements of scapular dyskinesia or protraction can be addressed with a periscapular strengthening regimen. For patients with symptoms due to GIRD, the "sleeper stretch" has been shown to be extremely effective in avoiding progression of symptoms or surgery. To perform this stretch, the patient lies on the injured side with the staple stabilized against a wall, the shoulder and elbow each flexed to 90°. The contralateral, nondominant arm applies passive internal rotation force to the wrist [22]. Nevertheless, some patients will not improve with therapy alone. Burkhead et al. showed that only 16 % of patients with traumatic posterior instability improved with therapy, versus nearly 80% resolution in patients with atraumatic instability [8, 53].

## 5.10 Surgical Treatment

Options for operative treatment of posterior instability are divided into two categories, based on the underlying type of lesion causing the instability. Procedures to correct or supplement osseous deficiencies of the glenoid or humerus address engaging reverse Hill-Sachs lesions, excessive glenoid retroversion, glenoid hypoplasia, or posterior glenoid deficiency. The other subgroup is procedures to correct soft tissue injuries of the rotator cuff or posterior capsulolabral complex.

## 5.11 Arthroscopic Treatment

Arthroscopic procedures for posterior instability have become the standard of care in the absence of severe bone deficiency. Surgical techniques address a spectrum of pathology in posteriorly unstable shoulders (Figs. 5.6, 5.7, and 5.8). The authors prefer a lateral decubitus position for arthroscopic labral repair and posterior capsular imbrication. Necessary portals include a high posterolateral portal and two anterior rotator interval portals, one high and one low. The angle of the glenoid makes anchor placement challenging, so placement of the posterior portal as lateral as possible facilitates the correct angle. An accessory portal in the far lateral position for anchor placement is often helpful.

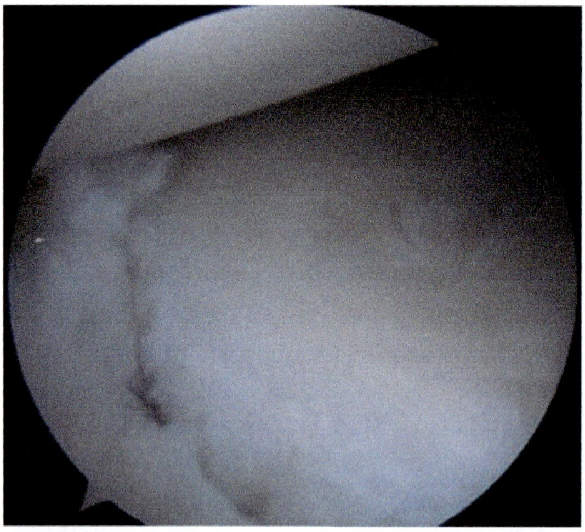

**Fig. 5.6** Arthroscopic view of an isolated posterior labral tear

For the repair, the high anterior portal is used for viewing and the lower rotator interval portal, just superior to the subscapularis, is used for shuttling. A large cannula is placed in the posterior portal. In the case of a labral tear, the labrum is mobilized with an arthroscopic elevator analogous to that for anterior labral repair. Anchors are placed in the posterior glenoid rim, sutures retrieved through the anterior portal. Sutures are subsequently shuttled through the soft tissue, a variety of devices are available to perform this. Capsular plication is dependent on the pathology – shoulders with traumatic labral tears can be treated with labral repair only; posterior instability resulting from laxity requires a more substantial imbrication of the posterior capsule. Posterior instability always has an inferior component, so a few plication sutures through the inferior and sometimes anteroinferior capsule are performed.

Postoperatively, patients should be immobilized with the arm in neutral rotation after poste-

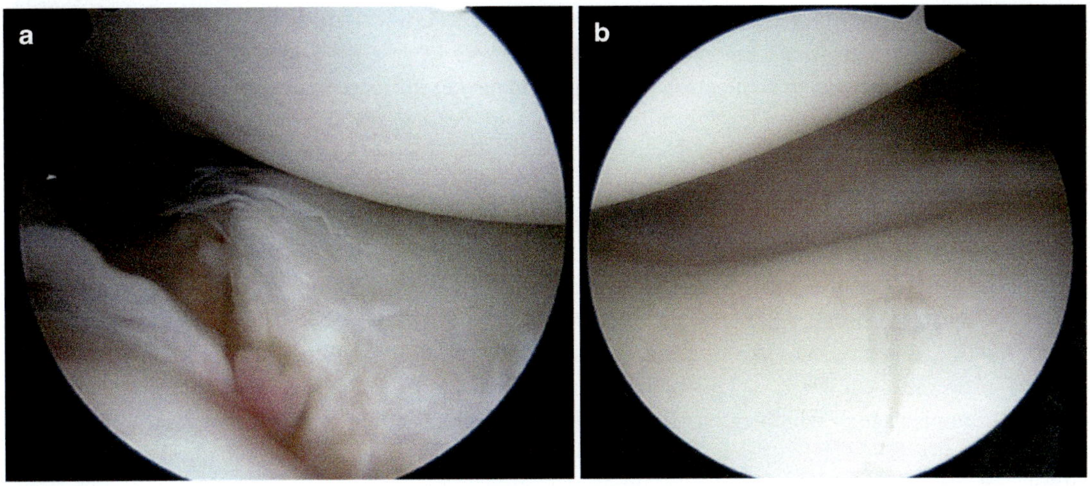


**Fig. 5.7** An arthroscopic view of a posterior labrum periosteal sleeve avulsion (POLPSA) lesion prior to repair. (**a**) Shows the periosteal sleeve layer separation along the posterior labrum. (**b**) Shows the posterior displacement of the capsulolabral complex along and posteroinferior glenoid neck, indicative of periosteal sleeve avulsion-type of injury that has retracted medially

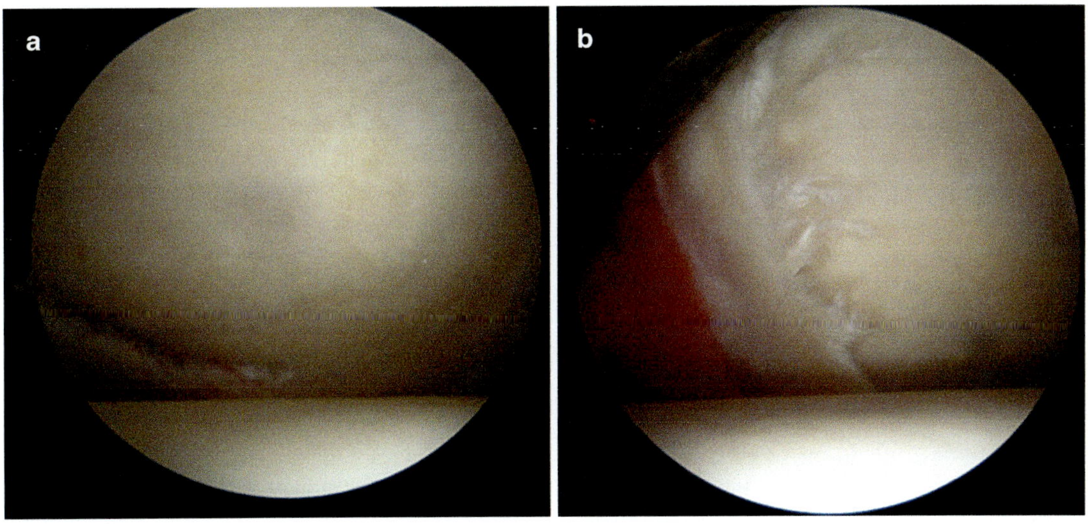


**Fig. 5.8** Arthroscopic view of the GLAD lesion (glenohumeral articular disruption) seen on MRI in Figure 4. (**a**) Shows the lesions initiation within the chondral layer of the glenoid surface. (**b**) Shows the complete separation of the posterior cartilage from the glenoid, along with the attached labrum. This correlates with the MRI image in Figure 4 showing contrast tracking underneath the chondral surface

rior instability surgery to keep the tension off the posterior repair. Four weeks of immobilization is usually sufficient with elbow, wrist, and hand motion during this early recovery; however, this is adjusted for patients with atraumatic etiology. The authors generally avoid internal rotation for at least 6 weeks.

## 5.12 Open Procedures for Bone Deficiency

Mclaughlin presented a technique to prevent the edges of a reverse Hill-Sachs lesion from engaging on the posterior glenoid rim by limiting maximal internal rotation. The subscapularis tendon is detached from the lesser tuberosity and retracted medially and then reattached into the defect with sutures [1]. The Neer modification of the McLaughlin procedure transfers the subscapularis tendon with the lesser tuberosity still attached via an osteotomy [8, 17, 55, 56]. Iliac crest bone graft has been used to fill small lesions of <25 % of the humeral articular surface, as well as allograft osteochondral bone plugs for larger defects of up to 40–50% of the articular surface [8, 17, 56–58]. Recently, a more common variant on this procedure for reverse Hill-Sachs is a reverse remplissage, which can be done arthroscopically [59]. The subscapularis muscle is sutured into the defect with suture anchors without detaching it from the lesser tuberosity. Duey et al. also described a technique to arthroscopically imbricate the middle glenohumeral ligament into the defect [60].

The deficient or retroverted glenoid can be corrected with a bone block procedure or a posterior glenoid neck opening wedge osteotomy [61–64]. A posterior bone block procedure was performed in the lateral position via an open, posterior deltoid-splitting approach, transferring a bicortical graft from posterior iliac crest to an extra-articular position on the posterior glenoid; unlike an anterior bone block, the capsule is intentionally left to interpose between the humeral head and the bone block [65]. Postoperatively, patients are able to regain full external rotation and return to sports at their prior level [64–66]. Millet et al. descried a technique to reconstruct posterior glenoid deficiency with a distal tibial osteoarticular allograft with good outcomes in two patients [67]. A systematic review of bone block procedures confirmed that bone grafting was a reliable procedure since significant improvement in outcomes scores was regularly reported. However, long-term studies showed a clear deterioration in outcomes over time, and the majority of studies reported high frequency of radiographic graft lysis, humeral head osteonecrosis, and advanced osteoarthritis [68].

Lafosse et al. [69] described a posterior bone block procedure analogous to the anterior arthroscopic Latarjet, and this may be appropriate in experienced hands.

## 5.13 Outcomes

Mauro et al. recently examined the effect of glenoid version and width on outcomes following arthroscopic posterior stabilization. In 118 MRAs on athletes with recurrent posterior unidirectional instability, patients with wider and more retroverted glenoid (mean glenoid version 10.8°, mean glenoid width 28.9 mm) had better mean preoperative pain and ASES than those with narrower and more anteverted glenoids. Postoperatively, the wider glenoids continued to have better pain and ASES scores and decreased risk of failure. No correlation was seen between chondral and labral width or version with any pre- or postoperative outcome measured. Thirteen patients who failed capsulolabral repair had 3.0 mm smaller labral width and 3° less labral retroversion, but no bony version differences [70].

In a large study of 200 shoulders (183 patients), Bradley et al. demonstrated excellent outcomes in athletes with unidirectional posterior instability. All patients underwent arthroscopic posterior capsulolabral repair with anchored or anchorless repair. At 36 months, mean ASES score improved 40 points, to 85.1. Stability, pain, and function scores were also improved. Sixty-four percent returned to their prior level of play, but 10 % were unable to return to their sport due to their shoulder injury. Twelve patients were failures by the ASES criteria of score <60, and 14 had a stability score >5; seven patients were failures by both scoring rubrics [71].

Arner et al. [72] showed excellent results of arthroscopic posterior capsulolabral repair in American football players with unidirectional posterior instability. In a group of 56 athletes, 93% returned to play, with 79% returning to the same level of competition at a mean of 44.7 months postoperatively. Significant improvements were seen in pain and ASES scores and 96% were satisfied. No patient was re-dislocated and no revision procedures were required. Baseball players have also shown excellent outcomes. Wanich et al. treated a series of baseball players with posterior labral tears of the lead shoulder. Eleven of 12 treated with surgery returned to previous level of play at 5.9 months postoperatively, and all patients regained full preoperative internal and external range of motion [73]. Wrestlers are also able to return to high levels of participation following arthroscopic posterior capsulolabral complex repair and do so without recurrence over the ensuring season [74].

In a comparison of overhead throwing athletes and non-throwing athletes who underwent capsulolabral repair, McClincy et al. showed no statistical differences in ASES scores, stability, strength, or range of motion at 37 months postoperatively. However, only 60% of throwers were able to return to preoperative level of play. Surgical repair that included discrete suture anchor placement showed a tenfold increase in likelihood of returning to play when compared with anchorless repairs. No variation between repair constructs was seen in return of non-throwing athletes. Additionally, true pitchers had worse return to play rates (50%) when compared with other types of throwers [75].

Pediatric athletes also have excellent results following arthroscopic repair when nonoperative treatment fails. In 25 cases under 18 years of age with unidirectional posterior instability, 92% of shoulders were stable at final follow-up, with two recurrent instability episodes. Equivalent level of play was achieved in 67 %. Outcomes were improved in males, contact athletes, and those with history of traumatic injury as cause of instability [76].

Voluntary dislocators commonly do poorly with surgical interventions [77, 78], and rehabilitation only is encouraged for a more prolonged period than the 6 months recommended for other patient groups. In a series of patients with multidirectional instability and ability to voluntarily dislocate posteriorly, DASH scores improved significantly at all time points with a three-phase rehabilitation program. Therapy focused on correction of abnormal muscle patterns, restoration of correct scapular kinetics, and strengthening [79].

### Conclusion

Posterior shoulder instability, whether due to traumatic events, accumulative microtrauma, or overhead throwing mechanics, can lead to pain, instability, mechanical symptoms, and inability to perform at a prior level of athletic performance. Historically, it was a commonly missed diagnosis, but can be strongly suspected on proper clinical exam and confirmed with focused imaging studies revealing specific spectrum of pathology. Nonoperative treatment is recommended first, especially in overhead athletes, but arthroscopic capsulolabral repair has shown excellent resolution of symptoms and return to play.

## References


1. McLaughlin H. Posterior dislocation of the shoulder. J Bone Joint Surg Am. 1952;24 A(3):584–90.
2. Antoniou J, Duckworth DT, Harryman 2nd DT. Capsulolabral augmentation for the management of posteroinferior instability of the shoulder. J Bone Joint Surg Am. 2000;82(9):1220–30.
3. Boyd HB, Sisk TD. Recurrent posterior dislocation of the shoulder. J Bone Joint Surg Am. 1972;54(4):779–86.
4. Pagnani MJ, Warren RF. Stabilizers of the glenohumeral joint. J Shoulder Elbow Surg. 1994;3(3):173–90.
5. Cole BJ, Rodeo SA, O'Brien SJ, Altchek D, Lee D, DiCarlo EF, Potter H. The anatomy and histology of the rotator interval capsule of the shoulder. Clin Orthop Relat Res. 2001;390:129–37.
6. Gaskill TR, Braun S, Millett PJ. Multimedia article. The rotator interval: pathology and management. Arthroscopy. 2011;27(4):556–67.
7. Bradley JP, Tejwani SG. Posterior shoulder instability. In: Delee & Drez orthopaedic sports medicine. 4th ed. Philadelphia: Elsevier; 2015. p. 517–31.
8. Tannenbaum EP, Sekiya JK. Posterior shoulder instability in the contact athlete. Clin Sports Med. 2013;32(4):781–96.
9. Blasier RB, Soslowsky LJ, Malicky DM, Palmer ML. Posterior glenohumeral subluxation: active and passive stabilization in a biomechanical model. J Bone Joint Surg Am. 1997;79(3):433–40.
10. Lippitt S, Matsen F. Mechanisms of glenohumeral joint stability. Clin Orthop Relat Res. 1993;291:20–8.
11. Lippitt SB, Vanderhooft JE, Harris SL, Sidles JA, Harryman 2nd DT, Matsen 3rd FA. Glenohumeral stability from concavity-compression: a quantitative analysis. J Shoulder Elb Surg. 1993;2(1):27–35.
12. Tibone JE, Bradley JP. The treatment of posterior subluxation in athletes. Clin Orthop Relat Res. 1993;291:124–37.
13. Delong JM, Bradley JP. Posterior shoulder instability in the athletic population: Variations in assessment, clinical outcomes, and return to sport. World J Orthop. 2015;6(11):927–34.
14. Cho JH, Chung NS, Song HK, Lee DH. Recurrent posterior shoulder instability after rifle shooting. Orthopedics. 2012;35(11):e1677–9.

15. Welch CM, Banks SA, Cook FF, Draovitch P. Hitting a baseball: a biomechanical description. J Orthop Sports Phys Ther. 1995;22(5):193–201.
16. Kang RW, Mahony GT, Harris TC, Dines JS. Posterior instability caused by batter's shoulder. Clin Sports Med. 2013;32(4):797–802.
17. Van Tongel A, Karelse A, Berghs B, Verdonk R, De Wilde L. Posterior shoulder instability: current concepts review. Knee Surg Sports Traumatol Arthrosc. 2011;19(9):1547–53.
18. Rebolledo BJ, Nwachukwu BU, Konin GP, Coleman SH, Potter HG, Warren RF. Posterior humeral avulsion of the glenohumeral ligament and associated injuries: assessment using magnetic resonance imaging. Am J Sports Med. 2015;43(12):2913–7.
19. Tibone JE, Jobe FW, Kerlan RK, Carter VS, Shields CL, Lombardo SJ, Yocum LA. Shoulder impingement syndrome in athletes treated by anterior acromioplasty. Clin Orthop Relat Res. 1985;198:134–40.
20. Kennedy JC, Hawkins RJ, Krusoff WB. Orthopedic manifestations of swimming. Am J Sports Med. 1978;6(6):309–22.
21. Perry J. Anatomy and biomechanics of the shoulder in throwing, swimming, gymnastics, and tennis. Clin Sports Med. 1983;2(2):247–70.
22. Burkhart SS, Morgan CD, Kibler WB. The disabled throwing shoulder: spectrum of pathology Part I: pathoanatomy and biomechanics. Arthroscopy. 2003;19(4):404–20.
23. Jobe CM. Posterior superior glenoid impingement: expanded spectrum. Arthroscopy. 1995;11(5):530–6.
24. Jobe FW, Giangarra CE, Kvitne RS, Glousman RE. Anterior capsulolabral reconstruction of the shoulder in athletes in overhead sports. Am J Sports Med. 1991;19(5):428–34.
25. Rubenstein DL, Jobe FW, Glousman RE, Kvitne RS, Pink M, Giangarra CE. Anterior capsulolabral reconstruction of the shoulder in athletes. J Shoulder Elb Surg. 1992;1(5):229–37.
26. Andrews JR, Carson Jr W, McLeod W. Glenoid labrum tears related to the long head of the biceps. Am J Sports Med. 1985;13(5):337–41.
27. Walch G, Boileau J, Noel E, Connell ST. Impingement of the deep surface of the supraspinatus tendon on the posterior superior glenoid rim: an arthroscopic study. Am J Sports Med. 1985;13(5):337–41.
28. Fessa CK, Peduto A, Linklater J, Tirman P. Posterosuperior glenoid internal impingement of the shoulder in the overhead athlete: pathogenesis, clinical features and MR imaging findings. J Med Imaging Radiat Oncol. 2015;59(2):182–7.
29. Chang ES, Greco NJ, McClincy MP, Bradley JP. Posterior shoulder instability in overhead athletes. Orthop Clin North Am. 2016;47(1):179–87.
30. O'Brien SJ, Neves MC, Arnoczky SP, Rozbruck SR, Dicarlo EF, Warren RF, Schwartz R, Wickiewicz TL. The anatomy and histology of the inferior glenohumeral ligament complex of the shoulder. Am J Sports Med. 1990;18(5):449–56.
31. Cyprien JM, Vasey HM, Burdet A, Bonvin JC, Kritsikis N, Vuagnat P. Humeral retrotorsion and glenohumeral relationship in the normal shoulder and in recurrent anterior dislocation (scapulometry). Clin Orthop Relat Res. 1983;175:8–17.
32. Pollock RG, Bigliani LU. Recurrent posterior shoulder instability: diagnosis and treatment. Clin Orthop Relat Res. 1993;(291):85–96.
33. Von Raebrox A, Campbell B, Ramesh R, Bunker T. The association of subacromial dimples with recurrent posterior dislocation of the shoulder. J Shoulder Elb Surg. 2006;15(5):591–3.
34. Barth JR, Burkhart SS, De Beer JF. The bear-hug test: a new and sensitive test for diagnosing a subscapularis tear. Arthroscopy. 2006;22(10):1076–84.
35. Pennock AT, Pennington WW, Torry MR, Decker MJ, Vaishnav SB, Provencher MT, Millett PJ, Hackett TR. The influence of arm and shoulder position on the bear-hug, belly-press, and lift-off tests: an electromyographic study. Am J Sports Med. 2011;39(11):2338–46.
36. Hawkins RJ, Koppert G, Johnston G. Recurrent posterior instability (subluxation) of the shoulder. J Bone Joint Surg Am. 1984;66(2):169–74.
37. Kim SH, Park JS, Jeong WK, Shin SK. The Kim test: a novel test for posteroinferior labral lesion of the shoulder – a comparison to the jerk test. Am J Sports Med. 2005;33(8):1188–92.
38. Owen JM, Boulter T, Walton M, Funk L, Mackenzie TA. Reinterpretation of O'Brien test in posterior labral tears of the shoulder. Int J Shoulder Surg. 2015;9(1):6–8.
39. Smith TO, Drew BT, Toms AP. A meta-analysis of the diagnostic test accuracy of MRA and MRI for the detection of glenoid labral injury. Arch Orthop Trauma Surg. 2012;132(7):905–19.
40. Kaplan LD, McMahon PJ, Towers J, Irrgang JJ, Rodosky MW. Internal impingement: findings on magnetic resonance imaging and arthroscopic evaluation. Arthroscopy. 2004;20(7):701–4.
41. Giaroli EL, Major NM, Higgins LD. MRI of internal impingement of the shoulder. AJR Am J Roentgenol. 2005;185(4):925–9.
42. Tuite MJ, Petersen BD, Wise SM, Fine JP, Kaplan LD, Orwin JF. Shoulder MR arthrography of the posterior labrocapsular complex in overhead throwers with pathologic internal impingement and internal rotation deficit. Skelet Radiol. 2007;36(6):495–502.
43. Yu JS, Ashman CJ, Jones G. The POLPSA lesion: MR imaging findings with arthroscopic correlation in patients with posterior instability. Skelet Radiol. 2002;31(7):396–9.
44. Ferrari JD, Ferrari DA, Coumas J, Pappas AM. Posterior ossification of the shoulder: the Bennett lesion. Etiology, diagnosis, and treatment. Am J Sports Med. 1994;22(2):171–5; discussion 175–6.
45. Nourissat G, Radier C, Aim F, Lacoste S. Arthroscopic classification of posterior labrum glenoid insertion. Orthop Traumatol Surg Res. 2014;100(2):167–70.

46. Kim SH, Ha KI, Park JH, Kim YM, Lee YS, Lee JY, Yoo JC. Arthroscopic posterior labral repair and capsular shift for traumatic unidirectional recurrent posterior subluxation of the shoulder. J Bone Joint Surg Am. 2003;85-A(8):1479–87.
47. Brewer BJ, Wubben RC, Carrera GF. Excessive retroversion of the glenoid cavity: a cause of non-traumatic posterior instability of the shoulder. J Bone Joint Surg Am. 1986;68(5):724–31.
48. Inui H, Sugamoto K, Miyamoto T, Yoshikawa H, Machida A, Hashimoto J, Nobuhara K. Glenoid shape in atraumatic posterior instability of the shoulder. Clin Orthop Relat Res. 2002;403:87–92.
49. Kim SH, Noh KC, Park JS, Ryu BD, Oh I. Loss of chondrolabral containment of the glenohumeral joint in atraumatic posteroinferior multidirectional instability. J Bone Joint Surg Am. 2005;87(1):92–8.
50. Hurley JA, Anderson TE, Dear W, Andrish JT, Bergfeld JA, Weiker GG. Posterior shoulder instability. Surgical versus conservative results with evaluation of glenoid version. Am J Sports Med. 1992;20(4):396–400.
51. Borrero CG, Casagranda BU, Towers JD, Bradley JP. Magnetic resonance appearance of posterosuperior labral peel back during humeral abduction and external rotation. Skelet Radiol. 2010;39(1): 19–26.
52. Probyn LJ, White LM, Salonen DC, Tomlinson G, Boynton EL. Recurrent symptoms after shoulder instability repair: direct MR arthrographic assessment: Correlation with second-look surgical evaluation. Radiology. 2007;245(3):814–23.
53. Burkhead Jr WZ, Rockwood Jr CA. Treatment of instability of the shoulder with an exercise program. J Bone Joint Surg Am. 1992;74(6):890–6.
54. Wilk KE, Macrina LC, Reinold MM. Non-operative rehabilitation for traumatic and atraumatic glenohumeral instability. N Am J Sports Phys Ther. 2006;1(1):16–31.
55. Cicak N. Posterior dislocation of the shoulder. J Bone Joint Surg Br. 2004;86(3):324–32.
56. Finkelstein JA, Waddell JP, O'Driscoll SW, Vincent G. Acute posterior fracture dislocations of the shoulder treated with the Neer modification of the McLaughlin procedure. J Orthop Trauma. 1995;9(3):190–3.
57. Checchia SL, Santos PD, Miyazaki AN. Surgical treatment of acute and chronic posterior fracture-dislocation of the shoulder. J Shoulder Elb Surg. 1998;7(1):53–65.
58. Connor PM, Boatright JR, D'Alessandro DF. Posterior fracture-dislocation of the shoulder: treatment with acute osteochondral grafting. J Shoulder Elb Surg. 1997;6(5):480–5.
59. Lavender CD, Hanzlik SR, Pearson SE, Caldwell 3rd PE. Arthroscopic reverse remplissage for posterior instability. Arthrosc Tech. 2016;5(1):e43–7.
60. Duey RE, Burkhart SS. Arthroscopic treatment of a reverse Hill-Sachs lesion. Arthrosc Tech. 2013;2(2):e155–9.
61. Barbier O, Ollat D, Marchaland JP, Versier G. Iliac bone-block autograft for posterior shoulder instability. Orthop Traumatol Surg Res. 2009;95(2):100–7.
62. Lévigne C, Garret J, Grosclaude S, Borel F, Walch G. Surgical technique arthroscopic posterior glenoidplasty for posterosuperior glenoid impingement in throwing athletes. Clin Orthop Relat Res. 2012;470(6):1571–8.
63. Meuffels DE, Schuit H, van Biezen FC, Reijman M, Verhaar JA. The posterior bone block procedure in posterior shoulder instability: a long-term follow-up study. J Bone Joint Surg Br. 2010;92(5):651–5.
64. Millett PJ, Clavert P, Hatch 3rd GF, Warner JJ. Recurrent posterior shoulder instability. J Am Acad Orthop Surg. 2006;14(8):464–76.
65. Servien E, Walch G, Cortes ZE, Edwards TB, O'Connor DP. Posterior bone block procedure for posterior shoulder instability. Knee Surg Sports Traumatol Arthrosc. 2007;15(9):1130–6.
66. Gosens T, van Biezen FC, Verhaar JA. The bone block procedure in recurrent posterior shoulder instability. Acta Orthop Belg. 2001;67(2):116–20.
67. Millett PJ, Schoenahl JY, Register B, Gaskill TR, van Deurzen DF, Martetschläger F. Reconstruction of posterior glenoid deficiency using distal tibial osteoarticular allograft. Knee Surg Sports Traumatol Arthrosc. 2013;21(2):445–9.
68. Cerciello S, Visonà E, Morris BJ, Corona K. Bone block procedures in posterior shoulder instability. Knee Surg Sports Traumatol Arthrosc. 2016;24(2): 604–11.
69. Lafosse L, Franceschi G, Kordasiewicz B, Andrews WJ, Schwartz D. Arthroscopic posterior bone block: surgical technique. Musculoskelet Surg. 2012;96(3):205–12.
70. Mauro CS, McClincy MP, Bradley JP. Effect of glenoid version and width on outcomes of arthroscopic posterior shoulder stabilization. Am J Sports Med. 2016;44(4):941–7.
71. Bradley JP, McClincy MP, Arner JW, Tejwani SG. Arthroscopic capsulolabral reconstruction for posterior instability of the shoulder: a prospective study of 200 shoulders. Am J Sports Med. 2013;41(9):2005–14.
72. Arner JW, McClincy MP, Bradley JP. Arthroscopic stabilization of posterior shoulder instability is successful in American football players. Arthroscopy. 2015;31(8):1466–71.
73. Wanich T, Dines J, Dines D, Gambardella RA, Yocum LA. 'Batter's shoulder': can athletes return to play at the same level after operative treatment? Clin Orthop Relat Res. 2012;470(6):1565–70.
74. Eckenrode BJ, Logerstedt DS, Sennett BJ. Rehabilitation and functional outcomes in collegiate wrestlers following a posterior shoulder stabilization procedure. J Orthop Sports Phys Ther. 2009;39(7):550–9.
75. McClincy MP, Arner JW, Bradley JP. Posterior shoulder instability in throwing athletes: a case-matched comparison of throwers and non-throwers. Arthroscopy. 2015;31(6):1041–51.

76. Wooten CJ, Krych AJ, Schleck CD, Hudgens JL, May JH, Dahm DL. Arthroscopic capsulolabral reconstruction for posterior shoulder instability in patients 18 years old or younger. J Pediatr Orthop. 2015;35(5):462–6.
77. Fuchs B, Jost B, Gerber C. Posterior-inferior capsular shift for the treatment of recurrent, voluntary posterior subluxation of the shoulder. J Bone Joint Surg Am. 2000;82(1):16–25.
78. Provencher MT, Bell SJ, Menzel KA, Mologne TS. Arthroscopic treatment of posterior shoulder instability: results in 33 patients. Am J Sports Med. 2005;33(10):1463–71.
79. Merolla G, De Santis E, Cools AM, Porcellini G. Functional outcome and quality of life after rehabilitation for voluntary posterior shoulder dislocation: a prospective blinded cohort study. Eur J Orthop Surg Traumatol. 2015;25(2):263–72.

# Management of Acute Shoulder Instability: Conservative Treatment

6

Rebecca A. Carr and Geoffrey D. Abrams

## Contents

6.1 **Background** ... 49
6.2 **Anatomy** ... 50
6.3 **Pathophysiology** ... 50
6.4 **Clinical Presentation** ... 51
6.5 **Radiographs** ... 51
6.6 **Reduction Techniques** ... 51
6.7 **Initial Postreduction Treatment** ... 52
6.8 **Rehabilitation and Physical Therapy** ... 52
**Conclusion** ... 54
**References** ... 54

R.A. Carr, BS (✉)
Royal College of Surgeons, Dublin, Ireland
e-mail: rebeccacarr88@gmail.com

G.D. Abrams
Department of Orthopedic Surgery, Stanford University, Veterans Administration, Palo Alto, USA
e-mail: gabrams@stanford.edu

## 6.1 Background

Shoulder instability is one of the most commonly diagnosed shoulder pathologies [1]. It describes a wide clinical spectrum that ranges from complete dislocation requiring mechanical reduction of the joint to shoulder subluxation in which some glenohumeral contact remains [2–6]. Anterior shoulder dislocations are the most common subtype, accounting for 98 % of cases [7–10], and are the most common large joint dislocation [11] with a reported prevalence of approximately 2 % within the general population [7, 10, 12, 13]. The incidence of anterior shoulder dislocation has a bimodal age distribution, with peaks occurring in the second and sixth decades; however, 90 % of cases occur in young individuals below the age of 30 years [14, 15]. Trauma is by far the most common cause of primary shoulder dislocation, accounting for 95 % of cases [9]. Other risk factors for shoulder dislocation include male sex and participation in contact sports [14].

Depending on the mechanism of injury, the humeral head may dislocate anteriorly, posteriorly, or inferiorly. Traumatic posterior dislocations are considerably more rare, accounting for approximately 2 % of cases [9, 15, 16], and are most frequently caused by direct trauma to the anterior shoulder or by an indirect force that is directed posteriorly through the arm to the shoulder [8]. Inferior dislocations are extremely rare, accounting for approximately 0.5 % of cases, and

© ISAKOS 2017
A.B. Imhoff, F.H. Savoie III (eds.), *Shoulder Instability Across the Life Span*,
DOI 10.1007/978-3-662-54077-0_6

are due to hyperabduction of the arm that forces the neck of the humerus against the acromion, resulting in displacement of the humeral head inferiorly [10].

## 6.2 Anatomy

The glenohumeral joint is a careful balance of mobility and stability [1, 17]. Glenohumeral mobility is the result of the small surface area of the humerus that articulates with the glenoid, the shape and minimal depth of the glenoid fossa, and the relative laxity of the surrounding joint capsule [18, 19]. Glenohumeral stability is the ability to keep the humeral head centered within the glenoid fossa and is achieved through the combined action of noncontractile, static stabilizers (such as the bony articulation) as well as more dynamic stabilizers [2, 20–22]. The inherent osseous stability of the shoulder is relatively small as only about 30 % of the humeral head articulates with the glenoid fossa at any one time [8, 22].

The primary dynamic stabilizers of the glenohumeral joint are the rotator cuff tendons and muscles, the biceps tendon, and the scapular muscles [1, 10, 13, 17, 22–24]. Coordinated muscle contraction of these dynamic stabilizers produces a synergistic effect that increases the compression of the humeral head against the glenoid fossa, resulting in an increase in the load required to translate the humeral head [17, 18, 21, 22, 25].

The primary static stabilizers of the glenohumeral joint are the osseous articulation, the glenoid labrum, and the capsuloligamentous structure [21, 22, 24]. The glenoid labrum is a rim of fibrocartilaginous tissue attached at the periphery of the glenoid that increases the depth of the socket by approximately 50 %, allowing for increased articulation between the humeral head and glenoid fossa. It also provides an attachment site for the long head of the biceps tendon and glenohumeral ligaments [13, 21, 22]. The superior, middle, and inferior glenohumeral ligaments are distinct capsular thickenings that limit excessive humeral translation at the extremes of motion [2, 21]. These ligaments only contribute to mechanical stability when stretched beyond their rest length; thus, depending on the humeral location within the glenoid, there is variable contribution of these ligaments to joint stability [2, 17, 18, 22, 25].

The inferior glenohumeral ligament is a complex of three distinct parts, the anterior and posterior bands and axillary pouch, all of which originate from the anteroinferior labrum and glenoid rim, and it is the most important stabilizing factor against anteroinferior shoulder dislocation [2, 13, 17, 24, 25]. Clinically, the anterior band is the most important because it is the primary stabilizer preventing excessive anterior glenohumeral translation when the shoulder is abducted and externally rotated, the same position that most anterior humeral dislocations occur [10, 13]. The superior glenohumeral ligament arises from the anterosuperior labrum and is the primary restraint of inferior translation when the shoulder is adducted and in a neutral position [20, 21]. The middle glenohumeral ligament arises adjacent to the superior glenohumeral ligament and is the most variable of the three [18]. The middle glenohumeral ligament prevents anterior glenohumeral translation when the shoulder is held in midrange abduction [20].

## 6.3 Pathophysiology

Glenohumeral joint instability occurs when excessive or repetitive force applied to the joint exceeds the force of these dynamic and static stabilizers, and depending on the mechanism of injury and the direction of dislocation, typically there is associated injury to one or more of these stabilizers [10, 22]. All dislocations have the potential to damage surrounding structures and cause various complications, such as neurological injury, vascular injury, fracture, and rotator cuff tears, which may negatively impair functional outcome and increase the risk of recurrence [25, 26]. Rotator cuff tears, fractures of the greater tuberosity, and neurological injuries are more common in women and in patients over the age of 60 [27].

Anterior shoulder dislocations are most often the result of forceful external rotation and abduction of the humerus [7, 9, 10, 13]. In this position, the excessive anterior glenohumeral translation commonly causes tear of the anterior-inferior labrum, referred to clinically as a Bankart lesion [10, 20, 22], which is seen in over 90 % of cases of traumatic humeral dislocations [10, 13]. When the humeral head dislocates anteriorly, impaction of the humeral head against the anteroinferior glenoid may cause a posterolateral humeral head compression fracture, referred to as a Hill-Sachs lesion [10, 13, 20, 25]. Furthermore, in adults over 40 years of age who sustain a shoulder dislocation, rotator cuff injury is a common sequela [26].

## 6.4 Clinical Presentation

Patients presenting with acute shoulder instability will typically have a clear history of trauma resulting in obvious dislocation of the joint requiring mechanical reduction or the subjective feeling of instability, indicating joint subluxation [13, 28, 29]. In contrast, patients who are not able to recall a definitive onset to their symptoms may have generalized laxity [10, 28]. When obtaining the patient history, it is critical to determine the mechanism of injury as well as the position of the arm during the injury, as this may help distinguish between an anterior or posterior dislocation [28]. Patients presenting with acute traumatic anterior dislocations typically describe the arm as being extended, abducted, and externally rotated at the time of injury. Other important components of the history include the number of previous episodes of subluxation or dislocation and the age at which these occurred, previous physical therapy or surgery to the shoulder, and the presence of pain or any other associated symptoms [13, 20, 30].

Physical examination should begin with general inspection for any gross abnormalities, especially if there is a history of trauma, followed by evaluation of active and passive range of movement [12]. In the setting of a dislocated shoulder, a visible deformity of the shoulder is often present. On examination, both active and passive movements are restricted due to pain, and the arm is typically held fixed in slight internal rotation and abduction, with resultant flattening of the shoulder contour [20]. A full neurovascular examination should be performed to assess the motor and sensory functions of the axillary, musculocutaneous, median, radial, and ulnar nerves and to palpate the radial and ulnar pulses [10, 13].

Patients presenting with acute traumatic posterior dislocations typically describe the arm as being forward flexed, adducted, and internally rotated at the time of injury and may have pain or a subjective feeling of instability when the arm is adducted and internally rotated [21, 28]. Athletes involved in blocking, such as football lineman and rugby players, are prone to this type of injury [16]. Additional features of the history that may suggest posterior dislocation include a history of epilepsy, electroconvulsive shock therapy, and alcohol withdrawal seizures [10, 21].

## 6.5 Radiographs

Following physical exam, conventional radiography is often the next step in evaluating most shoulder pathology. Plain films can be tailored according to the suspected condition [31, 32]. When evaluating shoulder instability, it is important to obtain orthogonal views, typically consisting of at least an anteroposterior (AP) and axillary lateral view [31]. Some clinicians may prefer a complete shoulder series including anterior-posterior views in both internal and external rotation, axillary, outlet, and 30 ° caudal tilt views.

## 6.6 Reduction Techniques

In most patients, acute shoulder dislocation causes significant pain and muscle spasm, particularly if it is a first-time dislocation, so it is important to offer the patient analgesia to reduce pain and promote muscle relaxation before attempting reduction [5, 11, 14, 20]. Intra-articular lidocaine (IAL) injection and intravenous analgesia with or without sedation provide effective analgesia and patient satisfaction during the reduction maneuver with equal rates of successful reduction; however, IAL is associated with less side effects and a shorter recovery time [10, 11, 13, 14]. Reduction with minimal or no analgesia may be attempted in patients presenting very soon after dislocation and/or in patients with recurrent dislocation only associated with moderate pain, as the most effective treatment is rapid reduction of the joint [11].

Once pain control is adequate and radiographs performed exclude the presence of an associated fracture, prompt joint reduction is necessary to minimize the risk of neurovascular compromise and soft tissue stretch [10, 14, 33]. Numerous reduction techniques can be used for closed reduction of anterior dislocations, and choice depends on physician preference. The most utilized techniques for anterior shoulder dislocations include the traction-countertraction, Milch, Stimson, and scapular manipulation techniques [33]. In general, these techniques move the humeral head, typically in an anterior-inferior position, into a more favorable position relative to the glenoid to facilitate reduction. Sometimes, a combination of techniques is utilized to achieve success. Closed reduction of posterior dislocations is considerably more difficult, and due to the risk of fracture, some authors recommend that closed reduction should only be attempted in patients with an associated humeral head defect comprising less than 20 % who are within a short time frame of the dislocation [10, 33].

Following reduction of the joint, a complete neurovascular exam should be conducted to ensure that the patient did not sustain any nerve or vessel injuries [14, 26]. Repeat radiographs should be obtained immediately after the procedure to confirm joint reduction and assess for any osseous lesions not present on initial radiographs [14]. Due to the significantly increased incidence of rotator cuff tears in patients over the age of 40, it is imperative that these patients undergo careful evaluation for possible rotator cuff lesions in the follow-up time frame [14].

## 6.7 Initial Postreduction Treatment

Following successful closed reduction of the joint, traditional management of a first-time dislocator is conservative, nonoperative treatment that aims to improve joint function while also reducing the rate of recurrent instability [10]. Typically, immediately following joint reduction, the arm is immobilized with the aim of reducing inflammation, controlling pain, restoring basic dynamic stability to the glenohumeral joint, and reducing the risk of further damage to the joint [5, 7, 10, 13].

Immobilization of anterior shoulder dislocations is traditionally with the arm in internal rotation and in adduction for a period of 1–4 weeks [11, 13, 34–36]; however, current research suggests that when immobilized in this position, there is no clinical benefit to immobilization longer than 1 week [5, 13]. Additionally, this arm position has recently been challenged by data from research studies on arm position using cadavers as well as MRI that proposed that there is better approximation of the Bankart lesion when the arm is immobilized in external rotation and abduction [37, 38]. Despite this proposed benefit of external rotation, the clinical significance remains controversial. While there have been several studies published reporting reduced incidence of recurrent shoulder instability when the arm is immobilized in external rotation [35, 36, 39, 40], other prospective studies have not found any significant difference in the recurrence rates between the two methods [41–43]. Furthermore, several reviews of the literature, including meta-analyses, have failed to show a statistically significant reduction in the rate of recurrence with either position [13, 34, 44]. Furthermore, the amount of external rotation needed has not been clearly defined, and a major drawback is patient adherence, as immobilization of the arm in external rotation and abduction is more cumbersome for the patient in terms of activities of daily living [10, 14].

## 6.8 Rehabilitation and Physical Therapy

Following immobilization, patients are typically enrolled into a rehabilitation program that consists of a variable number of sequential and progressive phases that each focus on specific goals and contain a protocol of exercises that gradually become more aggressive and demanding [45]. Progression through the program can be modified according to the degree of injury, premorbid activity level, and patient goals. The temporal framework of these phases is often useful to patients, as it provides them with a realistic timeline to recovery [46, 47]. The goal of rehabilitation is to reduce pain and restore full function of the joint, which is accomplished through exercises aimed to restore or improve range of motion and flexibility, muscle strength and power, proprioception, and endurance [7].

The acute phase can be clinically defined as the period beginning at the onset of the injury, and it typically lasts 4–6 days [47]. During this period, the emphasis for treatment is on controlling pain and reducing inflammation, while slowly restoring range of motion in the shoulder joint [45, 46, 48]. As stated previously, the acute phase of treatment typically begins with a short period of joint immobilization, at which time the patient is educated on activity modification. Following immobilization, the sling is removed and controlled, passive range of motion (PROM) exercises are initiated in order to restore physiologic joint motions, and these exercises are thought to promote healing and prevent contracture by enhancing collagen organization [5, 7, 49]. Systemic anti-inflammatories, cryotherapy, and electrical stimulation may be helpful in improving mobility by reducing inflammation and pain [5, 48, 50]. Light strengthening exercises focusing on the rotator cuff muscles and the muscles involved in scapula stabilization are utilized in order to inhibit muscular atrophy and improve dynamic stability and are performed through pain-free, submaximal, isometric contractions [5, 48, 50].

Once pain and inflammation are significantly reduced so that there is minimal pain on range of motion and there is an adequate level of muscle strength and scapular control, the patient is said to have entered the intermediate or early recovery phase, which focuses on regaining full range of motion, restoring neuromuscular control, and improving strength of the joint [5, 49, 51]. This phase of rehabilitation begins with active-assisted range of motion (AAROM) exercises, which require activation of the muscles surrounding the glenohumeral joint, such as active-assisted L-bar exercises and pendulum exercises [46]. During this time, shoulder mobilization is permitted within pain-free limits; however, external rotation and abduction past 90 ° is limited for the first 4–8 weeks in patients with anterior glenohumeral instability in order to promote healing of anterior capsuloligamentous structures [5, 7, 9], whereas internal rotation is limited in patients with posterior glenohumeral instability [33]. During this phase, patients progress from isometric to isotonic exercises that focus on improving strength of the internal and external rotators as well as the scapular muscles in order to restore muscle balance and maximize the dynamic stability of the joint [7, 45].

Patients are able to progress to the functional or advanced strengthening phase with achievement of pain-free, full range of motion, symmetric capsular mobility, and adequate strength [45, 48–50]. During this phase, aggressive strengthening exercises are initiated along with advanced functional drills, dynamic stabilization drills, and plyometric exercises in order to improve muscle power, strength, coordination, and endurance [48, 49, 51]. A shoulder stabilization brace may be utilized for support, but evidence for use of prosthetic devices such as these is lacking.

Recurrence of shoulder instability following an acute episode of glenohumeral instability is proportional to the activity level and inversely proportional to age at the time of the initial dislocation [12]. Despite increased rates of recurrent instability seen in younger patients, conservative treatment remains first-line treatment for most first-time anterior shoulder dislocations [12]. Some authors, however, recommend primary surgical repair for patients with acute traumatic anterior shoulder instability who are young and who participate in high-contact sports [52]. Additionally, a large Cochrane review evaluating the surgical and nonsurgical treatment for acute shoulder instability found that young, active males had statistically significant reduction in the rate of recurrent shoulder instability as well as an increase in subjective joint function when treated surgically [53].

## Conclusion

Glenohumeral joint dislocations are a common injury as the increased range of motion of the shoulder, compared to other joints, predisposes it to instability. Evaluation of the patient with an acute dislocation includes a history, physical exam, and high-quality radiographs. A variety of reduction maneuvers may be utilized to obtain reduction. First-line treatment for patients with an initial dislocation is typically nonoperative, with special attention paid to concomitant rotator cuff pathology in the elderly and consideration for early surgical intervention in young patients involved in contact sports.

## References


1. Matsen 3rd FA, Chebli CM, Lippitt SB. Principles for the evaluation and management of shoulder instability. Instr Course Lect. 2007;56:23–34.
2. Farrar NG, Malal JJ, Fischer J, Waseem M. An overview of shoulder instability and its management. Open Orthop J. 2013;7:338–46.
3. Bak K, Wiesler ER, Poehling GG. Consensus statement on shoulder instability. Arthroscopy. 2010;26:249–55.
4. Owens BD, Nelson BJ, Duffey ML, et al. Pathoanatomy of first-time, traumatic, anterior glenohumeral subluxation events. J Bone Joint Surg. 2010;92:1605–11.
5. Wilk KE, Macrina LC. Nonoperative and postoperative rehabilitation for glenohumeral instability. Clin Sports Med. 2013;32:865–914.
6. Lewis A, Kitamura T, Bayley JIL. (ii) The classification of shoulder instability: new light through old windows! Curr Orthop. 2004;18:97–108.
7. Karatsolis K, Athanasopoulos S. The role of exercise in the conservative treatment of the anterior shoulder dislocation. J Bodyw Mov Ther. 2006;10:211–9.
8. Tannenbaum EP, Sekiya JK. Posterior shoulder instability in the contact athlete. Clin Sports Med. 2013;32:781–96.
9. Hayes K, Callanan M, Walton J, Paxinos A, Murrell GA. Shoulder instability: management and rehabilitation. J Orthop Sports Phys Ther. 2002;32:497–509.
10. Rumian A, Coffey D, Fogerty S, Hackney R. Acute first-time shoulder dislocation. Orthop Trauma. 2011;25:363–8.
11. Hendey GW. Managing anterior shoulder dislocation. Ann Emerg Med. 2016;67:76–80.
12. Schrumpf MA, Maak TG, Delos D, et al. The management of anterior glenohumeral instability with and without bone loss: AAOS exhibit selection. J Bone Joint Surg Am. 2014;96:e12.
13. Dumont GD, Russell RD, Robertson WJ. Anterior shoulder instability: a review of pathoanatomy, diagnosis and treatment. Curr Rev Muscoskelet Med. 2011;4:200–7.
14. Khiami F, Gérometta A, Loriaut P. Management of recent first-time anterior shoulder dislocations. Orthop Traumatol Surg Res. 2015;101:S51–S7.
15. Lewis TL, Ferran NA, Gooding BWT. Current concepts in shoulder and elbow fractures and dislocations. Surgery (Oxford). 2016;34:122–8.
16. Van Lancker HP, Martineau PA. (i) The diagnosis and treatment of shoulder injuries in contact and collision athletes. Orthop Trauma. 2012;26:1–11.
17. Veeger HE, van der Helm FC. Shoulder function: the perfect compromise between mobility and stability. J Biomech. 2007;40:2119–29.
18. Pagnani MJ, Warren RF. Stabilizers of the glenohumeral joint. J Shoulder Elbow Surg. 1994;3:173–90.
19. Hurov J. Anatomy and mechanics of the shoulder: review of current concepts. J Hand Ther. 2009;22:328–42. quiz 43
20. Dodson CC, Cordasco FA. Anterior glenohumeral joint dislocations. Orthop Clin North Am. 2008;39:507–18. vii
21. Nguyen D. Anatomy, examination, and imaging of the shoulder. Oper Tech Orthop. 2008;18:2–8.
22. Lugo R, Kung P, Ma CB. Shoulder biomechanics. Eur J Radiol. 2008;68:16–24.
23. Labriola JE, Lee TQ, Debski RE, McMahon PJ. Stability and instability of the glenohumeral joint: the role of shoulder muscles. J Shoulder Elbow Surg. 2005;14:32s–8s.
24. Doukas WC, Speer KP. Anatomy, pathophysiology, and biomechanics of shoulder instability. Oper Tech Sports Med. 2000;8:179–87.
25. Murray IR, Goudie EB, Petrigliano FA, Robinson CM. Functional anatomy and biomechanics of shoulder stability in the athlete. Clin Sports Med. 2013;32:607–24.
26. Beeson MS. Complications of shoulder dislocation. Am J Emerg Med. 1999;17:288–95.
27. Robinson CM, Shur N, Sharpe T, Ray A, Murray IR. Injuries associated with traumatic anterior glenohumeral dislocations. J Bone Joint Surg Am. 2012;94:18–26.
28. Cadet ER. Evaluation of glenohumeral instability. Orthop Clin North Am. 2010;41:287–95.
29. Farber AJ, Castillo R, Clough M, Bahk M, McFarland EG. Clinical assessment of three common tests for traumatic anterior shoulder instability. J Bone Joint Surg Am. 2006;88:1467–74.
30. Hill AM, Bull AMJ, Richardson J, et al. The clinical assessment and classification of shoulder instability. Curr Orthop. 2008;22:208–25.
31. Goud A, Segal D, Hedayati P, Pan JJ, Weissman BN. Radiographic evaluation of the shoulder. Eur J Radiol. 2008;68:2–15.

32. Sanders TG, Jersey SL. Conventional radiography of the shoulder. Semin Roentgenol. 2005;40:207–22.
33. Youm T, Takemoto R, Park BK. Acute management of shoulder dislocations. J Am Acad Orthop Surg. 2014;22:761–71.
34. Smith TO. Immobilisation following traumatic anterior glenohumeral joint dislocation: a literature review. Injury. 2006;37:228–37.
35. Itoi E, Hatakeyama Y, Kido T, et al. A new method of immobilization after traumatic anterior dislocation of the shoulder: a preliminary study. J Shoulder Elbow Surg. 2003;12:413–5.
36. Itoi E, Hatakeyama Y, Sato T, et al. Immobilization in external rotation after shoulder dislocation reduces the risk of recurrence. A randomized controlled trial. J Bone Joint Surg Am. 2007;89:2124–31.
37. Itoi E, Sashi R, Minagawa H, Shimizu T, Wakabayashi I, Sato K. Position of immobilization after dislocation of the glenohumeral joint. A study with use of magnetic resonance imaging. J Bone Joint Surg Am. 2001;83-a:661–7.
38. Miller BS, Sonnabend DH, Hatrick C, et al. Should acute anterior dislocations of the shoulder be immobilized in external rotation? A cadaveric study. J Shoulder Elbow Surg. 2004;13:589–92.
39. Yamamoto N, Sano H, Itoi E. Conservative treatment of first-time shoulder dislocation with the arm in external rotation. J Shoulder Elbow Surg. 2010;19:98–103.
40. Heidari K, Asadollahi S, Vafaee R, et al. Immobilization in external rotation combined with abduction reduces the risk of recurrence after primary anterior shoulder dislocation. J Shoulder Elbow Surg. 2014;23:759–66.
41. Liavaag S, Brox JI, Pripp AH, Enger M, Soldal LA, Svenningsen S. Immobilization in external rotation after primary shoulder dislocation did not reduce the risk of recurrence. J Bone Joint Surg. 2011;93:897–904.
42. Finestone A, Milgrom C, Radeva-Petrova DR, et al. Bracing in external rotation for traumatic anterior dislocation of the shoulder. J Bone Joint Surg Br. 2009;91:918–21.
43. Heidari K, Asadollahi S, Vafaee R, Barfehei A, Kamalifar H, Chaboksavar ZA, Sabbaghi M. Immobilization with an external rotation brace was similar to an internal rotation sling for shoulder dislocation. J Bone Joint Surg. 2014;96:1398.
44. Vavken P, Sadoghi P, Quidde J, et al. Immobilization in internal or external rotation does not change recurrence rates after traumatic anterior shoulder dislocation. J Shoulder Elbow Surg. 2014;23:13–9.
45. Wilk KE, Hooks TR. Rehabilitation of the throwing athlete: where we are in 2014. Clin Sports Med. 2015;34:247–61.
46. Wilk KE, Macrina LC, Reinold MM. Non-operative rehabilitation for traumatic and atraumatic glenohumeral instability. N Am J Sports Phys Ther. 2006;1:16–31.
47. Dale RB. 4 – Principles of rehabilitation A2 – Andrews, James R. In: Harrelson GL, Wilk KE, editors. Physical rehabilitation of the injured athlete. 4th ed. Philadelphia: W.B. Saunders; 2012. p. 41–66.
48. Wilk KE, Williams Jr RA, Dugas JR, Cain Jr EL, Andrews JR. Current concepts in the assessment and rehabilitation of the thrower's shoulder. Oper Tech Sports Med. 2016;24:170–80.
49. Reinold MM, Gill TJ, Wilk KE, Andrews JR. Current concepts in the evaluation and treatment of the shoulder in overhead throwing athletes, part 2: injury prevention and treatment. Sports Health. 2010;2:101–15.
50. Stracciolini A, Meehan Iii WP, d'Hemecourt PA. Sports rehabilitation of the injured athlete. Clin Pediatr Emerg Med. 2007;8:43–53.
51. Rubin BD, Kibler WB. Fundamental principles of shoulder rehabilitation: conservative to postoperative management. Arthroscopy. 2002;18:29–39.
52. Kralinger FS, Golser K, Wischatta R, Wambacher M, Sperner G. Predicting recurrence after primary anterior shoulder dislocation. Am J Sports Med. 2002;30:116–20.
53. Handoll HH, Almaiyah MA, Rangan A. Surgical versus non-surgical treatment for acute anterior shoulder dislocation. Cochrane Database Syst Rev 2004;(1):Cd004325.

# Arthroscopic Repair for Initial Anterior Dislocation

7

Robert A. Arciero and Andreas Voss

## Contents


7.1 **Introduction** ... 57

7.2 **Pathology** ... 58
7.2.1 Natural History ... 58
7.2.2 Surgical Management ... 59
7.2.3 Author's Preferred Surgical Approach ... 60

**References** ... 63



R.A. Arciero (✉)
Department of Orthopaedic Surgery, University of Connecticut Health Center, Farmington, CT, USA
e-mail: arciero@uchc.edu

A. Voss
Department of Orthopaedic Sports Medicine, Technical University of Munich, Munich, Germany


## 7.1 Introduction

The aim of orthopedic surgeons with acute first-time shoulder dislocation is to prevent recurrence and restore the natural anatomy. Traditionally the initial management consists of reduction of the glenohumeral joint, immobilization, and a stepwise approach with physical therapy to prevent shoulder stiffness and restore muscle strength [3]. Many studies investigated the difference between conservative and operative management in young patients, depending on the level of activity due to the high recurrence rate reported in this young population of 60–100% [8, 9, 21, 25]. There are clear advantages for the early operative reconstruction with a reported decrease of dislocation with arthroscopic stabilization [1, 10, 11]. However, there is little information regarding a treatment algorithm for a population younger than 20 years. Most recent studies reporting about a young active population indicate a mean age between 20 and 30 years with a range from 12 to 40 years [9, 10, 12, 13, 31].

The purpose of this chapter is to review and assimilate the current literature on acute anterior shoulder instability and introduce the concept of acute arthroscopic stabilization to minimize recurrence, improve quality of life and sport, and decrease the risk of glenohumeral arthropathy in very young population.


© ISAKOS 2017


A.B. Imhoff, F.H. Savoie III (eds.), *Shoulder Instability Across the Life Span*,
DOI 10.1007/978-3-662-54077-0_7

## 7.2 Pathology

To maintain stability in the glenohumeral joint with a wide range of motion, there is an importance for static (bony, capsular, and ligamentous anatomy) and dynamic (rotator cuff muscles) stabilizers. To prevent antero-glenohumeral translation, the main restraint is the inferior glenohumeral complex with a maximum strength in abduction and external rotation. After an anterior glenohumeral dislocation, this balance between static and dynamic stabilizers can be interrupted, usually by a stretching or avulsion of the capsuloligamentous complex including detachment of the anteroinferior labrum, the so-called Bankart lesion [2]. Additional structural damages, such as SLAP and Hill-Sachs lesion, can be found. Major damages to the rotator cuff and the bony glenoid rim are more often found in the middle-age and older population [9]. A recent systematic review analyzed the management of primary acute anterior shoulder dislocations [14]. They included 31 studies, but none of them excluded patient older than 20 years, and the mean age ranges between 20 and 47. Only a few studies had a mean age about 20 years of age. Law et al. [12] operated 38 patients with a primary traumatic shoulder dislocation in patients between 16 and 30 (mean 21), and they radiologically found Bankart and Hill-Sachs leasing in all patients with none of them having bone loss more than 20%. Arthroscopically they also found nine SLAP lesions (seven by MRI).

A study by Arciero and Taylor investigating first-time traumatic shoulder dislocators less than 24 years old showed a high incidence of Bankart leasing of 97% with 89% having an additional Hill-Sachs lesion with no gross evidence of capsulary damages [24].

When considering operative treatment of first-time dislocators, it is always important to take the consequences of nonsurgical treatment into account. Basically there are two important facts that support early surgery:

First the soft tissue damage: Repetitive sub-failures using a cadaveric model showed a decreased ultimate load to failure after repetitive loading of the inferior glenohumeral ligament, as seen in overhead athletes [19]. These results were explained with an accumulation of microtrauma to the ligamentous structures leading to early failure. Additionally a study by Urayama et al. [27] showed an increased capsular elongation in patients with recurrent traumatic anteroinferior dislocations.

The second area of concern and rationale for early stabilization is progressive bone defects. It has been shown that there is a correlation between the number of preoperative dislocations and the development of postoperative arthritis risk, indication of a higher risk for patients with more frequent dislocations [5]. Additionally a glenoid rim lesion after a traumatic shoulder dislocation is associated with a higher risk of arthritis due to the loss of a passive stabilizer, resulting in an increased risk of recurrent dislocation [5].

Therefore the aim in surgery of first-time traumatic shoulder dislocators under the age of 20 is to prevent additionally instability events and to restore the anatomy of the capsulo-labral complex.

### 7.2.1 Natural History

For many years the recurrence rate was the only outcome measurement, but other factors have gained importance when considering the treatment opinions for a first-time traumatic shoulder dislocator such as continued apprehension, return to sports or work, and the development of a post-traumatic glenohumeral osteoarthritis. Therefore, it is very important to take all these conditions into account, as they should influence the treatment decisions for each individual patient.

Children with an open physis showed a higher recurrence rate after first-time traumatic shoulder dislocation with a rate up to 100% [15], and this rate was confirmed by Rowe et al. [21] who found the same rate with children younger than 10 years of age. First-time dislocator between the age of 10 and 20 showed a rate of 60–94% [8, 9, 21].

Due to this high recurrence rate, it is important to clarify which patient population would benefit from early operation after first-time traumatic shoulder dislocation. One of the best known predictors is age and activity level. A study by Sachs et al. [22] followed a first-time dislocator population for 5 years and found a high recurrence rate for collusion sports athletes and those patients who used their arms above the chest level with a rate of 55% and 51%, respectively. According to these numbers, less than 50% of this high-risk population underwent surgical stabilization, which raises the question of the necessity of an early operation. However, the authors noted that patients, who did not follow surgical intervention, had lower outcome scores (WOSI, ASES).

Once a conservative treatment was chosen, there is a debate about the rotational rest position of the upper limb. A systematic review by Longo et al. [14] has shown that immobilization with external rotation was associated with a significant lower rate of recurrence when compared with patient immobilized with internal rotation. Interestingly a recent study by Whelan et al. [29] could not show any statistical significant comparing those two arm positions. Additionally there was no difference in patient's compliance comparing external to internal rotation immobilization.

So there is still a big controversy about the immobilization with open questions regarding the optimum position of external rotation, the acceptance of external rotation by patients, and the difference in recurrence rate [17]. A study by Chong et al. [7] showed that approximately 7% of orthopedic surgeons in England prefer external rotation immobilization for their patients after anterior shoulder dislocation.

Besides the short-term outcomes which are mostly related to recurrence rate, return to sport and work, as well as wellness, the long-term outcome for degenerative changes to the glenohumeral joint due to dislocation and instability has been investigated by Hovelius et al. They could show that 25 years after first-time dislocation, arthropathy was significantly more in patients with recurrent instability (40%) compared to patients without recurrent dislocation (18%). Similar results have been reported by Plath et al. [18] and Buscayret et al. [5] which found older age at initial dislocation and surgery, the number of preoperative dislocations, and the number of anchors used to be the most important risk factors for osteoarthritis.

Summarizing these findings the recent literature proposes early surgical stabilization to prevent recurrent dislocations and instability and to reduce osteoarthritis.

### 7.2.2 Surgical Management

Many different techniques and outcomes have been reported for first-time traumatic shoulder dislocators varying from a simple lavage to an open stabilization procedure.

#### 7.2.2.1 Lavage

Wintzell et al. [30] prospectively compared non-operative treatment to simple lavage and found a lower recurrence rate with the lavage (13%) compared to the non-operative treatment group (43%) after a follow-up of 1 year. Interestingly these results are even more evident in a younger population (<25 years) with a re-dislocation rate of 12% in the lavage group and 65%, respectively. However, 1 year might be too short to draw conclusions, as a study of Slaa et al. [25] found similar results to Wintzell after 1 year with a recurrence rate of 7%, but when following their lavage patients for another 4 years, they found an overall instability rate of 55%.

In a level I study comparing lavage to arthroscopic Bankart repair after first-time traumatic shoulder dislocation, the Bankart repair group showed a risk of recurrent instability reduction of 76% [20]. Furthermore there was significant difference between the recurrence rate of 38% with lavage and 7% with Bankart repair. Additionally the repair group had better functional outcome scores, higher satisfaction, and a better cost-effectiveness with lower treatment costs. These findings are supported by a meta-analysis of four studies (three randomized, one quasi-randomized), which showed that the rate of recurrent instability was significantly lower among patients undergoing arthroscopic Bankart repair compared with those undergoing simple lavage [6].

Taking into account the results and literature reports, the lavage procedure has become obsolete, and surgical stabilization shows excellent outcome measures.

#### 7.2.2.2 Arthroscopic Transglenoid Repair

Prior to the evolving advantages of suture anchor fixation, Bankart repair was performed through an open or arthroscopic transglenoidal technique. A study by Boszotta et al. [4] who prospectively followed a population of 72 first-time shoulder dislocators using a transglenoidal technique with two drill holes (3 and 5 o'clock position) reported excellent outcome with a recurrence rate of only 6.9%. The results indicated that this technique was effective for young patients to resume sporting activity (85%). In contrast to this result, a study by Söderlund et al. [23] who retrospectively analyzed 312 patients (mean age of 20 years) after transglenoidal Bankart repair with a mean follow-up of 6.4 years reported a high recurrence rate of 56%. However, it must be mentioned that the study did not only include first-time dislocators but also patients with over 20 events of dislocations before surgery, which might explain their findings. Therefore the authors did not recommend this technique for young athletic patients with glenohumeral instability.

#### 7.2.2.3 Open Versus Arthroscopic Repair

Recent studies evaluating the outcomes of stabilization techniques have evolved to where arthroscopy should be the preferred method of repair for anterior first-time traumatic instability, because the results show equal stability, better range of motion, and improved functional outcomes with early return to sports and work [26].

Waterman et al. [28] retrospectively analyzed all army patients who underwent arthroscopic or open Bankart repair in the time between 2003 and 2010. During their study period, a total of 3854 patients (mean age 28.0 years) underwent surgical treatment, most of them arthroscopic (84%). They observed a very low rate of recurrence for patients treated with arthroscopic Bankart repair (4.5%) compared to those treated with an open repair (7.7%). Additionally they found that younger age, higher facility volume, open repair, and postoperative inpatient disposition were significant factors associated with recurrent instability.

These low rates are confirmed by Milchteim et al. [16], who presented a recurrence rate of 6.4% (mean follow-up of 5 years, mean age of 21.9 years) with improved outcome measurement scores and an 82.5% return to sports rate for arthroscopic primary and revision surgery.

However studies investigating the functional outcomes and recurrence rates only including a population younger than 20 years with reliable data are still missing. Therefore the authors propose to transfer the recent evidence for a young active population to patients younger than 20 years of age with an early surgical arthroscopic treatment after a traumatic first-time shoulder dislocation.

### 7.2.3 Author's Preferred Surgical Approach

After summarizing the recent literature and concerning the pathomechanism, the natural history, as well as the surgical management, the authors believe that an early surgical treatment for patients less than 20 years old, who sustained a traumatic first-time shoulder dislocation, will benefit from early arthroscopic Bankart repair. This is not only based on the recurrence rate but also on the improved quality of life and the return to sports and work.

The authors prefer to perform an arthroscopic Bankart repair within 2 weeks after trauma due to the still good tissue conditions in this time frame. The patient is brought into a lateral decubitus position with the arm in an abduction device, which allows for longitudinal (5 lb) and lateral traction (7 lb) (Fig. 7.1).

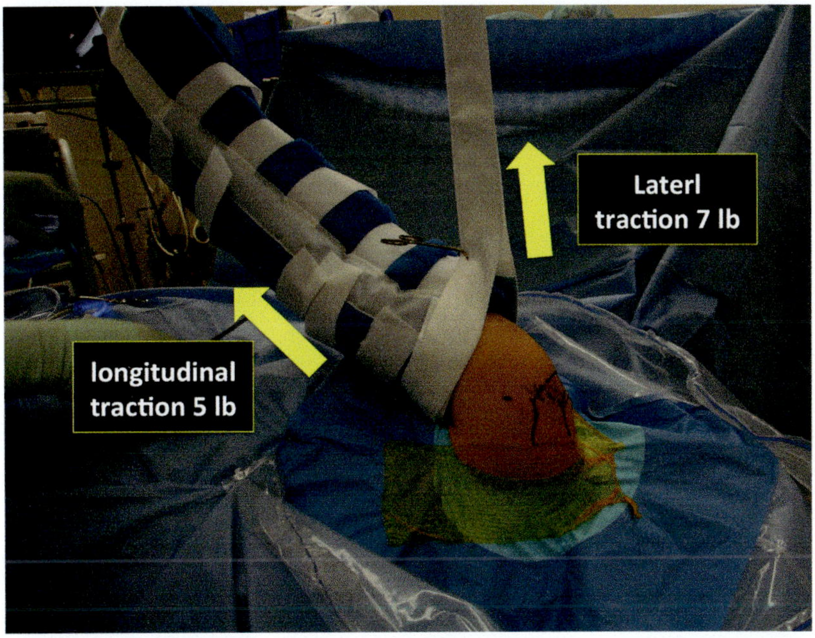


**Fig. 7.1** Lateral decubitus position with abduction and lateral traction arm holder

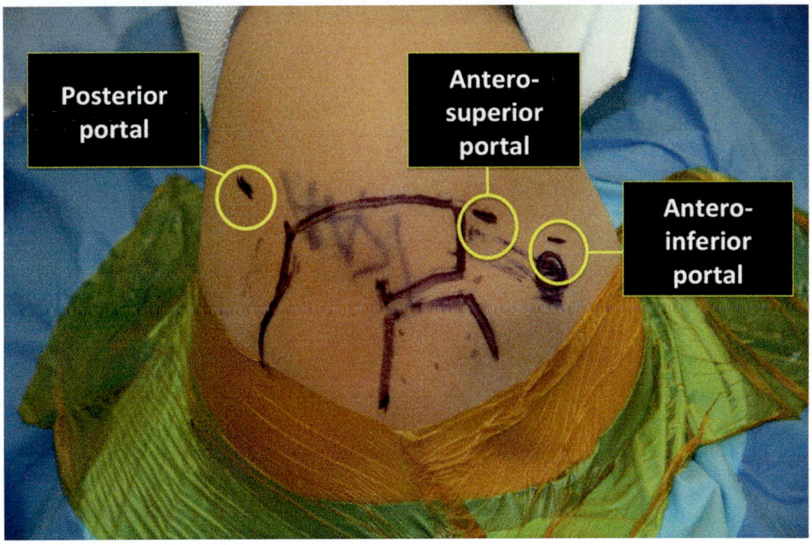


**Fig. 7.2** Anatomical landmarks and arthroscopic portals for a left shoulder

Additionally a role is placed in the axilla to enable the surgeon to have a clear and good view to the 6 o'clock position and an overview over the rest of glenoid, labrum, and capsule.

For a better orientation, the anatomical landmarks are marked, and a posterior standard portal is created first to insert the scope (Fig. 7.2).

Under visualization the anterosuperior and anteroinferior portals are generated using a spinal needle. This allows for accurate portal placement. After a diagnostic overview, the displaced labrum is visualized, and a probe is used to determine the size of the defect, followed by neck roughening to support healing with a rasp or burr (Figs. 7.3 and 7.4).

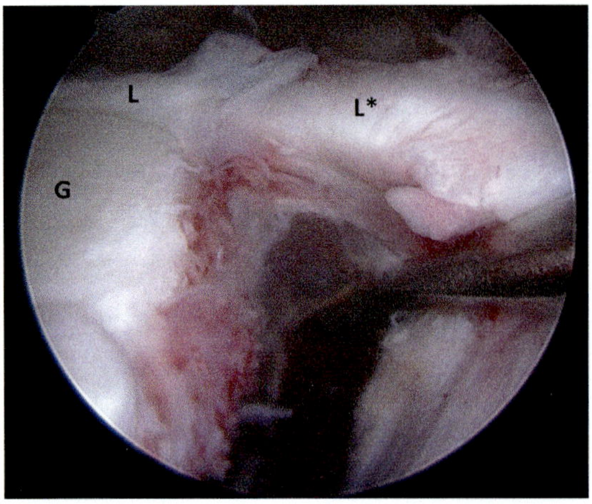


**Fig. 7.3** Arthroscopic view of Bankart lesion (*L* inferior labrum, *L** anteroinferior labrum, *G* glenoid)

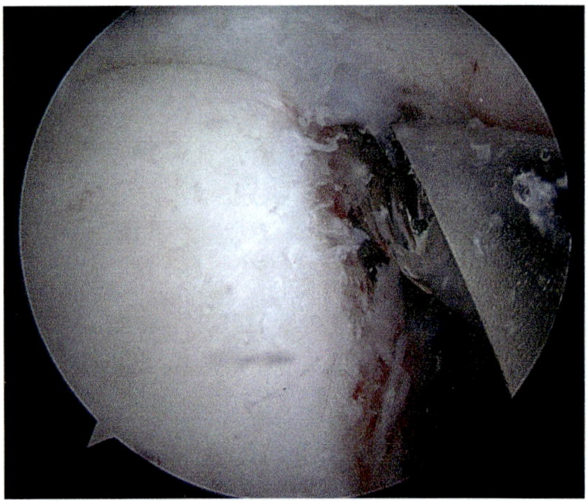

**Fig. 7.4** Glenoid decortication for improved healing using a shaver

To refix and reduce the capsule, a "suture fist" technique is used in which a PDS-0 is passed through the labrum and capsule at the 6 o'clock position. A suture anchor is then placed at the 7 o'clock position (left shoulder), and a high strained number 2 suture is then shuttled through the labrum and capsule by using the PDS (Fig. 7.5). If a double-loaded suture anchor is used, this can be repeated to even more the IGHL retention. If necessary a mattress stitch configuration can be performed (Fig. 7.6). Depending on the size of the Bankart lesion, two to three anchors are placed in the same technique for labral refixation (Fig. 7.7). It is very important to take normal variations of labral configurations, such as a Buford complex or a cord-like MGHL. Postoperative protocol is shown in Table 7.1.

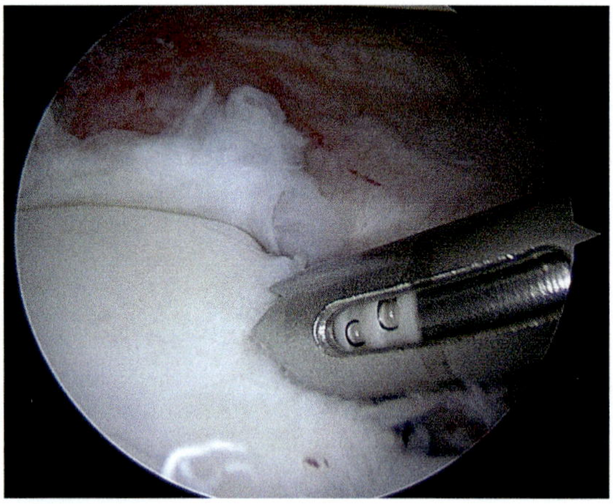

**Fig. 7.5** First anchor placement at the 7 o'clock position

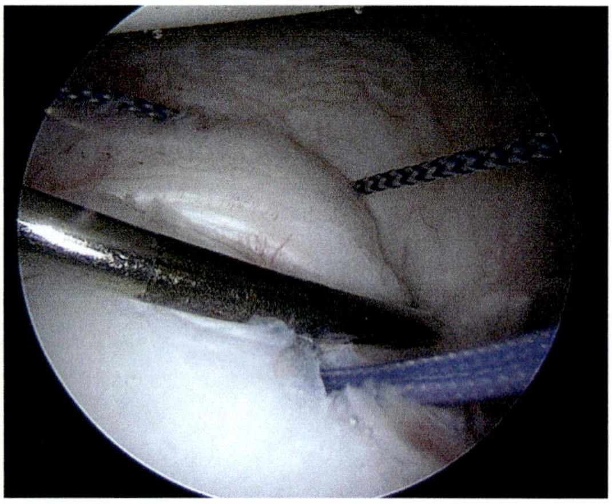

**Fig. 7.6** Mattress stitches for IGHL retention to address capsular stretching

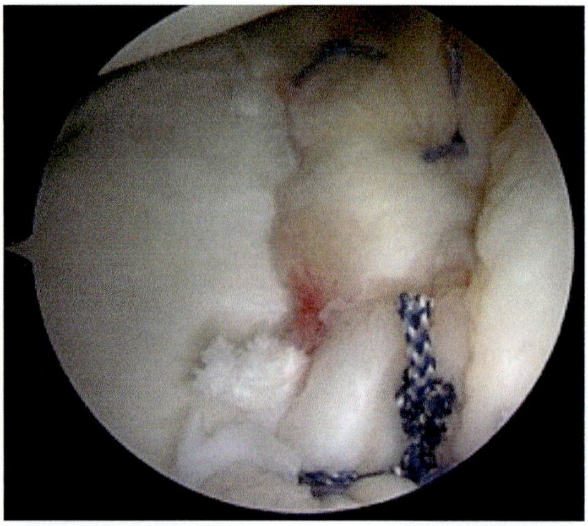

**Fig. 7.7** Final repair with optimal labrum reposition and posterior knot position to prevent cartilage damage

**Table 7.1** Postoperative protocol for arthroscopic Bankart repair

| Postoperative treatment | Range of motion |
|---|---|
| 1–4 weeks | Immobilizer<br>Immediate initiation of pendulum exercise<br>Codman's only<br>Rotator cuff isometrics |
| 4–6 weeks | AROM and AAROM<br>Forward elevation: 90°<br>Abduction: 90°<br>External rotation: 30° |
| 6–8 weeks | Full active range of motion exercise and scapula setting |
| >8 weeks | Strengthening but defer military press, bench press, incline press for 3 months |
| 4–5 months | Sports-specific training |
| 5–6 months | Return to full and contact sports |

*AROM* active range of motion, *AAROM* active-assisted range of motion

## References


1. Arciero RA, Wheeler JH, Ryan JB, McBride JT. Arthroscopic Bankart repair versus nonoperative treatment for acute, initial anterior shoulder dislocations. Am J Sports Med. 1994;22(5):589–94.
2. Bigliani LU, Pollock RG, Soslowsky LJ, Flatow EL, Pawluk RJ, Mow VC. Tensile properties of the inferior glenohumeral ligament. J Orthop Res. 1992;10(2):187–97.
3. Boone JL, Arciero RA. First-time anterior shoulder dislocations: has the standard changed? Br J Sports Med. 2010;44(5):355–60.
4. Boszotta H, Helperstorfer W. Arthroscopic transglenoid suture repair for initial anterior shoulder dislocation. Arthroscopy. 2000;16(5):462–70.
5. Buscayret F, Edwards TB, Szabo I, Adeleine P, Coudane H, Walch G. Glenohumeral arthrosis in anterior instability before and after surgical treatment: incidence and contributing factors. Am J Sports Med. 2004;32(5):1165–72.
6. Chahal J, Marks PH, Macdonald PB, Shah PS, Theodoropoulos J, Ravi B, Whelan DB. Anatomic Bankart repair compared with nonoperative treatment and/or arthroscopic lavage for first-time traumatic shoulder dislocation. Arthroscopy. 2012;28(4):565–75.
7. Chong M, Karataglis D, Learmonth D. Survey of the management of acute traumatic first-time anterior shoulder dislocation among trauma clinicians in the UK. Ann R Coll Surg Engl. 2006;88(5):454–8.
8. Deitch J, Mehlman CT, Foad SL, Obbehat A, Mallory M. Traumatic anterior shoulder dislocation in adolescents. Am J Sports Med. 2003;31(5):758–63.
9. Hovelius L, Olofsson A, Sandstrom B, Augustini BG, Krantz L, Fredin H, Tillander B, Skoglund U, Salomonsson B, Nowak J, Sennerby U. Nonoperative treatment of primary anterior shoulder dislocation in patients forty years of age and younger. a prospective twenty-five-year follow-up. J Bone Joint Surg Am. 2008;90(5):945–52.
10. Jakobsen BW, Johannsen HV, Suder P, Sojbjerg JO. Primary repair versus conservative treatment of first-time traumatic anterior dislocation of the shoulder: a randomized study with 10-year follow-up. Arthroscopy. 2007;23(2):118–23.
11. Kirkley A, Werstine R, Ratjek A, Griffin S. Prospective randomized clinical trial comparing the effectiveness of immediate arthroscopic stabilization versus immobilization and rehabilitation in first traumatic anterior dislocations of the shoulder: long-term evaluation. Arthroscopy. 2005;21(1):55–63.
12. Law BK, Yung PS, Ho EP, Chang JJ, Chan KM. The surgical outcome of immediate arthroscopic Bankart repair for first time anterior shoulder dislocation in young active patients. Knee Surg Sports Traumatol Arthrosc. 2008;16(2):188–93.
13. Liavaag S, Brox JI, Pripp AH, Enger M, Soldal LA, Svenningsen S. Immobilization in external rotation after primary shoulder dislocation did not reduce the risk of recurrence: a randomized controlled trial. J Bone Joint Surg Am. 2011;93(10):897–904.
14. Longo UG, Loppini M, Rizzello G, Ciuffreda M, Maffulli N, Denaro V. Management of primary acute anterior shoulder dislocation: systematic review and quantitative synthesis of the literature. Arthroscopy. 2014;30(4):506–22.
15. Marans HJ, Angel KR, Schemitsch EH, Wedge JH. The fate of traumatic anterior dislocation of the shoulder in children. J Bone Joint Surg Am. 1992;74(8):1242–4.
16. Milchteim C, Tucker SA, Nye DD, Lamour RJ, Liu W, Andrews JR, Ostrander RV. Outcomes of Bankart repairs using modern arthroscopic technique in an athletic population. Arthroscopy. 2016;32(7):1263–70.
17. Momenzadeh OR, Pourmokhtari M, Sefidbakht S, Vosoughi AR. Does the position of shoulder immobilization after reduced anterior glenohumeral dislocation affect coaptation of a Bankart lesion? An arthrographic comparison. J Orthop Traumatol. 2015;16(4):317–21.
18. Plath JE, Aboalata M, Seppel G, Juretzko J, Waldt S, Vogt S, Imhoff AB. Prevalence of and risk factors for dislocation arthropathy: radiological long-term outcome of arthroscopic Bankart repair in 100 shoulders at an average 13-year follow-up. Am J Sports Med. 2015;43(5):1084–90.
19. Pollock RG, Wang VM, Bucchieri JS, Cohen NP, Huang CY, Pawluk RJ, Flatow EL, Bigliani LU, Mow VC. Effects of repetitive subfailure strains on the mechanical behavior of the inferior glenohumeral ligament. J Shoulder Elbow Surg. 2000;9(5):427–35.
20. Robinson CM, Jenkins PJ, White TO, Ker A, Will E. Primary arthroscopic stabilization for a first-time anterior dislocation of the shoulder. A ran-

domized, double-blind trial. J Bone Joint Surg Am. 2008;90(4):708–21.
21. Rowe CR. Prognosis in dislocations of the shoulder. J Bone Joint Surg Am. 1956;38-A(5):957–77.
22. Sachs RA, Lin D, Stone ML, Paxton E, Kuney M. Can the need for future surgery for acute traumatic anterior shoulder dislocation be predicted? J Bone Joint Surg Am. 2007;89(8):1665–74.
23. Soderlund T, Mattila VM, Visuri TI, Pihlajamaki HK. Long-term outcome of a transglenoid suture technique for anterior shoulder instability in young adults. J Bone Joint Surg Br. 2008;90(2):189–93.
24. Taylor DC, Arciero RA. Pathologic changes associated with shoulder dislocations. Arthroscopic and physical examination findings in first-time, traumatic anterior dislocations. Am J Sports Med. 1997;25(3):306–11.
25. te Slaa RL, Brand R, Marti RK. A prospective arthroscopic study of acute first-time anterior shoulder dislocation in the young: a five-year follow-up study. J Shoulder Elbow Surg. 2003;12(6):529–34.
26. Tjoumakaris FP, Bradley JP. The rationale for an arthroscopic approach to shoulder stabilization. Arthroscopy. 2011;27(10):1422–33.
27. Urayama M, Itoi E, Sashi R, Minagawa H, Sato K. Capsular elongation in shoulders with recurrent anterior dislocation. Quantitative assessment with magnetic resonance arthrography. Am J Sports Med. 2003;31(1):64–7.
28. Waterman BR, Burns TC, McCriskin B, Kilcoyne K, Cameron KL, Owens BD. Outcomes after bankart repair in a military population: predictors for surgical revision and long-term disability. Arthroscopy. 2014;30(2):172–7.
29. Whelan DB, Kletke SN, Schemitsch G, Chahal J. Immobilization in external rotation versus internal rotation after primary anterior shoulder dislocation: a meta-analysis of randomized controlled trials. Am J Sports Med. 2016;44(2):521–32.
30. Wintzell G, Haglund-Akerlind Y, Ekelund A, Sandstrom B, Hovelius L, Larsson S. Arthroscopic lavage reduced the recurrence rate following primary anterior shoulder dislocation. A randomised multicentre study with 1-year follow-up. Knee Surg Sports Traumatol Arthrosc. 1999;7(3):192–6.
31. Wintzell G, Haglund-Akerlind Y, Tidermark J, Wredmark T, Eriksson E. A prospective controlled randomized study of arthroscopic lavage in acute primary anterior dislocation of the shoulder: one-year follow-up. Knee Surg Sports Traumatol Arthrosc. 1996;4(1):43–7.

# Management of Acute Shoulder Instability: The Combined Lax Shoulder with Added Acute Trauma

**8**

S.C. Petterson, A.M. Green, and Kevin D. Plancher

## Contents


| | | |
|---|---|---|
| 8.1 | **Introduction** | 65 |
| 8.2 | **Anatomy, Examination, and Imaging** | 66 |
| 8.2.1 | Anatomy | 66 |
| 8.2.2 | Examination | 66 |
| 8.2.3 | Imaging | 66 |
| 8.3 | **Indications and Technique** | 67 |
| 8.3.1 | Indications | 67 |
| 8.3.2 | Technique | 67 |
| 8.4 | **Rehabilitation** | 69 |
| 8.5 | **Results** | 70 |
| 8.6 | **Complications and Tips to Avoid Them** | 70 |
| 8.6.1 | Significant Bone Loss | 70 |
| 8.6.2 | Postoperative Loss of External Rotation or Stiffness | 70 |
| 8.6.3 | Insufficient Anchors or Incorrect Anchor Placement | 70 |
| **Conclusion** | | 71 |
| **References** | | 71 |


S.C. Petterson, MPT, PhD • A.M. Green, PhD
Orthopaedic Foundation, Stamford, CT, USA

K.D. Plancher, MD (✉)
Orthopaedic Foundation, Stamford, CT, USA

Plancher Orthopaedics and Sports Medicine, New York, NY, USA

Albert Einstein College of Medicine, New York, NY, USA
e-mail: kplancher@plancherortho.com

## 8.1 Introduction

Less than 10% of patients with shoulder instability have multidirectional instability (MDI) [1, 2]. While generalized joint laxity does not necessarily translate to shoulder laxity, approximately 50% of patients with MDI of the shoulder also have generalized ligamentous laxity. Furthermore, while the distribution of MDI between the sexes is almost equal, functional deficits and symptoms may be magnified in the female population [3].

As first described by Neer and Foster in 1980, the term MDI encompasses the patient with symptomatic laxity in more than one direction [4]. Classification of multidirectional instability is inconsistent in the literature and comprises three different groups [5]. The classic patient with Atraumatic, Multidirectional, frequently Bilateral, responds to Rehabilitation and rarely requires an Inferior capsular shift (AMBRI) presents with excessive laxity in multiple joints (e.g., fingers, elbows, ankles). The second group consists primarily of patients with MDI due to overuse syndromes (e.g., swimmers, gymnasts), who also may not require surgical intervention, whereas the third group develops MDI as a result of sustaining multiple injuries. Treatment for each of these cases varies. This chapter will focus on the patient with atraumatic MDI that sustains an acute anterior shoulder dislocation (i.e., group 3).

© ISAKOS 2017
A.B. Imhoff, F.H. Savoie III (eds.), *Shoulder Instability Across the Life Span*,
DOI 10.1007/978-3-662-54077-0_8

## 8.2 Anatomy, Examination, and Imaging

### 8.2.1 Anatomy

The static and dynamic constraints of the bony geometry of the glenohumeral joint contribute to glenohumeral joint stability. While the glenoid labrum increases the contact area for the humeral head, it is still relatively smaller and shallower leading to an increased propensity for dislocation. In addition to the glenoid labrum, the glenohumeral ligaments provide static restraints to excessive joint motion, whereas the musculature of the rotator cuff, deltoid, long head of the biceps, and periscapular muscles provide dynamic stabilization. The shoulder is most vulnerable to anterior subluxation or dislocation at 45° of abduction because the capsuloligamentous structures are lax in this position, therefore, the dynamic muscular restraints provide joint stability in these midranges of motion through joint compression (concavity compression mechanism).

Small capsular and labral deficiencies are thought to be of primary importance in the shoulder with MDI. At the extremes of ranges of motion, these static capsuloligamentous structures become taught, providing joint stability. The inferior glenohumeral ligament (IGHL) is the thickest of the glenohumeral ligaments with an anterior band, posterior band, and axillary pouch. The IGHL is the primary restraint against anterior glenohumeral translation when the shoulder is abducted to 90° and externally rotated [6, 7]. As the arm adducts, the middle glenohumeral ligament (MGHL) becomes taught providing restraint, and when the arm is completely adducted at the side, the superior glenohumeral ligament (SGHL) contributes. Posterior glenohumeral translation is limited by the posterior band of the IGHL as well as the rotator interval capsule in a position of 90° abduction [8]. Inferior glenohumeral translation at 90° of abduction is limited by the SGHL as well as the rotator interval capsule.

### 8.2.2 Examination

A diagnosis of MDI is often exclusively made on history and physical examination. In the patient with atraumatic MDI that sustains an acute anterior shoulder dislocation, a detailed history of the shoulder before the traumatic event is essential and must be collected in addition to the specific details of the injury and any subsequent subluxation or dislocation events [9]. Common complaints in patients with MDI include shoulder weakness, fatigue, joint looseness, and possible reports of transient neurologic symptoms. Any repetitive activities such as overhead throwing, swimming, and volleyball or even activities of lifting a heavy suitcase should also be noted as these activities are sufficient to cause symptoms as a result of microtrauma. Activities that elicit the patient's symptoms as well as arm positions of subluxation or dislocation events should be documented and are typically reported to occur in the mid-glenohumeral ROM in the patient with MDI. Assessment of generalized ligamentous laxity should also be completed using the Beighton scale [10]. The Beighton scale is a 5-point, validated measure for ligamentous laxity testing the ability to (1) dorsiflex the fifth digit beyond 90°, (2) oppose the first digit to the ipsilateral forearm, (3) hyperextend the elbow beyond 10°, (4) hyperextend the knee beyond 10°, and (5) trunk flexion with the knees extended so the palms of the hand lie flat on the floor. The examiner must inquire about a familial history of hereditary collagen disorders (e.g., Ehlers-Danlos syndrome, Marfan syndrome) as patients with these disorders do not respond well to soft tissue instability repairs.

Clinical evaluation should include assessment of neurovascular integrity, periscapular atrophy, shoulder ROM, and strength, particularly of the rotator cuff. Shoulder instability should be examined using the apprehension test, augmentation-relocation test, load and shift test, sulcus sign, and lag sign (Fig. 8.1). Comparison to the contralateral side is essential in these individuals to determine the presence of pathology. Patients with a large sulcus sign and no history of traumatic event precipitating instability most likely suffer from multidirectional shoulder instability.

### 8.2.3 Imaging

Radiographic imaging should include a standard instability series including an anterior-posterior

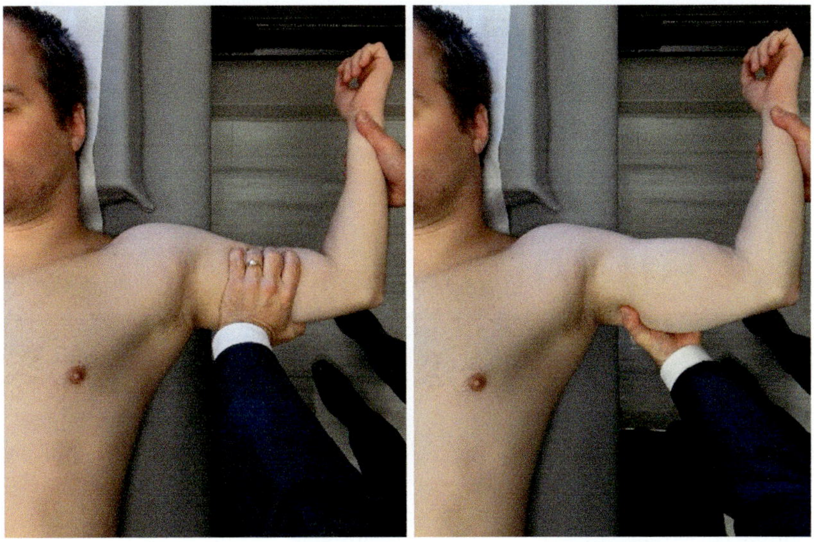

**Fig. 8.1** Apprehension and relocation tests. The involved arm is carefully placed in a position of abduction and external rotation. Symptoms of anterior instability or pain or both that resolve with a posteriorly directed force by the examiner indicate a positive finding of anterior shoulder instability. Copyright Kevin D. Plancher, MD

(AP), scapular-Y, Bergeneau, and axillary views to assess for concomitant bony injuries as well as alignment. The axillary view can detect anterior or posterior glenoid rim fractures and assists in the detection of AP subluxation or dislocation. Magnetic resonance imaging (MRI) and/or computed tomography (CT) scans can also aid in the detection of concomitant soft tissue pathologies and assist in quantifying bony lesions when present.

## 8.3 Indications and Technique

### 8.3.1 Indications

The inferior capsular shift in patients with MDI has been the gold standard treatment to restore function with less than 10% recurrence. In the setting of the patient with MDI that sustains an acute anterior shoulder dislocation with radiographic evidence of Bankart lesion, the authors recommend an arthroscopic Bankart repair with a modified inferior capsular shift to restore shoulder stability in these challenging patients.

### 8.3.2 Technique

An interscalene block supplemented with general endotracheal anesthesia can be used for most surgical patients. An intraoperative examination of shoulder stability and ROM should be conducted on both limbs to confirm preoperative impressions. Patients can then be positioned in the lateral decubitus position with the arm secured in a holder in approximately 45° of abduction and 15° of forward flexion with neutral rotation under seven to ten pounds of traction. Bankart surgery can be performed in the beach chair or lateral decubitus position; however, in the senior author's experience, the lateral decubitus position allows for superior access to the 6 o'clock position of the shoulder and aids in positioning the glenoid parallel to the floor, creating a standard reference point and allowing for excellent visualization of the glenohumeral joint during surgery [11].

A modified 3-portal technique similar to that previously described by Nebelung should be utilized [12]. Posterior, anteroinferior, and anterosuperior portals are established using an outside-in technique and 18-gauge spinal needles for optimal positioning. The posterior portal is the primary viewing portal; the anterosuperior portal is used to visualize the pathology, prepare the glenoid rim, and perform the Bankart repair; and the anteroinferior portal provides access to the glenoid for optimal anchor placement. A thorough arthroscopic examination inspecting the 15 points originally described by Snyder and identifying associated glenoid or humeral defects, anterior labral lesions, and capsular tissue quality should be performed [13]. The extent of the labral tear is documented using a clock-face model as previously described [14].

Following confirmation of less than 20% glenoid bone loss, an arthroscopic shaver and hooded 3.5 mm burr are used to expose an area of bleeding cortical bone on the anterior aspect of the glenoid for anchor placement (Fig. 8.2). Two

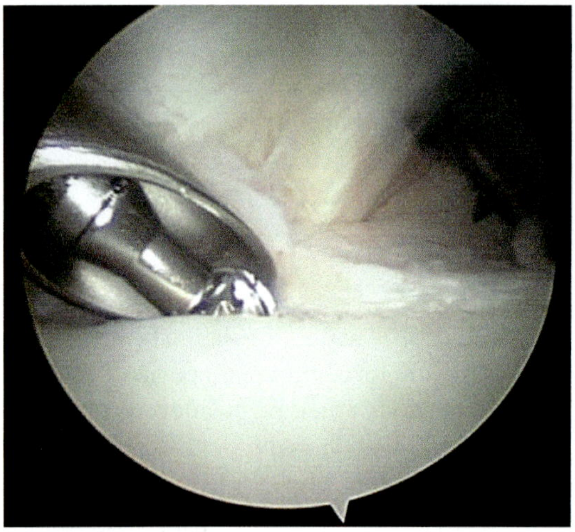

**Fig. 8.2** Burr in place. The anterior glenoid rim is debrided to create a bleeding bony bed. Copyright Kevin D. Plancher, MD

or three anchors are placed below the 3-o'clock position, perpendicular to the glenoid rim, and at least 3 mm inside the edge of the glenoid rim (Fig. 8.3a, b). A suture-passing instrument or suture shuttle device is used to pass sutures through the capsular tissue and labrum in an inferior to superior fashion (Fig. 8.4). Sutures should be secured on the nonarticular side of the repair with a modified sliding locking Weston knot or bioknotless anchor. A minimum of three additional anchors based on the size of the lesion should be placed from inferior to superior. High-strength suture either single- or double-loaded with bioabsorbable anchors or PLA-composite bioabsorbable suture anchors should be used to secure capsular imbrication, and this inferior capsular shift should be employed in patients at a high risk for recurrence. The authors also recommend an arthroscopic rotator interval closure using polydioxanone (PDS) sutures when these patients previously admitted to dislocating in their sleep. The need to prevent recurrence of instability or any subluxations is essential (Fig. 8.5a–c). Surgical incisions are closed using Vicryl and Monocryl sutures followed by infiltration of the joint with 10 mL of 0.25% Marcaine without epinephrine.

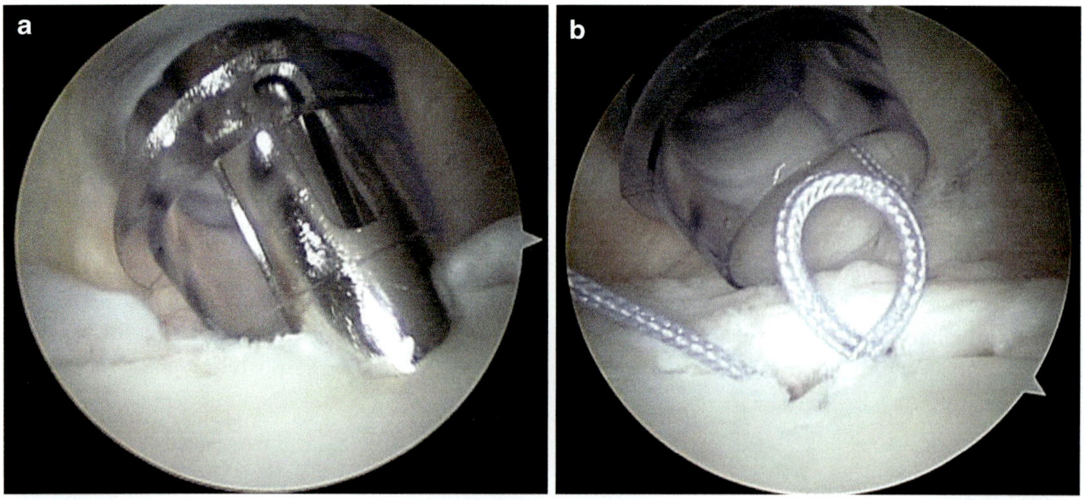


**Fig. 8.3** (**a**) An arthroscopic guide placed on the glenoid bumper for accurate placement. (**b**) An anchor in place with suture ready for lasso passer. Copyright Kevin D. Plancher, MD

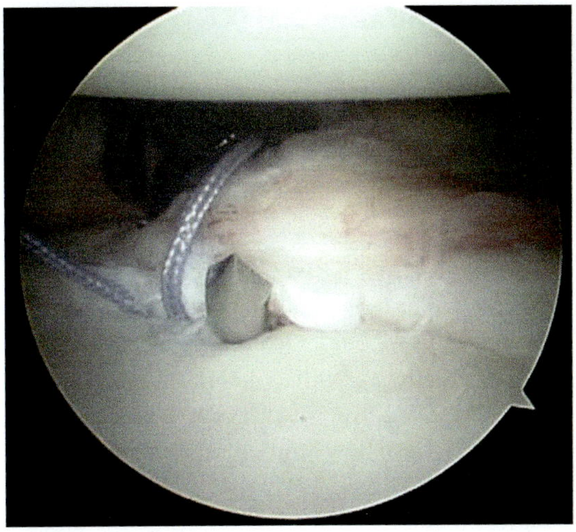

**Fig. 8.4** Arthroscopic suture lasso placed under the labrum to reconstruct for stability. Copyright Kevin D. Plancher, MD

## 8.4 Rehabilitation

Following surgery, a conservative rehabilitation protocol should be followed to avoid stressing the repaired capsuloligamentous structures [9]. Patients should be placed in an immobilizing sling in neutral rotation for 4 weeks. The patient is permitted to remove the sling and let the arm hang by the side three times daily for 5 minutes. After 2 weeks, the sutures are removed, and active-assisted flexion ROM exercises in a supine position only are initiated. If the patient is not able to achieve 90° active-assisted supine forward flexion (FF) at 2 weeks, an adjusted rehab program is instituted. External rotation (ER) beyond 10° should be prohibited until 4 weeks postoperatively. After 4 weeks, the immobilizing abduction sling

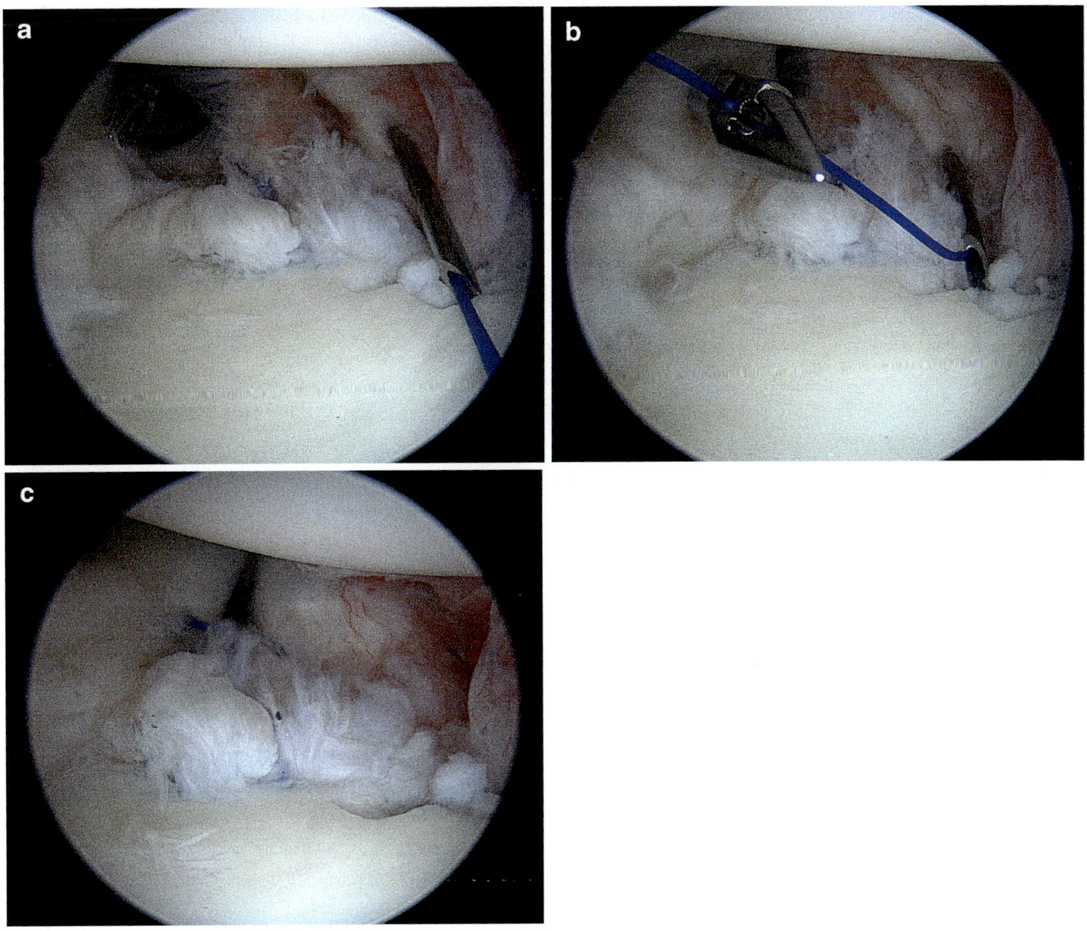


**Fig. 8.5** Rotator interval closure. (**a**) Spinal needles are placed through the upper border of the subscapularis. (**b**) A piercing instrument is used to close the rotator interval through the superior glenohumeral ligament. (**c**) The rotator interval is tied extraarticularly and now seen after arthroscopic closure. Copyright Kevin D. Plancher, MD

device is discontinued, and the use of a soft sling is introduced to be worn during sleep and when out in public for safety. Supine, active-assisted FF exercises to 120°, progressing to 160° while avoiding end range forced flexion, are also initiated. Light, end range stretching exercises are begun at week 5 with internal rotation behind the back. Proprioceptive and scapular-stabilization exercises are initiated at 6 weeks, and strengthening exercises are initiated at 8 weeks with progression until week 12 when isokinetics and sport-specific activities are introduced. Return to sports is permitted at 3 months for noncontact athletes, at 4–5 months for contact athletes depending on their position, and at 9 months for athletes participating in overhead sports.

## 8.5 Results

Recent systematic reviews have demonstrated that both arthroscopic capsular plication and open capsular shift are the best surgical procedures for treatment of MDI following a failed 6-month course of physical therapy [15, 16]. In 2016, Witney-Lagen and colleagues reported a 4% recurrence rate and 100% rate of return to sport and work in 50 patients that underwent arthroscopic plication for symptomatic MDI with no labral lesion [17]. In the setting of the patients with MDI that sustains an acute shoulder dislocation with radiographic evidence of a Bankart lesion with less than 20% bone loss, the senior author recommends the described arthroscopic Bankart repair technique with a modified inferior capsular shift with suture anchors and plication sutures. To date, the senior author has seen excellent outcomes with low recurrence rate and return to pre-injury sports without loss of external rotation ROM.

## 8.6 Complications and Tips to Avoid Them

There are several possible complications of arthroscopic Bankart repair which have been associated with repair failure or nonoptimal outcomes.

### 8.6.1 Significant Bone Loss

Glenoid bone loss greater than 25% or humeral bone loss resulting in an engaging Hill-Sachs lesion place patients at higher risk for recurrence of instability following arthroscopic Bankart repair [18]. If significant osseous lesions are present in addition to a Bankart lesion, they must also be addressed at the time of capsulolabral repair in order to restore shoulder stability. Potential procedures for patients with concomitant significant bone loss in addition to a Bankart lesion include the Latarjet-Bristow procedure, remplissage, humeral head osteotomy, and osteochondral allograft transplantation depending on the size of the lesion.

### 8.6.2 Postoperative Loss of External Rotation or Stiffness

In patients at a high risk for recurrence in which rotator interval closure is employed, postoperative loss of ER or stiffness has been reported [19]. To minimize the risk of reduced motion, correct positioning of the arm during interval closure is imperative. The arm must be abducted to 45° with 45° of ER in the lateral decubitus position.

### 8.6.3 Insufficient Anchors or Incorrect Anchor Placement

Several studies have reported that an insufficient number of anchors results in an increased risk of anterior instability recurrence [19–21]. Specifically, use of less than four anchors, regardless of the size of initial Bankart lesion, has been associated with a higher incidence of arthroscopic Bankart repair failure. Incorrect placement of anchors can also influence repair failure, as placement of anchors less than 3 mm from the glenoid rim can result in an insufficient amount of tissue being incorporated into the imbrication. A minimum of four anchors placed at least 3 mm from the glenoid edge should be used for labral repair during Bankart surgery.

**Conclusion**

The management of patients with MDI that have sustained an acute traumatic dislocation is a challenging population. Arthroscopic Bankart repair with a modified inferior capsular shift with suture anchors and plication sutures is recommended for these patients to return them to their prior activities with low recurrence rates of instability.

## References

1. Altchek DW, Warren RF, Skyhar MJ, Ortiz G. T-plasty modification of the Bankart procedure for multidirectional instability of the anterior and inferior types. J Bone Joint Surg Am. 1991;73(1):105–12.
2. Cooper RA, Brems JJ. The inferior capsular-shift procedure for multidirectional instability of the shoulder. J Bone Joint Surg Am. 1992;74(10):1516–21.
3. Hiemstra LA, Kirkley A. Shoulder instability in female athletes. Sports Med Arthrosc Rev. 2002;10(1):50–7.
4. Neer 2nd CS, Foster CR. Inferior capsular shift for involuntary inferior and multidirectional instability of the shoulder. A preliminary report. J Bone Joint Surg Am. 1980;62(6):897–908.
5. Matsen FA. Glenohumeral instability. In: Rockwood CA, Matsen FA, Wirth MA, et al. e, eds. The shoulder. Philadelphia: Saunders/Elsevier; 2009:617–770.
6. Kuhn JE, Huston LJ, Soslowsky LJ, Shyr Y, Blasier RB. External rotation of the glenohumeral joint: ligament restraints and muscle effects in the neutral and abducted positions. J Shoulder Elbow Surg. 2005;14(1 Suppl S):39S–48S.
7. O'Connell PW, Nuber GW, Mileski RA, Lautenschlager E. The contribution of the glenohumeral ligaments to anterior stability of the shoulder joint. Am J Sports Med. 1990;18(6):579–84.
8. O'Brien SJ, Neves MC, Arnoczky SP, et al. The anatomy and histology of the inferior glenohumeral ligament complex of the shoulder. Am J Sports Med. 1990;18(5):449–56.
9. Plancher KD, Petterson SC. Arthroscopic Bankart repair with suture anchors: tips for success. Oper Tech Sports Med. 2013;21(4):192–200.
10. Beighton P, Solomon L, Soskolne CL. Articular mobility in an African population. Ann Rheum Dis. 1973;32(5):413–8.
11. Peruto CM, Ciccotti MG, Cohen SB. Shoulder arthroscopy positioning: lateral decubitus versus beach chair. Arthroscopy. 2009;25(8):891–6.
12. Nebelung W, Ropke M, Urbach D, Becker R. A new technique of arthroscopic capsular shift in anterior shoulder instability. Arthroscopy. 2001;17(4):426–9.
13. Snyder SJ, Fasulo GJ. Shoulder arthroscopy: surgical technique. Surg Technol Int. 1993;2:447–53.
14. Voos JE, Livermore RW, Feeley BT, et al. Prospective evaluation of arthroscopic bankart repairs for anterior instability. Am J Sports Med. 2010;38(2):302–7.
15. Chen D, Goldberg J, Herald J, Critchley I, Barmare A. Effects of surgical management on multidirectional instability of the shoulder: a meta-analysis. Knee Surg Sports Traumatol Arthrosc. 2016;24(2):630–9.
16. Longo UG, Rizzello G, Loppini M, et al. Multidirectional instability of the shoulder: a systematic review. Arthroscopy. Dec 2015;31(12):2431–43.
17. Witney-Lagen C, Hassan A, Doodson A, Venkateswaran B. Arthroscopic plication for multidirectional instability: 50 patients with a minimum of 2 years of follow-up. J Shoulder Elbow Surg. 2017;26(2):e29–e36.
18. Boileau P, Villalba M, Henry JY, Balg F, Ahrens P, Neyton L. Risk factors for recurrence of shoulder instability after arthroscopic Bankart repair. J Bone Joint Surg Am. 2006;88(8):1755–63.
19. Plausinis D, Bravman JT, Heywood C, Kummer FJ, Kwon YW, Jazrawi LM. Arthroscopic rotator interval closure: effect of sutures on glenohumeral motion and anterior-posterior translation. Am J Sports Med. 2006;34(10):1656–61.
20. Randelli P, Ragone V, Carminati S, Cabitza P. Risk factors for recurrence after Bankart repair a systematic review. Knee Surg Sports Traumatol Arthrosc. 2012;20(11):2129–38.
21. Kim SH, Ha KI, Kim YM. Arthroscopic revision Bankart repair: a prospective outcome study. Arthroscopy. 2002;18(5):469–82.

# Stabilization Options in the Adolescent: Open Bankart Repair

**9**

Stephen C. Weber

## Contents

9.1 **Brief Introduction** ... 73
9.2 **Literature Overview Summary** ... 73
9.3 **Anatomy, Examination, and Imaging** ... 74
9.4 **Indication and Technique** ... 75
9.5 **Specific Points in Rehabilitation** ... 76
9.6 **Results** ... 76
9.7 **Complications and Tips to Avoid Them** ... 76
9.8 **Conclusion Summary** ... 77
**References** ... 77

## 9.1 Brief Introduction

Shoulder instability is a common injury, with an incidence of 23.9 per 100,000 [1]. While the peak incidence of shoulder instability is at 20 years of age, shoulder instability under the age of twenty is still common and represents about 20% of all dislocations [1]. While historic reviews of surgical management of shoulder instability have shown rates of recurrence from 2 to 5% [2, 3], more recent studies have shown recurrence rates of over 25% at long-term follow-up [4, 5]. While arthroscopic stabilization has generally been successful in the over 30-year-old age group, recurrence rates in the younger old group have been disturbingly high [4, 6, 7]. This has been especially problematic in the under 18-year-old contact athlete [6]. For this reason, treatment alternatives to traditional arthroscopic Bankart repair have been reexamined. One option has been open Bankart repair.

## 9.2 Literature Overview Summary

The historic recurrence rates associated with open Bankart repair reported by Rowe [2] and Thomas and Matsen [3] have been difficult to reproduce in later studies. Functional outcomes have also been difficult to evaluate, as traditional shoulder scoring systems have often not corre-

S.C. Weber, MD
Johns Hopkins Department of Orthopedics, Baltimore, Maryland, USA
e-mail: webersc@earthlink.net

© ISAKOS 2017
A.B. Imhoff, F.H. Savoie III (eds.), *Shoulder Instability Across the Life Span*,
DOI 10.1007/978-3-662-54077-0_9

lated with return to play, especially with overhead sports [8]. Arthroscopic stabilization was hoped to resolve these issues by maintaining the low recurrence rates of prior open procedures and still allow return to overhead sports. While arthroscopic repair has generally shown equivalent recurrence rates to open repair in the over 30-year-old population, the younger patient have often not shown equivalent results. Bacilla et al. were one of the first to recognize age as a potential risk factor for arthroscopic shoulder stabilization [9]. Several subsequent studies have since supported this as a risk factor for high rates of recurrence [1, 7, 10, 11]. Several related variables also affect the recurrence rates in this age group, including the higher percentage of participation in contact sports [6, 12]. At least one study showed that the most significant variable was postoperative activity score and that age alone was not as significant in predicting outcome [12]. Given the higher failure rates in this population, several alternatives to arthroscopic Bankart repair have been reevaluated. These include treatment of first-time dislocators [13], open repair [14], and differing types of bone-block procedures [15]. The subject of this review will be open Bankart repair in the adolescent shoulder.

It should be understood that the adolescent shoulder with instability has more recently been divided into two subgroups: (1) patients under 14 years of age, with open epiphyses, and (2) patients in the 15- to 18-year-old group with closed epiphyses [1, 7]. Several studies have shown that recurrent instability falls off dramatically in the under 14-year-old population and can often be treated initially nonoperatively [1]. The pathology in this age group is also different, with a disproportionately higher percentage of multidirectional instability, and a far lesser percentage of Bankart lesions [1]. With the presence of closed epiphyses, the injury patterns more mimic adult pathologic anatomy. It is the adolescent with closed or nearly closed physes that has been the subject of several recent studies.

Unfortunately, no large, prospective, randomized studies are available to definitively answer the question of what procedure to perform to stabilize the shoulder in this age group. Given the relatively poor results of arthroscopic treatment of shoulder instability in this age group, open Bankart repair seems like a viable option. In a systematic review, Randelli et al. recommended that in young (<22 year of age) high-demand male athletes consider open stabilization due to the higher risk of recurrence after an arthroscopic stabilization [16]. Recent articles regarding stabilization of young patients are summarized in Table 9.1.

## 9.3 Anatomy, Examination, and Imaging

Examination of the adolescent shoulder seeks to evaluate similar issues to those present in adult shoulder instability. Careful examination of the unclothed shoulder bilaterally is critical, as scapular dyskinesia and multidirectional instability will be present to a greater degree than with adults. Range of motion should be checked and compared with the unaffected side, with careful attention to loss of internal rotation or GIRD syndrome. Profound loss of motion or significant strength deficits can indicate a need for a preoperative course of physical therapy. Again, asymptomatic laxity can be difficult to separate from pathologic instability, and careful check for anterior and posterior apprehension tests and load and shift test are critical. Pathologically increased shoulder motion or a large sulcus sign should prompt the examiner to consider multidirectional instability, and all patients should be asked about any voluntary instability, which may recommend pursuing a course of nonoperative treatment due to the inferior success rates with surgical repair of multidirectional instability [21] although recent experiences have been more successful [22]. Especially in the under 14 age group, voluntary instability can be otherwise asymptomatic and has been shown by Neer and others to often correct with time [23]. Significant hyperlaxity of the shoulder can also be the initial presentation of several hereditary musculoskeletal conditions such as Ehlers-Danlos or Marfan's syndrome in this age group, with significantly poorer outcomes with surgical repair, and may require con-

**Table 9.1** Recent literature on the use of open Bankart repair in adolescent patients

| Author, year | Age range | Recurrence rate | Follow-up | Technique variants | Outcome measures | Comments |
|---|---|---|---|---|---|---|
| Hatch et al. 2016 [10] | 14–18 | 0% | >2 year | Open repair Detached subscap | Rowe, UCLA | 34% lost ave 11 degrees ER |
| Kraus et al. 2010 [11] | 11–15 | 0% | 6–48 months | Arthroscopic and Open all with open physes | Rowe, Constant | Constant score 92, Rowe score 97.5 |
| Mazzocca et al. 2005 [17] | Age<20 | 11% | 24–66 months | Arthroscopic repair only | ASES, SST, SF-36, Rowe | All contact/collision athletes |
| Uhorchak et al. 2000 [18] | 18–24 | 11% recurrent subluxation or dislocation | 24–72 months | Open repair, subscapularis incised, capsulorrhaphy | ASES, Rowe | Rare subluxation did not affect clinical outcome |
| Owens et al. 2009 [19] | 17–23 | 21.4% recurrent subluxation, 14.3% revision rate | 9.1–13.9 years | Arthroscopic repair only | SANE, WOSI, SST, Rowe ASES, SF-36,Tegner | Long-term follow-up of results of first time dislocator repair |
| Jones et al. 2007 [20] | 11–18 | 18.75% | 24 months | Arthroscopic repair | SANE | Mixed group primary and secondary repair |

sideration of other associated disorders such as cardiac and ocular conditions.

Radiographs should include at least standard AP and axillary view; a Grashey view can also be helpful [24]. While large bone defects are less common in this age group, they are not unheard of, and significant bone defects such as large Hill-Sachs lesions or glenoid defects may require bone-block-type procedures [25]. Rotator cuff pathology in this group is distinctly uncommon and does not require special preoperative imaging, and so plain arthrograms are not normally indicated. While CT scanning can more reliably measure bone loss, the risks of the required radiation is not insignificant, especially as the field involves the breast and thyroid tissues [26]. For this reason, MRI scanning may be a more appropriate imaging study if bone loss is to be assessed in this age group.

## 9.4 Indication and Technique

The indication for an open Bankart repair in the adolescent is the presence of recurrent instability failing conservative management in an appropriate patient with significant limitations of activities. The presence of neurologic deficits, large bone defects, and profound stiffness or marked weakness contraindicates this procedure. While universal success of surgical treatment is not common, nonoperative treatment fails in a substantial number of patients [13], and primary open repair for the first-time dislocator has become a reasonable option. The presence of a significant component of multidirectional instability will at least require a change in technique to incorporate some component of capsular tightening, and marked voluntary instability with significant ligament laxity should give the surgeon pause.

The technique is much the same as for adult Bankart repair. Because of the risk of unrecognized associated intraarticular pathology, complete, thorough arthroscopic evaluation of the shoulder should be done prior to proceeding with the open repair, and any associated pathology, such as superior labral lesions, articular cartilage injuries, loose bodies, and rotator cuff injuries can be addressed arthroscopically prior to the open repair. This can be done in the beach chair position, with the advantage of easy conversion to the open repair, or in the lateral decubitus position and then re-prepping and redraping the patient.

With the arthroscopic examination completed, attention can be directed to the open repair. A low axillary incision has been shown to improve the cosmesis of the scar [10]. A standard deltopectoral approach with preservation of the cephalic vein is performed. Management of the subscapularis is controversial, with a subscapularis split felt by some [27] to improve overhead function and others [10] finding reasonable results with a negative postoperative lift off test with detachment. As these younger patients rarely get stiff, immobilization after repair is reasonable and may permit the greater exposure afforded by detachment of the subscapularis without causing postoperative weakness. Once exposed, the Bankart lesion can be prepared by abrading the glenoid. At least three suture anchors should be placed at roughly the one, three, and five o'clock position and used to reattach the labrum to the bone. A Heaney needle holder can be very helpful in placing these sutures anatomically. Traditionally, the rotator interval has been closed, although recently some surgeons have suggested that leaving this open might improve external rotation [10]. Meticulous hemostasis should be assured prior to skin closure, and a thorough check of the neurologic status should be performed in the recovery room prior to discharge, an advantage of general anesthesia over intrascalene block.

## 9.5 Specific Points in Rehabilitation

Open Bankart surgery can generally be performed outpatient without undue difficulty. Compliance with postoperative restrictions, as any parent knows, can be difficult in this patient population. Both the patient and parents need to be well aware that failure to comply with postoperative restrictions can negatively impact the results of the surgery. For this reason, it has seemed easier over the years to insist on continuous use of a sling for six weeks postoperatively, as this seems to create an easily understandable demarcation between appropriate and inappropriate activities. Driving should be avoided for six weeks as well and should be clearly understood preoperatively, as this is often a significant issue postoperatively. Hand, wrist, and elbow exercises can start immediately, with pendulum exercises starting at three weeks.

Gentle physical therapy can be started at six weeks, with formal strengthening starting at three months. Rarely, patients will have significant restriction of motion at three months, which can usually be addressed with vigorous physical therapy and rarely requires arthroscopic release in this age group. At six months, sports-specific rehabilitation can be started. For most athletes, resumption of previous sports will be with the following season, although multi-sport athletes can make this decision difficult. Isokinetic testing to confirm the restoration of full strength prior to resuming activities can be helpful, as it provides an objective, measurable goal that parents, coaches, and athletes can all understand.

## 9.6 Results

Results of recent publications regarding adolescent Bankart repair are shown in Table 9.1. As can be seen, most of these are relatively short-term level four studies of this specific technique. Despite this, results of open repair are generally superior to arthroscopic Bankart repair at similar follow-up times and present a low rate of complications. It should be noted that none of these studies specifically address the outcome of the open Bankart repair in the elite overhead athlete, and while stability can be reasonably assured to the patient and family in a high percentage of patients, unrestricted return to activities such as pitching, due to the loss of external rotation [10], can be problematic.

## 9.7 Complications and Tips to Avoid Them

Complications with open Bankart repair are generally uncommon. None of the articles referenced here had any significant complications other than recurrence. That said, bleeding and neurologic injury are not impossible, and careful check and palpation of at least the axillary and musculocutaneous nerve should be performed prior to closure. Unrecognized loose hardware, either metal or resorbable, can create profound articular cartilage injury and can be avoided by meticulous placement and traction on suture anchor sutures prior to refixing the labrum. Meticulous closure of the subscapularis regardless of the chosen technique of incision can prevent later problems of weakness and instability. Most of the complications relate to failure to comply with restrictions and appropriate rehabilitation in this age group, while not avoidable, ensuring that the patient, family, coach, and athletic trainer are all on the same page in recognizing that this is not "band aid surgery" goes a long way to safeguard compliance.

## 9.8 Conclusion Summary

In conclusion, open Bankart repair is a viable option for the adolescent patient with primarily unidirectional anterior instability. Recent studies however have suggested that patients under 14 years of age with open physes should have at least primary conservative treatment due to substantially lower recurrence rates in this age group. Primary fixation of the first-time dislocator may further improve these results, but reasonable expectation for outcome and time to return to play is especially important in this age group. Complications are uncommon, and recurrent instability rates with open Bankart repair remain lower than reported recurrence rates for arthroscopic Bankart repair. Good results have been obtained with a variety of techniques involving the handling of the subscapularis, and no single technique appears to offer substantial superiority. Data on return to high-demand overhead sports remains limited, however, and the prognosis for unrestricted return to sport for these athletes remains guarded. Further prospective, randomized studies may further elucidate treatment options in this difficult population.

## References

1. Li X, Ma R, Nielsen NM, Gulotta LV, Dines JS, Owens BD. Management of shoulder instability in the skeletally immature patient. J Am Acad Orthop Surg. 2013;21(9):529–37.
2. Rowe CR, Patel D, Southmayd WW. The Bankart procedure: a long-term end-result study. J Bone Joint Surg Am. 1978;60(1):1–16.
3. Thomas SC, Matsen 3rd FA. An approach to the repair of avulsion of the glenohumeral ligaments in the management of traumatic anterior glenohumeral instability. J Bone Joint Surg Am. 1989;71(4):506–13.
4. Castagna A, Markopoulos N, Conti M, Delle Rose G, Papadakou E, Garofalo R. Arthroscopic bankart suture-anchor repair: radiological and clinical outcome at minimum 10 years of follow-up. Am J Sports Med. 2010;38(10):2012–6.
5. Plath JE, Aboalata M, Seppel G, Juretzko J, Waldt S, Vogt S, et al. Prevalence of and risk factors for dislocation arthropathy: radiological long-term outcome of arthroscopic Bankart repair in 100 shoulders at an average 13-year follow-up. Am J Sports Med. 2015;43(5):1084–90.
6. Castagna A, Delle Rose G, Borroni M, Cillis BD, Conti M, Garofalo R, et al. Arthroscopic stabilization of the shoulder in adolescent athletes participating in overhead or contact sports. Arthroscopy. 2012;28(3):309–15.
7. Longo UG, van der Linde JA, Loppini M, Coco V, Poolman RW, Denaro V. Surgical versus nonoperative treatment in patients up to 18 years old with traumatic shoulder instability: a systematic review and quantitative synthesis of the literature. Arthroscopy. 2016;32(5):944–52.
8. Kraeutler MJ, Ciccotti MG, Dodson CC, Frederick RW, Cammarota B, Cohen SB. Kerlan-Jobe orthopaedic clinic overhead athlete scores in asymptomatic professional baseball pitchers. J Shoulder Elbow Surg. 2013;22(3):329–32.
9. Bacilla P, Field LD, Savoie 3rd FH. Arthroscopic Bankart repair in a high demand patient population. Arthroscopy. 1997;13(1):51–60.
10. Hatch MD, Hennrikus WL. The open Bankart repair for traumatic anterior shoulder instability in teenage athletes. J Pediatr Orthop 2016 doi:10/1097/BPO.0000000000000744.
11. Kraus R, Pavlidis T, Heiss C, Kilian O, Schnettler R. Arthroscopic treatment of post-traumatic shoulder instability in children and adolescents. Knee Surg Sports Traumatol Arthrosc. 2010;18(12):1738–41.
12. Weber S. Arthroscopic Bankart repair: Minimum 10-year follow-up with emphasis on suvivorship. Arthroscopy. 2014;30(6):e4.
13. Arciero RA, Taylor DC. Primary anterior dislocation of the shoulder in young patients. A ten-year prospective study. J Bone Joint Surg Am. 1998;80(2):299–300.

14. Pagnani MJ. Open capsular repair without bone block for recurrent anterior shoulder instability in patients with and without bony defects of the glenoid and/or humeral head. Am J Sports Med. 2008;36(9):1805–12.
15. Hovelius L, Vikerfors O, Olofsson A, Svensson O, Rahme H. Bristow-Latarjet and Bankart: a comparative study of shoulder stabilization in 185 shoulders during a seventeen-year follow-up. J Shoulder Elbow Surg. 2011;20(7):1095–101.
16. Randelli P, Ragone V, Carminati S, Cabitza P. Risk factors for recurrence after Bankart repair a systematic review. Knee Surg Sports Traumatol Arthrosc. 2012;20(11):2129–38.
17. Mazzocca AD, Brown Jr FM, Carreira DS, Hayden J, Romeo AA. Arthroscopic anterior shoulder stabilization of collision and contact athletes. Am J Sports Med. 2005;33(1):52–60.
18. Uhorchak JM, Arciero RA, Huggard D, Taylor DC. Recurrent shoulder instability after open reconstruction in athletes involved in collision and contact sports. Am J Sports Med. 2000;28(6):794–9.
19. Owens BD, DeBerardino TM, Nelson BJ, Thurman J, Cameron KL, Taylor DC, et al. Long-term follow-up of acute arthroscopic Bankart repair for initial anterior shoulder dislocations in young athletes. Am J Sports Med. 2009;37(4):669–73.
20. Jones KJ, Wiesel B, Ganley TJ, Wells L. Functional outcomes of early arthroscopic bankart repair in adolescents aged 11 to 18 years. J Pediatr Orthop. 2007;27(2):209–13.
21. Kuroda S, Sumiyoshi T, Moriishi J, Maruta K, Ishige N. The natural course of atraumatic shoulder instability. J Shoulder Elbow Surg. 2001;10(2):100–4.
22. Greiwe RM, Galano G, Grantham J, Ahmad CS. Arthroscopic stabilization for voluntary shoulder instability. J Pediatr Orthop. 2012;32(8):781–6.
23. Neer 2nd CS, Foster CR. Inferior capsular shift for involuntary inferior and multidirectional instability of the shoulder: a preliminary report. 1980. J Bone Joint Surg Am. 2001;83-A(10):1586.
24. Koh KH, Han KY, Yoon YC, Lee SW, Yoo JC. True anteroposterior (Grashey) view as a screening radiograph for further imaging study in rotator cuff tear. J Shoulder Elbow Surg. 2013;22(7):901–7.
25. Burkhart SS, Debeer JF, Tehrany AM, Parten PM. Quantifying glenoid bone loss arthroscopically in shoulder instability. Arthroscopy. 2002;18(5):488–91.
26. Schenkman L. Radiology. Second thoughts about CT imaging. Science. 2011;331(6020):1002–4.
27. Montgomery 3rd WH, Jobe FW. Functional outcomes in athletes after modified anterior capsulolabral reconstruction. Am J Sports Med. 1994;22(3):352–8.

# Part II

# The Young Athletic High Risk Patient with Shoulder Instability (Age 18–30)

# Spectrum of Instability in the Athletic Young Adult

# 10

K. Beitzel, A.B. Imhoff, and A. Voss

## Content

References .................................................................... 82

The population between 18 and 30 years is the most discussed collective for shoulder instabilities. This young and active generation shows the highest incidence rate over all generations. According to Zacchilli et al. [15] who investigated 8940 shoulder dislocations, the incidence rate was 47.76 per 100,000 person-years at risk in the age between 20 and 30 compared to the reported general incidence rate of 3.1–23.9 [4, 6, 13, 15]. A much higher incidence rate was noted for male patients (79.2) when compared to females (14.8) [15]. Overall sports (especially football and basketball) and recreation-related dislocations caused 48.3% of all injuries with a significant higher rate for males [15]. It is still unknown why there is such a big difference between male and female and if neuromuscular factors, the mechanism of dislocation, or the type of repositioning may have an influence [10]. It has to be noted that most of the contact and collision sports may be affected by a gender bias, as most of them are performed by male athletics and some contact sports do have sex-modified regulations for women [5, 10].

Due to the high incidence rate, the recurrence rate of conservative treated patients in these active populations is high, too, with a rate up to 56% (range 23–29 years of age) [2, 3, 9, 11], but the systematic review by Olds et al. [9] found that this rate might be too high, due to very strict inclusion and exclusion criteria, which may not represent the general population. Additionally it

K. Beitzel (✉) • A.B. Imhoff • A. Voss
Department of Orthopaedic Sports Medicine, Technical University of Munich, Munich, Germany
e-mail: beitzelknut@tum.de

© ISAKOS 2017
A.B. Imhoff, F.H. Savoie III (eds.), *Shoulder Instability Across the Life Span*,
DOI 10.1007/978-3-662-54077-0_10

has been shown that surgical stabilization is significantly reducing the recurrence rate, and therefore it is necessary to identify which patient would benefit from early surgical treatment compared to conservative treatment [3, 12, 14].

Several studies have tried to identify the risk factors, but due the inhomogeneous reported data of dislocation direction, time to first presentation, mechanism of injury, and many more factors, it is hard to compare the results. To encounter this challenge, several scores have been developed such as the instability severity index score or the FEDS (frequency, etiology, direction, and severity) classification system with good intra- and inter-rater reliability in order to simplify the documentation of a shoulder instability event and to achieve comparable data [1, 7]. Interestingly the FEDS classification did correlate with patient requiring surgical stabilization [8]. In the same study, the risk factors for recurrent instability established by the instability severity index score were similar to the reported factors such as involvement in contact sports, hyperlaxity, Hill-Sachs lesions, or loss of inferior glenoid bone after arthroscopic treatment. Especially frequency and etiology showed to be good predictors for surgery [8].

The following chapter will comment on surgical treatment within this active and young population with shoulder instability and address the surgical demands for this group.

## References


1. Balg F, Boileau P. The instability severity index score. A simple pre-operative score to select patients for arthroscopic or open shoulder stabilisation. J Bone Joint Surg Br. 2007;89(11):1470–7.
2. Hovelius L, Augustini BG, Fredin H, Johansson O, Norlin R, Thorling J. Primary anterior dislocation of the shoulder in young patients. A ten-year prospective study. J Bone Joint Surg Am. 1996;78(11):1677–84.
3. Jakobsen BW, Johannsen HV, Suder P, Sojbjerg JO. Primary repair versus conservative treatment of first-time traumatic anterior dislocation of the shoulder: a randomized study with 10-year follow-up. Arthroscopy. 2007;23(2):118–23.
4. Kardouni JR, McKinnon CJ, Seitz AL. Incidence of shoulder dislocations and the rate of recurrent instability in soldiers. Med Sci Sports Exerc. 2016;48:2150–6.
5. Keeler LA. The differences in sport aggression, life aggression, and life assertion among adult male and female collision, contact, and non-contact sport athletes. J Sport Behav. 2007;30:57–76.
6. Kroner K, Lind T, Jensen J. The epidemiology of shoulder dislocations. Arch Orthop Trauma Surg. 1989;108(5):288–90.
7. Kuhn JE. A new classification system for shoulder instability. Br J Sports Med. 2010;44(5):341–6.
8. Lebus GF, Raynor MB, Nwosu SK, Wagstrom E, Jani SS, Carey JL, Hettrich CM, Cox CL, Kuhn JE, Group MS. Predictors for surgery in shoulder instability: a retrospective cohort study using the FEDS system. Orthop J Sports Med. 2015;3(10):2325967115607434.
9. Olds M, Ellis R, Donaldson K, Parmar P, Kersten P. Risk factors which predispose first-time traumatic anterior shoulder dislocations to recurrent instability in adults: a systematic review and meta-analysis. Br J Sports Med. 2015;49(14):913–22.
10. Owens BD, Agel J, Mountcastle SB, Cameron KL, Nelson BJ. Incidence of glenohumeral instability in collegiate athletics. Am J Sports Med. 2009;37(9):1750–4.
11. Robinson CM, Howes J, Murdoch H, Will E, Graham C. Functional outcome and risk of recurrent instability after primary traumatic anterior shoulder dislocation in young patients. J Bone Joint Surg Am. 2006;88(11):2326–36.
12. Sachs RA, Lin D, Stone ML, Paxton E, Kuney M. Can the need for future surgery for acute traumatic anterior shoulder dislocation be predicted? J Bone Joint Surg Am. 2007;89(8):1665–74.
13. Simonet WT, Melton 3rd LJ, Cofield RH, Ilstrup DM. Incidence of anterior shoulder dislocation in Olmsted County, Minnesota. Clin Orthop Relat Res. 1984;186:186–91.
14. te Slaa RL, Brand R, Marti RK. A prospective arthroscopic study of acute first-time anterior shoulder dislocation in the young: a five-year follow-up study. J Shoulder Elbow Surg. 2003;12(6):529–34.
15. Zacchilli MA, Owens BD. Epidemiology of shoulder dislocations presenting to emergency departments in the United States. J Bone Joint Surg Am. 2010;92(3):542–9.

# 11 Overview of Evaluation and Management of the Unstable Shoulder With and Without Bone Loss: Definition, Measurement, and Guidelines on Treatment

Eiji Itoi, Nobuyuki Yamamoto, Taku Hatta, and Jun Kawakami

## Contents


| | | |
|---|---|---|
| 11.1 | **Introduction** | 83 |
| 11.2 | **Evaluation of Glenoid Bony Lesion** | 83 |
| 11.2.1 | Prevalence and Location of the Glenoid Bony Defect | 83 |
| 11.2.2 | X-Ray Methods | 84 |
| 11.2.3 | CT Methods | 84 |
| 11.2.4 | MRI Method | 85 |
| 11.2.5 | Arthroscopic Bare Spot Method | 85 |
| 11.3 | **Critical Size of the Glenoid Bony Defect** | 85 |
| 11.4 | **Hill-Sachs Lesion** | 86 |
| 11.4.1 | Incidence and Prevalence | 86 |
| 11.4.2 | Critical Size of the Hill-Sachs Lesion | 86 |
| 11.5 | **Risk Assessment of Shoulders with a Bipolar Lesion** | 87 |
| 11.6 | **Guidelines on Treatment** | 88 |
| **References** | | 89 |



E. Itoi, MD, PhD (✉) • N. Yamamoto, MD, PhD
T. Hatta, MD, PhD • J. Kawakami, MD, PhD
Department of Orthopaedic Surgery, Tohoku University School of Medicine,
1-1 Seiryo-machi, Aoba-ku, Sendai 980-8574, Japan
e-mail: itoi-eiji@med.tohoku.ac.jp


## 11.1 Introduction

Shoulders with anterior instability often have bony defects of the glenoid and the humeral head. Kurokawa et al. reported that 86% of patients with recurrent anterior dislocation of the shoulder had a glenoid bony defect, whereas 94% had a Hill-Sachs lesion [1]. A bipolar lesion, combination of glenoid defect and Hill-Sachs lesion, is observed in 81% of patients with anterior instability. Therefore, it is extremely important to evaluate the risk of instability caused by the bipolar lesion. In this chapter, we introduce various methods of evaluating the bone loss of the glenoid and the humeral head, how to assess the risk of instability, and how to select the treatment option.

## 11.2 Evaluation of Glenoid Bony Lesion

### 11.2.1 Prevalence and Location of the Glenoid Bony Defect

The prevalence of glenoid bony defect ranges between 66 and 90% [1–5]. There are two types of lesion: a fragment type and an erosion type. The fragment type is more common than the erosion type [2, 4, 5].


© ISAKOS 2017


A.B. Imhoff, F.H. Savoie III (eds.), *Shoulder Instability Across the Life Span*,
DOI 10.1007/978-3-662-54077-0_11

The glenoid bony lesions had been neglected due to difficulty in making a diagnosis by plain X-rays [6]. Kummel reported two cases of chronic shoulder dislocation caused by an antero-inferior glenoid rim fracture [7]. Aston and Gregory reported three cases of anterior shoulder dislocation caused with the arm in adduction [8]. They speculated that the fragment was more anterior in their series because of the uncommon mechanism of injury, whereas the fragments were anteroinferior in Kummel's series because they were caused by the common mechanism of injury. Largely due to a paucity of studies regarding the location of the defect, some biomechanical studies were performed with the glenoid defect created at anteroinferior rim of the glenoid [9, 10]. However, precise assessment of the lesion revealed that the average orientation of the glenoid bony defects defined as a line passing through the center of the glenoid and perpendicular to the rim of the bony defect was pointing toward 3:01 on the clock face of the glenoid, which means the glenoid defects are anterior, not anteroinferior, to the glenoid [11].

### 11.2.2 X-Ray Methods

There are several glenoid profile X-ray views to visualize the anterior rim of the glenoid, such as the West-Point view [12], Bernageau view [13], and apical oblique view [14]. With these specific views, it is possible to obtain a tangential view of the anterior rim of the glenoid. Edwards et al. reported that they found glenoid bony lesions in 87% of patients with anterior shoulder instability (fragment type 49%, erosion type 38%) with the use of anteroposterior and Bernageau views [5]. The prevalence of these lesions is quite similar to the one using CT images [2]. Pansard et al. also reported the Bernageau profile view was a valid and reliable method for visualizing the glenoid bony defect [15]. Thus, specific X-ray views would be sensitive enough to detect the presence of bony defect at the anterior rim of the glenoid. However, with 2D images, it is difficult to assess the extent or size of the lesion.

### 11.2.3 CT Methods

Measurements using CT images are by far the most commonly used method these days. Of course, even with the CT images, eyeballing the defect is not accurate: it should be precisely measured [16]. With the use of an en face view of the glenoid, a bony defect can easily be identified and measured. There are mainly two methods of assessing the size of bony defect.

One is to use linear measurements. With the use of the glenoid width as a reference, the width of the defect relative to the glenoid width is measured [3, 9, 17–20]. There are various methods reported such as the width-to-length ratio [3], which is the same as the glenoid index [20], and the ratio method [21]. The basic concepts of these methods are the same. The advantage of using the linear measurement is easiness of measurement. Using a ruler, the width can very easily be measured.

The other method is to use area measurements. Using a best-fit inscribed circle to the inferior part of the glenoid, the area of the defect relative to the whole circle area is measured [2, 16, 22]. Baudi et al. reported a method called "Pico method" to measure the areas of the defect and the circle using 2D sagittal multiplanar reconstructions instead of 3D reconstructions [23]. They recommended this method as a simple and easy one. The reliability of this measurement method was reported to be very good [24]. However, 3D reconstruction CT images provide the most accurate assessment of bone deficiency [25]. We need a special software to measure the area. As opposed to the linear measurement, the area measurement cannot always be possible without an area measurement software.

The very basic question is this: how can we estimate the original shape of the glenoid when it is already gone? There are several studies to provide a CT-based formula to estimate the lost glenoid size [26, 27]. However, estimation by these formulae may not be accurate if the glenoid shape deviates from the average shape. The best-fit circle gives us an estimated shape of the original glenoid [2, 16, 22]. The diameter of this circle can be used as the width of the original glenoid.

Another method is to use the contralateral shoulder. When we take CT scan, not only the involved shoulder but also the contralateral shoulder is simultaneously scanned because both shoulders are in the CT gantry. The data of the contralateral glenoid are always available without additional scanning. The side-to-side differences in the glenoid length, width, and area are all less than 1% [28]. Thus, it is quite reasonable, legitimate, and precise to use the contralateral shoulder as a reference when using CT [3, 29].

### 11.2.4 MRI Method

Considering radiation exposure, MRI is more preferable. Huijsmans et al. compared the area of the glenoid defect relative to the best-fit circle area measured with 3D-CT images and MR images [22]. Both methods showed high reliability without any significant difference between them. They concluded that measurement of glenoid bone loss could be done with 3D-CT scans as well as MRI. However, a more recent study showed that the correlation between MRI and CT scans was only moderate [30]. Bishop et al. compared X-ray, CT, 3D-CT, and MRI and concluded that 3D-CT was the most reliable imaging modality for measuring glenoid bone loss [31]. When we use MRI, we need to obtain the reference either using a best-fit circle method or MRI-based formula [32].

### 11.2.5 Arthroscopic Bare Spot Method

Burkhart et al. proposed a method to measure the size of the glenoid defect during arthroscopy [17]. They reported that the bare spot was located near the center of the best-fit circle of the inferior portion of the glenoid. The length between the bare spot and the posterior rim of the glenoid was close to the diameter of the best-fit circle. The difference between this diameter and the length from the bare spot to the anterior rim of the glenoid was supposed to be equal to the size of the anterior glenoid defect. This method is called "arthroscopic bare spot method." Later, anatomical studies have shown that the bare spot is located slightly anterior and inferior to the center of the circle [33, 34]. Provencher et al. showed in a cadaveric study that a bone loss measurement using the arthroscopic bare spot method overestimated the amount of bone loss located anteroinferiorly more than the one located anteriorly due to this off-center location of the bare spot [35]. More recently, Barcia et al. reported that the bare spot was visible in 48% of the shoulders without a diagnosis of instability, and it was at the center of the glenoid in 37% of the time [36]. Therefore, the bare area may not always be a reliable reference point during arthroscopic surgery.

## 11.3 Critical Size of the Glenoid Bony Defect

Rowe et al. were the first to describe the relationship between the glenoid defect and the surgical outcome of Bankart repair [37]. They reported that there were no significant differences in the outcome of Bankart repair when the bony defect of the glenoid was between 1/6 and 1/3 of the glenoid. Based on this observation, a glenoid defect greater than 1/3 of the glenoid is reported to be an indication for bone grafting [38, 39]. Itoi et al. clearly showed for the first time the relationship between the glenoid defect and shoulder stability in a cadaveric study [9]. They created an anteroinferior bony defect of the glenoid stepwise, repaired the Bankart lesion, and measured shoulder stability. They concluded that with a defect equal to or greater than 21% of the glenoid length, shoulder stability could not be restored after the Bankart repair. Later, Montgomery et al. reported that a contoured iliac bone graft to a defect of this critical size could fully restore shoulder stability [10]. These experiments were performed with a bony defect created at the anteroinferior portion of the glenoid. However, the glenoid defects are located more anteriorly rather than anteroinferiorly [11]. Yamamoto et al. performed similar biomechanical studies but with a defect created anteriorly [18, 19]. These studies showed that the critical defect size of the glenoid was 25% of the glenoid width or 20% of the glenoid length. This critical size was also confirmed by the clinical studies [40–42]. One limitation of the previous biomechanical studies is that the bony defects were created with an increment of 2 mm [18, 19]. With this method, the 6 mm defect (25% of the glenoid width) or greater caused instability, whereas the 4 mm defect (17.5% of the glenoid width) or less caused no instability. Thus, all we can say is that the critical size of the glenoid defect is 25% of the glenoid width and the safe size is 17.5% or less. The zone between 17.5 and 25% is a gray zone. Recently, Shaha et al. showed that when a defect was more than 20% of the glenoid width, the recurrent dislocation was the problem after arthroscopic Bankart repair in the military patients [43]. However, when a defect was between 13.5 and 20%, the recurrence was not a problem, but the WOSI scores were less satisfactory due to remnant pain or positive apprehension in this group than those with smaller bony defects. They defined this bone loss as a "subcritical bone loss," which also needs to be considered when dealing with high-risk patients. Their subcritical bone loss obtained from the clinical study (13.5–20%) was slightly smaller than the one observed in the cadaveric studies (17.5–25%), probably due to the difference in patient's background and risks. The subcritical bone loss needs to be further clarified.

## 11.4 Hill-Sachs Lesion

### 11.4.1 Incidence and Prevalence

This is a compression fracture of the humeral head created by the anterior rim of the glenoid when the humeral head dislocates anteriorly. This lesion was first reported by Malgaigne in 1847 [44]. Later, Hill and Sachs published a comprehensive review article of this lesion, by which this lesion carries their names these days [45]. The incidence of this lesion ranges 65–67% after initial dislocation, and the prevalence increases to 84–93% after recurrent dislocations [46, 47]. The lesion is located at the posterior lateral aspect of the humeral head articular surface, extending from 0 to 24 mm from the top of the humeral head, with an average width of 22 mm and an average depth of 5 mm [48].

### 11.4.2 Critical Size of the Hill-Sachs Lesion

Regarding the critical size of the Hill-Sachs lesion, Rowe et al. reported that moderate (4 cm long × 0.5 cm deep) to severe (4 cm long × 1 cm deep) Hill-Sachs lesion might be a risk factor to cause recurrent dislocation following a Bankart repair [49]. Others recommended skeletal reconstruction for a Hill-Sachs lesion greater than 20–25% of the articular surface of the humeral head to obtain clinical stability [50, 51]. Later, Sommaire et al. also quantitatively measured the depth or volume of the Hill-Sachs lesion to determine the critical size [52]. These investigators focused on the size of the Hill-Sachs lesion alone, and none of them took the size of the glenoid into consideration.

However, different from the critical size of the glenoid bone loss, the critical size of the Hill-Sachs lesion cannot be determined by the size of the Hill-Sachs lesion alone: it also needs to be determined by the glenoid bone loss [53, 54]. This is because a Hill-Sachs lesion which does not engage with the intact glenoid could engage with the glenoid with an anterior bone loss. Thus, it is not the absolute size of the Hill-Sachs lesion but the relative size of the lesion to the glenoid that determines whether it would engage with the glenoid.

In order to assess the Hill-Sachs lesion together with the glenoid, a new concept, the "glenoid track," has been introduced [55]. The glenoid track is the contact area between the glenoid and the humeral head when the arm is moved along the posterior end range of motion. If the Hill-Sachs lesion stays on the glenoid track, there is no chance that this lesion engages with the anterior rim of the glenoid. On the other hand, if the Hill-Sachs lesion is extending more medially over the medial margin of the glenoid track, the lesion has a chance to engage with the anterior rim of the glenoid at the zone where the Hill-Sachs lesion overrides the medial margin of the glenoid track. The existence of the glenoid track was first confirmed in cadaveric shoulders [55]. The medial margin of the glenoid track was found to be located at a distance equivalent to 84% of the glenoid width from the medial margin of the footprint of the rotator cuff. Later, the size and location of the glenoid track were measured in live shoulders, which revealed that the medial margin of the glenoid track was located at a distance equivalent to 83% of the glenoid width at 90° of arm abduction, which slightly increased with the arm less than 90° of abduction and decreased with the arm more than 90° of abduction [56].

Not only the location of the Hill-Sachs lesion but also the orientation of the lesion seems to affect the risk of engagement. Burkhart and De Beer were the first to pay attention to the orientation of the Hill-Sachs lesion [41]. They defined an engaging Hill-Sachs lesion as the one that presents the long axis of the Hill-Sachs lesion parallel to the anterior rim of the glenoid with the arm in a functional position of abduction and external rotation. It was likely that an engaging Hill-Sachs lesion was created with the arm in abduction and external rotation, whereas a non-engaging Hill-Sachs lesion was created with the arm in adduction. Cho et al. quantified the orientation of the Hill-Sachs lesion by measuring the Hill-Sachs angle, which was between the longitudinal axis of the humeral shaft and the axis of the deepest groove of the Hill-Sachs lesion on the frontal plane of 3D reconstructed image [57]. They reported that the average Hill-Sachs angle was 25.6° for engaging Hill-Sachs lesion and 13.8° for non-engaging Hill-Sachs lesion. More recently, Di Giacomo et al. also measured the orientation of the Hill-Sachs lesion in patients after initial shoulder dislocation [58]. They divided the patients into two groups: those whose initial dislocation had occurred with the arm less than 60° of abduction (ADD group) and those whose initial dislocation had occurred with the arm more than 60° of abduction (ABD group). The Hill-Sachs angle was 32.4° in ABD group and 16.1° in ADD group. Although all the Hill-Sachs lesions were on-track in their series, they speculated that the Hill-Sachs lesion in ABD group was more likely to engage because the Hill-Sachs lesion was closer to parallel to the glenoid rim with the arm in a functional position. The orientation of the Hill-Sachs lesion is solely determined by the position of the arm when the lesion was created. It may or may not be the same as the position of dislocation [41]. If the lesion is in parallel with the glenoid rim in a functional arm position, the engagement is more likely to occur in that functional arm position.

## 11.5 Risk Assessment of Shoulders with a Bipolar Lesion

As mentioned previously, the risk of instability after a Bankart repair can be precisely assessed with the use of the glenoid track concept. In the clinical setting, however, many surgeons prefer to use dynamic examination. Most surgeons do dynamic examination as follows. During arthroscopic operation, they move the arm to an anterior apprehension position of abduction and external rotation. If they observe an engagement of the Hill-Sachs lesion with the anterior rim of the glenoid, it is assessed as an "engaging" lesion, and remplissage procedure may be indicated. However, this is not the correct way to assess the risk of engagement. Many Hill-Sachs lesions (theoretically all lesions) show engagement during this maneuver due to anterior instability of the humeral head. After the Bankart repair, most of them do not engage anymore because the humeral head is well centered after the Bankart repair. During arthroscopic operation, the prevalence of engaging Hill-Sachs lesion ranges greatly between 15 and 52% of all the cases who underwent arthroscopic Bankart repair: all the dynamic examinations were done before the Bankart repair [57, 59–63]. There is only one study, in which the authors performed dynamic examination after the Bankart repair (Parke CS, et al. Read at the 39th Annual Meeting of Japan Shoulder Society, 2012). They found 72 cases with an engaging Hill-Sachs lesion out of 983 cases treated with arthroscopic Bankart repair: the prevalence of engaging Hill-Sachs lesion was 7%. In order to avoid the confusion and misunderstanding of engaging lesions, the term "on-track/off-track" lesion was coined by Di Giacomo et al. [29]. If a Hill-Sachs lesion stays on the glenoid track (on-track lesion), there is no risk of engagement. If a Hill-Sachs lesion stays out of the glenoid track (off-track lesion), there is a risk of engagement. It is interesting that Kurokawa et al. reported the prevalence of off-track Hill-Sachs lesion to be 7% using the glenoid track concept [1], which is exactly the same as the one reported by Parke et al. (2012) with the use of dynamic examination after the Bankart repair. A more recent study using MRI or CT for the assessment of on-track/off-track lesion showed that the prevalence of off-track lesion was 12% [64]. Therefore, the prevalence of so-called engaging lesion assessed before the Bankart repair ranges 15–52%, whereas that of the off-track lesion or "true" engaging lesion ranges 7–12% [57, 59–63].

## 11.6 Guidelines on Treatment

Based on this on-track/off-track concept together with the critical size of the glenoid defect, we can divide the unstable shoulders into four categories: #1 on-track lesion with a glenoid defect less than 25% of the glenoid defect, #2 on-track lesion with a glenoid defect equal to or greater than 25%, #3 off-track lesion with a glenoid defect less than 25%, and #4 off-track lesion with a glenoid defect equal to or greater than 25% (Table 11.1) [29]. For Category #1, we do not need to worry about the bony lesions. Soft tissue repair such as arthroscopic Bankart repair would be just sufficient. For Category #2, only a large glenoid defect needs to be treated. Coracoid transfer such as the Latarjet procedure is commonly performed. For Category #3, a glenoid bony defect can be ignored, but the Hill-Sachs lesion is off-track, so it needs to be treated either by remplissage or coracoid transfer such as the Latarjet procedure depending upon the patient's sport activity. If the patient is a collision or contact athlete, the risk of recurrence is higher than noncollision, noncontact athletes. In such cases, the Latarjet procedure, which is supposed to provide an additional stability, may be preferable [65, 66]. If the patient is a baseball pitcher, they require maximum amount of external rotation with the arm in abduction. However, remplissage procedure is known to reduce the range of external rotation in abduction (Kelly, Tokish et al. AJSM 2016 In Press) [67]. In such cases, the Latarjet procedure seems to be more preferable than remplissage. For Category #4, a large glenoid defect needs to be fixed by bone grafting such as the Latarjet procedure. After this procedure, remplissage may need to be added if the engagement still remains. With this treatment paradigm, satisfactory outcomes of surgical treatment have been reported. Locher et al. reported that the recurrence rate after the Bankart repair was 6% (5/88) of those with an on-track Hill-Sachs lesion and 33% (4/12) of those with an off-track lesion [64]. The odds ratio of recurrence for those with an off-track lesion was 8.3 (95% CI: 1.85–37.26). Shaha et al. also reported a validation study of on-track/off-track concept [68]. The recurrence rate was 8% (4/49) of on-track patients and 75% (6/8) of off-track patients. The positive predictive value of 75% using the off-track concept was significantly higher than that using the bone loss size >20%. They concluded that application of the glenoid track concept was superior to using glenoid bone loss alone.

**Table 11.1** Treatment paradigm

| | On-track Hill-Sachs lesion | Off-track Hill-Sachs lesion |
|---|---|---|
| Glenoid <25% | Arthroscopic Bankart repair | Arthroscopic Bankart repair + remplissage or Latarjet procedure |
| Glenoid ≥25% | Latarjet procedure | Latarjet procedure w/ or w/out remplissage |

Modified from the Ref. [29]

The outcome of the Latarjet procedure was also assessed with the use of the glenoid concept. Mook et al. reported that failure after the Latarjet procedure occurred in 50% (4/8) of those whose

Hill-Sachs lesion was located more medially than the grafted coracoid process (off-track lesion), but only in 16% (4/25) of those with an on-track lesion [69]. The patients with an off-track lesion after the Latarjet procedure were 4.0 times more likely to experience postoperative instability than those without. They concluded that the glenoid track concept may be predictive of stability after the Latarjet procedure.

One thing we need to consider is the fragment type of glenoid bony defect. It is more frequently observed than erosion-type lesions [2, 4, 5]. Sugaya et al. performed bony Bankart repair in patients with an average bone loss of 24.8% (range: 11.4–38.6%) and an average fragment size of 9.2% (range, 2.1–20.9%) of the glenoid fossa [69]. All the fragments were in the capsulolabral complex and were fixed back to the glenoid with the use of suture anchors. With an average 34-month follow-up, 39/42 (93%) were rated good or excellent. Two patients (5%) had recurrent dislocations due to reinjury during sports. They concluded that arthroscopic bony Bankart repair yielded a successful outcome even in shoulders with a large bony defect >25%.

The fragment may be absorbed gradually if you leave it alone [4]. Nakagawa et al. reported that all the fragments underwent absorption to some extent: <50% in 32 shoulders, >50% in 45, and 100% in 15. Most fragments showed absorption during the first year after the primary dislocation. Thus, by the time the fragment is fixed to the glenoid by means of osseous Bankart repair, there is a significant discrepancy between the size of the glenoid defect and the size of the fragment as shown in the previous study [70]. This discrepancy could be a concern when performing bony fragment fixation. After the midterm to long-term follow-up, however, the original glenoid defect was well remodeled, and the gap between the fragment and the glenoid became much smaller with new bone formation [71]. On the other hand, Nakagawa et al. reported that the bone union was not always observed and the outcome was affected by bone union [72]. On the contrary, Jiang et al. reported that the size of the reconstructed glenoid, not the bone union, affected the outcome [73]. The indication and efficacy of bony fragment fixation are still controversial and need to be determined by clarifying the outcomes and factors affecting the outcomes.

## References


1. Kurokawa D et al. The prevalence of a large Hill-Sachs lesion that needs to be treated. J Shoulder Elbow Surg. 2013;22(9):1285–9.
2. Sugaya H et al. Glenoid rim morphology in recurrent anterior glenohumeral instability. J Bone Joint Surg Am. 2003;85-a(5):878–84.
3. Griffith JF et al. Anterior shoulder dislocation: quantification of glenoid bone loss with CT. AJR Am J Roentgenol. 2003;180(5):1423–30.
4. Nakagawa S et al. Absorption of the bone fragment in shoulders with bony Bankart lesions caused by recurrent anterior dislocations or subluxations: when does it occur? Am J Sports Med. 2013;41(6):1380–6.
5. Edwards TB, Boulahia A, Walch G. Radiographic analysis of bone defects in chronic anterior shoulder instability. Arthroscopy. 2003;19(7):732–9.
6. Rowe CR, Sakellarides HT. Factors related to recurrences of anterior dislocations of the shoulder. Clin Orthop. 1961;20:40–8.
7. Kummel BM. Fractures of the glenoid causing chronic dislocation of the shoulder. Clin Orthop Relat Res. 1970;69:189–91.
8. Aston Jr JW, Gregory CF. Dislocation of the shoulder with significant fracture of the glenoid. J Bone Joint Surg Am. 1973;55(7):1531–3.
9. Itoi E et al. The effect of a glenoid defect on anteroinferior stability of the shoulder after Bankart repair: a cadaveric study. J Bone Joint Surg Am. 2000;82(1):35–46.
10. Montgomery Jr WH et al. Anteroinferior bone-grafting can restore stability in osseous glenoid defects. J Bone Joint Surg Am. 2005;87(9):1972–7.
11. Saito H et al. Location of the glenoid defect in shoulders with recurrent anterior dislocation. Am J Sports Med. 2005;33(6):889–93.
12. Rokous JR, Feagin JA, Abbott HG. Modified axillary roentgenogram. A useful adjunct in the diagnosis of recurrent instability of the shoulder. Clin Orthop Relat Res. 1972;82:84–6.
13. Bernageau J et al. Value of the glenoid profil in recurrent luxations of the shoulder. Rev Chir Orthop Reparatrice Appar Mot. 1976;62(2 suppl):142–7.
14. Garth Jr WP, Slappey CE, Ochs CW. Roentgenographic demonstration of instability of the shoulder: the apical oblique projection. A technical note. J Bone Joint Surg Am. 1984;66(9):1450–3.

15. Pansard E et al. Reliability and validity assessment of a glenoid bone loss measurement using the Bernageau profile view in chronic anterior shoulder instability. J Shoulder Elbow Surg. 2013;22(9):1193–8.
16. Huijsmans PE et al. Recurrent anterior shoulder instability: accuracy of estimations of glenoid bone loss with computed tomography is insufficient for therapeutic decision-making. Skeletal Radiol. 2011; 40(10):1329–34.
17. Burkhart SS et al. Quantifying glenoid bone loss arthroscopically in shoulder instability. Arthroscopy. 2002;18(5):488–91.
18. Yamamoto N et al. Effect of an anterior glenoid defect on anterior shoulder stability: a cadaveric study. Am J Sports Med. 2009;37(5):949–54.
19. Yamamoto N et al. Stabilizing mechanism in bone-grafting of a large glenoid defect. J Bone Joint Surg Am. 2010;92(11):2059–66.
20. Chuang TY, Adams CR, Burkhart SS. Use of preoperative three-dimensional computed tomography to quantify glenoid bone loss in shoulder instability. Arthroscopy. 2008;24(4):376–82.
21. Barchilon VS et al. A simple method for quantitative evaluation of the missing area of the anterior glenoid in anterior instability of the glenohumeral joint. Skeletal Radiol. 2008;37(8):731–6.
22. Huijsmans PE et al. Quantification of a glenoid defect with three-dimensional computed tomography and magnetic resonance imaging: a cadaveric study. J Shoulder Elbow Surg. 2007;16(6):803–9.
23. Baudi P et al. How to identify and calculate glenoid bone deficit. Chir Organi Mov. 2005;90(2):145–52.
24. Magarelli N et al. Intra-observer and interobserver reliability of the 'Pico' computed tomography method for quantification of glenoid bone defect in anterior shoulder instability. Skeletal Radiol. 2009;38(11):1071–5.
25. Provencher MT et al. Recurrent shoulder instability: current concepts for evaluation and management of glenoid bone loss. J Bone Joint Surg Am. 2010;92(Suppl 2):133–51.
26. Giles JW, Owens BD, Athwal GS. Estimating glenoid width for instability-related bone loss: a CT evaluation of an MRI formula. Am J Sports Med. 2015;43(7):1726–30.
27. Ohl X et al. 3D morphometric analysis of 43 scapulae. Surg Radiol Anat. 2012;34(5):447–53.
28. Shi L et al. Excellent side-to-side symmetry in glenoid size and shape. Skeletal Radiol. 2013;42(12):1711–5.
29. Di Giacomo G, Itoi E, Burkhart SS. Evolving concept of bipolar bone loss and the Hill-Sachs lesion: from "engaging/non-engaging" lesion to "on-track/off-track" lesion. Arthroscopy. 2014;30(1):90–8.
30. Friedman LG et al. Glenoid bone loss measurement in recurrent shoulder dislocation: assessment of measurement agreement between CT and MRI. Orthop J Sports Med. 2014;2(9):2325967114549541.
31. Bishop JY et al. 3-D CT is the most reliable imaging modality when quantifying glenoid bone loss. Clin Orthop Relat Res. 2013;471(4):1251–6.
32. Owens BD et al. Simple method of glenoid bone loss calculation using ipsilateral magnetic resonance imaging. Am J Sports Med. 2013;41(3):622–4.
33. Aigner F et al. Anatomical considerations regarding the "bare spot" of the glenoid cavity. Surg Radiol Anat. 2004;26(4):308–11.
34. Kralinger F et al. Is the bare spot a consistent landmark for shoulder arthroscopy? A study of 20 embalmed glenoids with 3-dimensional computed tomographic reconstruction. Arthroscopy. 2006;22(4):428–32.
35. Provencher MT et al. Measurement of glenoid bone loss: a comparison of measurement error between 45 degrees and 0 degrees bone loss models and with different posterior arthroscopy portal locations. Am J Sports Med. 2008;36(6):1132–8.
36. Barcia AM et al. Glenoid bare area: arthroscopic characterization and its implications on measurement of bone loss. Arthroscopy. 2013;29(10):1671–5.
37. Rowe CR, Patel D, Southmayd WW. The Bankart procedure: a long-term end-result study. J Bone Joint Surg Am. 1978;60(1):1–16.
38. Matsen III FA, Thomas SC. Glenohumeral instability. In: Evarts CMC, editor. Surgery of the musculoskeletal system. 2nd ed. New York: Churchill Livingstone; 1990. p. 1439–69.
39. Matsen III FA et al. Glenohumeral instability. In: Rockwood Jr CA, Matsen III FA, editors. The shoulder. 2nd ed. Philadelphia: W. B. Saunders; 1998. p. 611–754.
40. Bigliani LU et al. Glenoid rim lesions associated with recurrent anterior dislocation of the shoulder. Am J Sports Med. 1998;26(1):41–5.
41. Burkhart SS, De Beer JF. Traumatic glenohumeral bone defects and their relationship to failure of arthroscopic Bankart repairs: significance of the inverted-pear glenoid and the humeral engaging Hill-Sachs lesion. Arthroscopy. 2000;16(7):677–94.
42. Lo IK, Parten PM, Burkhart SS. The inverted pear glenoid: an indicator of significant glenoid bone loss. Arthroscopy. 2004;20(2):169–74.
43. Shaha JS et al. Redefining "critical" bone loss in shoulder instability: functional outcomes worsen with "subcritical" bone loss. Am J Sports Med. 2015;43(7):1719–25.
44. Malgaigne JF. Traité des fractures et luxations. Paris: JB Baillière; 1847.
45. Hill HA, Sachs MD. The grooved defect of the humeral head: a frequently unrecognized complication of dislocations of the shoulder joint. Radiology. 1940;35(6):690–700.
46. Spatschil A et al. Posttraumatic anterior-inferior instability of the shoulder: arthroscopic findings and clinical correlations. Arch Orthop Trauma Surg. 2006;126(4):217–22.
47. Yiannakopoulos CK, Mataragas E, Antonogiannakis E. A comparison of the spectrum of intra-articular lesions in acute and chronic anterior shoulder instability. Arthroscopy. 2007;23(9):985–90.

48. Saito H et al. Location of the Hill-Sachs lesion in shoulders with recurrent anterior dislocation. Arch Orthop Trauma Surg. 2009;129(10):1327–34.
49. Rowe CR, Zarins B, Ciullo JV. Recurrent anterior dislocation of the shoulder after surgical repair. Apparent causes of failure and treatment. J Bone Joint Surg Am. 1984;66(2):159–68.
50. Buhler M, Gerber C. Shoulder instability related to epileptic seizures. J Shoulder Elbow Surg. 2002; 11(4):339–44.
51. Miniaci A, Berlet G. Recurrent anterior instability following failed surgical repair: Allograft reconstruction of large humeral head defects. J Bone Joint Surg Br. 2001;83(Suppl 1):19–20.
52. Sommaire C et al. Recurrence after arthroscopic Bankart repair: is quantitative radiological analysis of bone loss of any predictive value? Orthop Traumatol Surg Res. 2012;98(5):514–9.
53. Itoi E et al. Bone loss in anterior instability. Curr Rev Musculoskelet Med. 2013;6(1):88–94.
54. Itoi E, Yamamoto N. Shoulder instability: treating bone loss. Curr Orthop Pract. 2012;23(6):609–15.
55. Yamamoto N et al. Contact between the glenoid and the humeral head in abduction, external rotation, and horizontal extension: a new concept of glenoid track. J Shoulder Elbow Surg. 2007;16(5):649–56.
56. Omori Y et al. Measurement of the glenoid track in vivo as investigated by 3-dimensional motion analysis using open MRI. Am J Sports Med. 2014;42(6):1290–5.
57. Cho SH, Cho NS, Rhee YG. Preoperative analysis of the Hill-Sachs lesion in anterior shoulder instability: how to predict engagement of the lesion. Am J Sports Med. 2011;39(11):2389–95.
58. Di Giacomo G et al. Radiographic analysis of the Hill-Sachs lesion in anteroinferior shoulder instability after first-time dislocations. Arthroscopy. 2016;32:1509–14.
59. Haviv B, Mayo L, Biggs D. Outcomes of arthroscopic "remplissage": capsulotenodesis of the engaging large Hill-Sachs lesion. J Orthop Surg Res. 2011;6:29.
60. Zhu YM et al. Arthroscopic Bankart repair combined with remplissage technique for the treatment of anterior shoulder instability with engaging Hill-Sachs lesion: a report of 49 cases with a minimum 2-year follow-up. Am J Sports Med. 2011;39(8):1640–7.
61. Merolla G et al. Outcomes of arthroscopic Hill-Sachs remplissage and anterior Bankart repair: a retrospective controlled study including ultrasound evaluation of posterior capsulotenodesis and infraspinatus strength assessment. Am J Sports Med. 2015;43(2):407–14.
62. Garcia GH et al. Outcomes of the remplissage procedure and its effects on return to sports: average 5-year follow-up. Am J Sports Med. 2016;44(5):1124–30.
63. Cho NS et al. Anterior shoulder instability with engaging Hill-Sachs defects: a comparison of arthroscopic Bankart repair with and without posterior capsulodesis. Knee Surg Sports Traumatol Arthrosc. 2016;24:3801–8.
64. Locher J et al. Hill-Sachs off-track lesions as risk factor for recurrence of instability after arthroscopic bankart repair. Arthroscopy. 2016;32:1993–9.
65. Neyton L et al. Surgical treatment of anterior instability in rugby union players: clinical and radiographic results of the Latarjet-Patte procedure with minimum 5-year follow-up. J Shoulder Elbow Surg. 2012;21(12):1721–7.
66. Yamamoto N et al. The stabilizing mechanism of the Latarjet procedure: a cadaveric study. J Bone Joint Surg Am. 2013;95(15):1390–7.
67. Omi R et al. The effect of the remplissage procedure on shoulder range of motion: a cadaveric study. Arthroscopy. 2014;30(2):178–87.
68. Shaha JS et al. Clinical validation of the glenoid track concept in anterior glenohumeral instability. J Bone Joint Surg Am. 2016;98(22):1918–23.
69. Mook WR et al. Clinical and anatomic predictors of outcomes after the latarjet procedure for the treatment of anterior glenohumeral instability with combined glenoid and humeral bone defects. Am J Sports Med. 2016;44(6):1407–16.
70. Sugaya H et al. Arthroscopic osseous Bankart repair for chronic recurrent traumatic anterior glenohumeral instability. J Bone Joint Surg Am. 2005;87(8):1752–60.
71. Kitayama S et al. Clinical outcome and glenoid morphology after arthroscopic repair of chronic osseous bankart lesions: a five to eight-year follow-up study. J Bone Joint Surg Am. 2015;97(22):1833–43.
72. Nakagawa S et al. Bone fragment union and remodeling after arthroscopic bony bankart repair for traumatic anterior shoulder instability with a glenoid defect: influence on postoperative recurrence of instability. Am J Sports Med. 2015;43(6):1438–47.
73. Jiang CY et al. Do reduction and healing of the bony fragment really matter in arthroscopic bony Bankart reconstruction?: a prospective study with clinical and computed tomography evaluations. Am J Sports Med. 2013;41(11):2617–23.

# Arthroscopic Soft Tissue Repair: Bankart Repair and Remplissage Procedure

# 12

Jiwu Chen

## Contents

12.1 **Overview** 93

12.2 **Bankart Lesion and Hill-Sachs Lesion** 94
12.2.1 Bankart Lesion 94
12.2.2 Hill-Sachs Lesion 94

12.3 **Arthroscopic Soft Tissue Repair** 95
12.3.1 Indications 95
12.3.2 Preoperative Evaluation 95
12.3.3 Operative Technique 96
12.3.4 Arthroscopic Bankart Repair and Remplissage Technique 96

**Conclusion** 100

**References** 100

J. Chen, MD, PhD
Department of Sports Medicine, Huashan Hospital, Fudan University, Shanghai, China
e-mail: jeevechen@gmail.com

## 12.1 Overview

Traumatic anterior shoulder instability is a common sports injury with high risk of recurrence in young and active patients [1]. Many factors have been evaluated to analyze their correlation with the recurrence of instability, including age, sports participation, immobilization, rehabilitative exercises, and time before return to sports or full activity.

McLaughlin and MacLellan [2] reported a 95% recurrence rate in 181 patients aged ≤20 years and 96% recurrence within the 265 cases starting the first dislocation before age 30 years. The recurrence rates in Rowe's study [3] were 94% in 53 patients aged <20 years and 79% in 64 patients aged 21–30 years. The study of Henry and Genung [4] showed 88% in 121 athletes aged<32 years had the recurrent instability. Hoelen et al. [5] reported the highest recurrence was found in 64% in 168 patients aged ≤30 years. Therefore, it can be concluded that the most important prognostic factor correlated with recurrence was the age at the time of the first dislocation.

Besides the age, athletic activity was another important factor in relation with the recurrence of shoulder instability. Simonet and Cofield [6] reported the recurrence rate was 82% in 33 athletes aged <30 years as compared with 30% in 27 nonathletes of similar age. The study of Henry and Genung [4] showed a recurrent dislocation rate of 88% in 121 athletes aged<32 years. The

© ISAKOS 2017
A.B. Imhoff, F.H. Savoie III (eds.), *Shoulder Instability Across the Life Span*,
DOI 10.1007/978-3-662-54077-0_12

high incidence of shoulder instability in athletes was also evidenced by the study in the military population [7, 8].

Currently, no consensus has been reached on whether to treat a first-time anterior shoulder dislocation surgically. A study of the long-term prognosis in 257 first-time anterior shoulder dislocations (255 patients, aged 12–40 years) at follow-up of 25 years showed that almost 50% of all first-time dislocations at the age of <25 years will be treated by surgery and 61% will develop different stages of arthropathy within 25 years [10]. It was also noticed that the number of dislocations correlated with the evolution of the labrum-ligament complex lesions and the Hill-Sachs lesion [11, 12]. Yiannakopoulos et al. [13] reported that associated and secondary intra-articular lesions, including anterior labroligamentous periosteal sleeve avulsion (ALPSA) lesion, Hill-Sachs lesion, partial-thickness articular rotator cuff tear, and inverted pear-shaped glenoid, are more frequent in patients with chronic compared with acute shoulder instability. A systemic review of five randomized controlled trials supported surgical stabilization as a reasonable alternative to nonoperative treatment for first-time shoulder dislocation in young, active adults participating in highly demanding physical activities [9].

Due to the high risk of failure of conservative management and the secondary lesions followed, particularly among young patients participating in sports activities [14, 15], early surgical shoulder stabilization is generally recommended for traumatic anterior shoulder instability in the young athletes involved in shoulder demanding activities [14, 16–19].

## 12.2 Bankart Lesion and Hill-Sachs Lesion

### 12.2.1 Bankart Lesion

Bankart lesion (Perthes-Bankart lesion) was first described by Perthes [20] as an avulsion of the anterior inferior labrum from the glenoid rim in shoulder dislocation. Bankart [21] described that "no tendency whatever for the detached capsule to unite spontaneously with the fibro-cartilage" following an anterior shoulder dislocation in 1923. With the development of arthroscopic surgery, Bankart lesion was confirmed to be the most common pathologic finding in shoulder instability. Taylor and Arciero [22] reported that Bankart lesion was observed in 97% of the 67 patients with first-time traumatic anterior dislocations. With an arthroscopic evaluation of 212 unstable shoulders, 87% in 184 cases was confirmed to have labrum tear [23]. With the analysis of intra-articular lesions in 127 patients with acute and chronic traumatic anterior instability, Yiannakopoulos et al. [13] reported that the incidence of Bankart lesions was 78.2% (18/23) in patients with acute dislocations, whereas the incidence of Bankart or ALPSA lesions was 97.11% (101/104) in chronic cases. Since the high incidence of Bankart lesion, Bankart repair have been widely used to address the lesion of capsule-ligament-labrum complex in anterior shoulder instability. Several studies have reported on the return to sporting activity after arthroscopic Bankart repair compared with the pre-trauma activity level [24–27].

### 12.2.2 Hill-Sachs Lesion

Hill-Sachs lesion, first documented in 1940 by Hill and Sachs [28], is a posterolateral compression fracture in the humeral head, which results from the glenoid rim impacts the humeral head during an anterior dislocation [29, 30]. It is another common pathologic finding in traumatic anterior shoulder instability, which was found in 65–71% of initial glenohumeral dislocations [13, 29, 31, 32] and in 93–100% of patients with recurrent dislocations [13, 33, 34]. Moreover, subsequent dislocation and subluxation events increase the size of the Hill-Sachs lesion, increasing the risk of recurrence [35].

It has been noticed that a severe Hill-Sachs lesion was a risk factor for recurrent dislocation after an isolated Bankart repair [36, 37]. The size and location of the lesion are important factors in strong relation to the degree of instability and the risk of engagement of the defect on the glenoid rim during shoulder movement [38, 39]. Thus, several concepts have been developed to define what condition Hill-Sachs lesion is critical and needs to be treated.

If its long axis of the defect parallel to the anterior glenoid with the shoulder in abduction and external rotation, the Hill-Sachs lesion will engage the corner of the glenoid and result in re-dislocation following the labrum repair. This condition was defined as an engaging Hill-Sachs lesion by Burkhart and Debeer [37] and suggested to be treated if it could be observed under arthroscopy.

Some authors try to define the engaging lesion through radiographic evaluation. With measurements on three-dimensional computed tomography, Hill-Sachs lesion was classified as "on-track" and "off-track" lesions according to their locations with respect to the glenoid track [40]. Off-track lesions are at greatest risk of engagement [40–42].

Various techniques were introduced to address the Hill-Sachs lesion, including open capsular shift to restrict external rotation [43], rotational proximal humeral osteotomy [44], percutaneous humeroplasty [45], bone graft or coracoid transfer to the anterior part of the glenoid rim [37], and osteoarticular allograft transplantation [46, 47].

Since the "remplissage" technique was introduced, it has been the most used arthroscopic technique in case of humeral bone defects. The technique of remplissage, which means "to fill" in French, involves imbrication of the posterior capsule and infraspinatus tendon into the humeral head defect [48]. In a systemic review, Longo et al. [49] concluded that arthroscopic remplissage is the safest technique for the patients with shoulder instability with humeral bone loss.

## 12.3 Arthroscopic Soft Tissue Repair

The goal is to avoid further injury to the shoulder joint and promise shoulder stability, improved shoulder function, and a successful return to sports [24, 25].

### 12.3.1 Indications

#### 12.3.1.1 Bankart Repair

1. First-time traumatic anterior shoulder dislocation in young patients with high demands of shoulder activities without significant bony lesion
2. Recurrent traumatic anterior shoulder instability without significant bony lesion

#### 12.3.1.2 Bankart Repair + Remplissage

1. First-time traumatic anterior shoulder dislocation in young patients with high demands of shoulder activities with engaging Hill-Sachs lesion
2. Recurrent traumatic anterior shoulder instability with <25% glenoid bone loss

### 12.3.2 Preoperative Evaluation

#### 12.3.2.1 History

The individual factors including age, gender, affected side, mechanism and direction of the first dislocation, the reduction method (spontaneous, patient himself, external), the number of recurrence, time between initial injury and surgery, demands of shoulder activity, and type of sports should be documented. Relevant comorbidities (e.g., epilepsy, Marfan syndrome, Ehlers-Danlos syndrome, psychological disorders) should be excluded, which may be relative contraindication for arthroscopic soft tissue stabilization.

#### 12.3.2.2 Physical Examination

In the recurrent cases, besides the routine examination (e.g., shoulder range of motion, strength, scapular kinesis), apprehension tests, relocation test, load-and-shift test, sulcus sign, and Gagey hyperabduction test will be performed to define the instability and evaluate the capsular laxity.

#### 12.3.2.3 Imaging

The shoulders were evaluated preoperatively with anteroposterior, axillary, and scapular-Y X-ray images for the presence of bony lesions in the glenoid or humeral head (glenoid fractures, bony Bankart lesion, Hill-Sachs lesions).

Magnetic resonance imaging (MRI) or magnetic resonance arthrogram (MRA) is obtained to assess the size and extent of Bankart lesions and screen for any associated lesions (e.g., SLAP lesion, rotator cuff tear).

3D-CT scan is a very important tool for evaluation of traumatic shoulder instability, to assess the glenoid bone defect or Hill-Sachs lesion.

### 12.3.3 Operative Technique

#### 12.3.3.1 Anesthesia, Positioning, and Preparation

1. *Anesthesia*: General anesthesia or regional anesthesia with sedation can be selected depending on the preference of the surgeon.
2. *Position*: Beach chair position or lateral decubitus position can be used according to the surgeon's preference.

The introduced techniques in this chapter are performed with the patient placed in lateral decubitus position and are similar to that in beach chair position.

The patient is placed in the lateral decubitus position, leaned back about 30° with the shoulder in approximately 30°of abduction and 15°of forward flexion. The arm is initially suspended with 15 pounds of distal traction. A secondary lateral traction is added later in the procedure for the Bankart repair, but only after the remplissage has been completed.

3. *Examination under anesthesia (EUA)*

Before the surgery, physical examination should be performed again to evaluate the degree and direction of shoulder instability, capsular laxity, and passive range of motion, to confirm the preoperative diagnosis and modify the surgical strategy if necessary.

### 12.3.4 Arthroscopic Bankart Repair and Remplissage Technique

1. *Portals*: Three portals, e.g., posterior portal, anterolateral superior portal, and anterior portal, are produced and always enough for all procedures.
2. *Surgical sequence*:
   - To establish a standard posterior portal
   - Diagnostic arthroscopy through posterior portal
   - To establish an anterior portal close to the upper border of the subscapularis tendon (Fig. 12.1)
   - To establish an anterolateral superior portal at the anterolateral corner of the acromion (Fig. 12.2a, b)
   - Repair of the SLAP lesion, if it is confirmed under arthroscope (Fig. 12.3)
   - Diagnostic arthroscopy through anterolateral superior portal
   - Releasing the detached and displaced labrum
   - Remplissage technique
   - Bankart repair from inferior to superior
3. *Bankart Repair* [27, 50]

In the view from the anterolateral superior portal, the detached labrum, especially the ALPSA lesion, can be easily recognized (Fig. 12.4a–c) and is released by an elevator through the anterior portal. It is mandatory to release scar tissue between torn labrum and scapular until the subscapularis muscle belly can be visualized (Fig. 12.5), then the labrum can be easily repositioned.

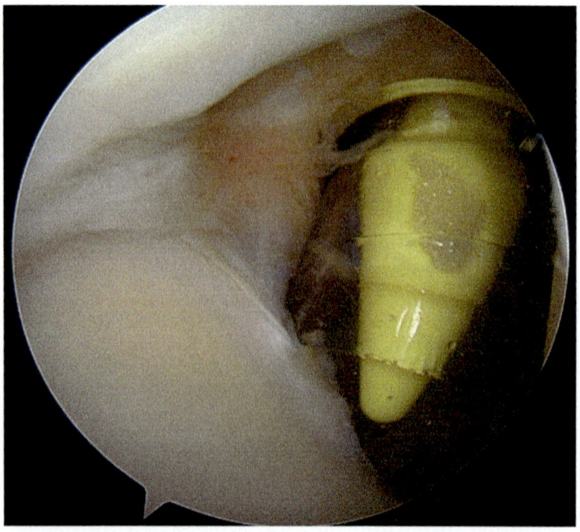

**Fig. 12.1** The canula through anterior portal

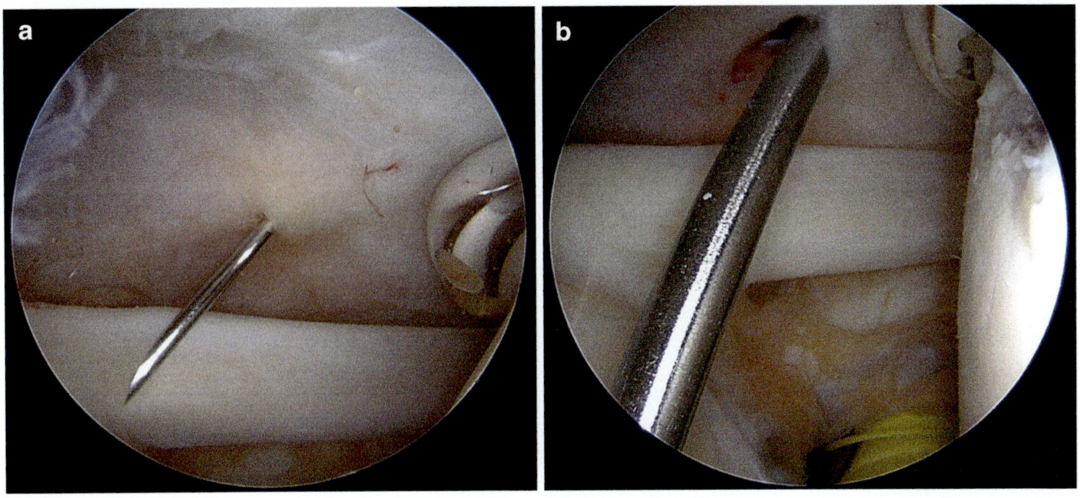


**Fig. 12.2** To establish the anterolateral superior portal. (**a**) a spine needle anterior to the supraspinatus tendon; (**b**) a switching stick through the anterolateral superior portal

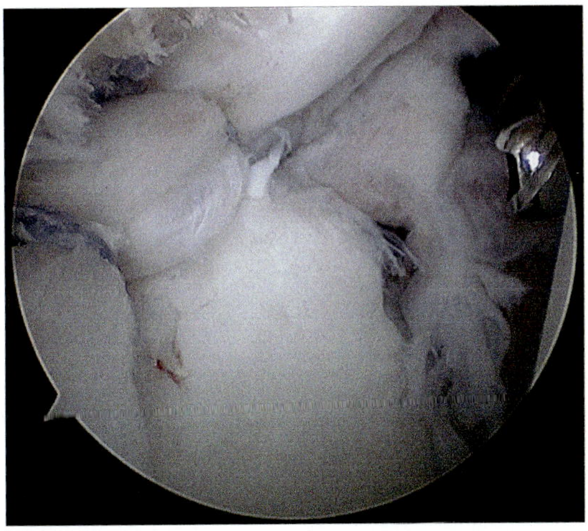

**Fig. 12.3** SLAP repair with suture anchor

The glenoid rim is debrided with a shaver and freshened with the rasp to create a bleeding bone surface for healing.

Usually, three to four anchors are used to repair the Bankart lesion and are inserted from inferior to superior through the anterior portal. The implant choice is made based on each surgeon's preference and familiarity with any of the available 2.8- to 3.5-mm anchors.

For the first suture anchor at the 5:30 o'clock position, some authors recommend to create the deep anteroinferior portal through the lower third of the subscapularis.

The first suture anchor is implanted at the 5:30 o'clock position of the glenoid. From the anterior portal (Fig. 12.6), a suture passer is then used to pass a shuttling suture through the capsule, anterior bundle of the inferior glenohumeral ligament, and labrum about 6–7 mm inferior to the previously placed anchor, so that the whole capsulolabral complex including the aIGHL is incorporated. The goal is to get a healthy capsular bite, grabbing inferior to the anchor in an effort to shift the tissue superiorly, reducing capsular volume (Fig. 12.7).

The sutures were shuttled and tied arthroscopically in a simple or mattress fashion. Afterward, other anchors are implanted sequentially to repair the labrum in the same manner. The capsulorrhaphy is routinely incorporated into labral repair in the recurrent cases.

4. *Remplissage technique* [51]

The remplissage technique is used to address the engaging Hill-Sachs lesion. The goal of remplissage technique is to fix the conjoined infraspinatus tendon and posterior capsule to the Hill-Sachs lesion. The procedures of anchor implanting and suture passing must be completed before Bankart repair. Otherwise, the reduced capsular volume will compromise the visualization of Hill-Sachs lesion.

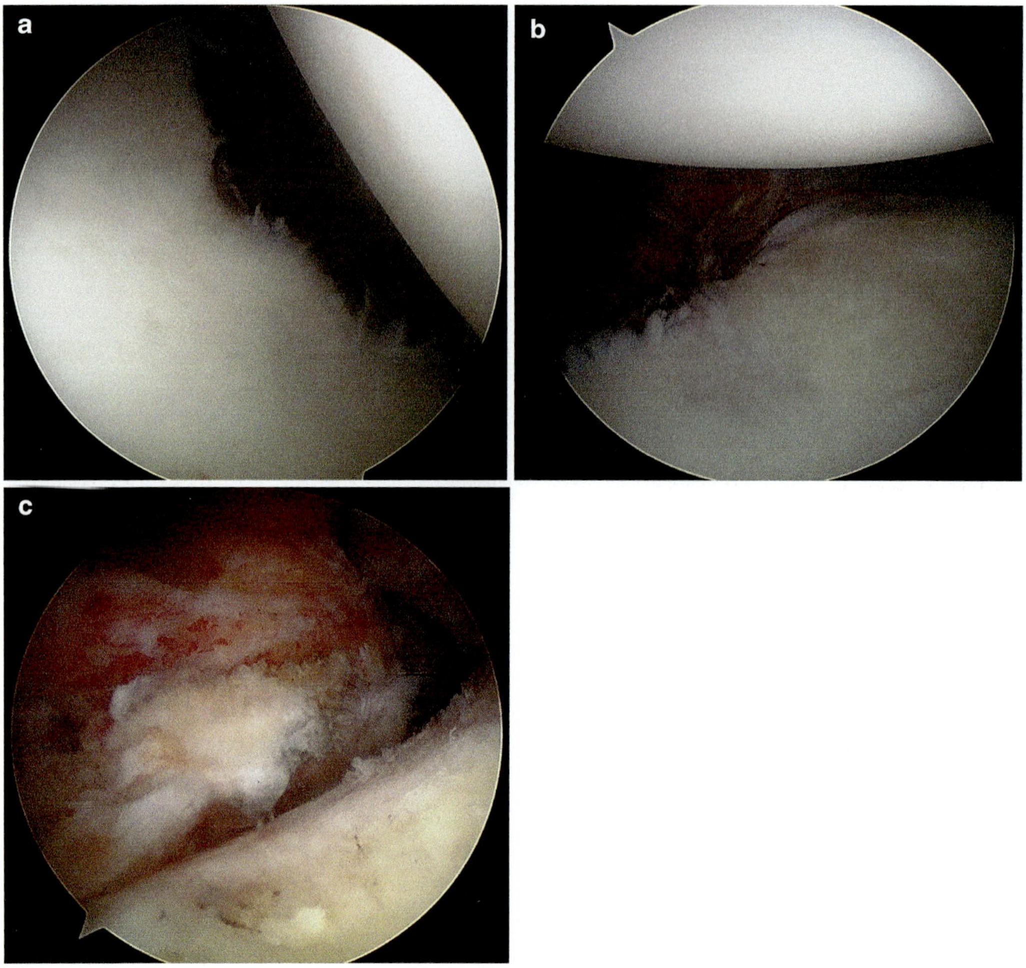


**Fig. 12.4** ALPSA lesion. (**a**) the labrum in ALPSA lesion cannot be found from posterior view; (**b**) the labrum was found from anterolateral superior portal; (**c**) the labrum was released

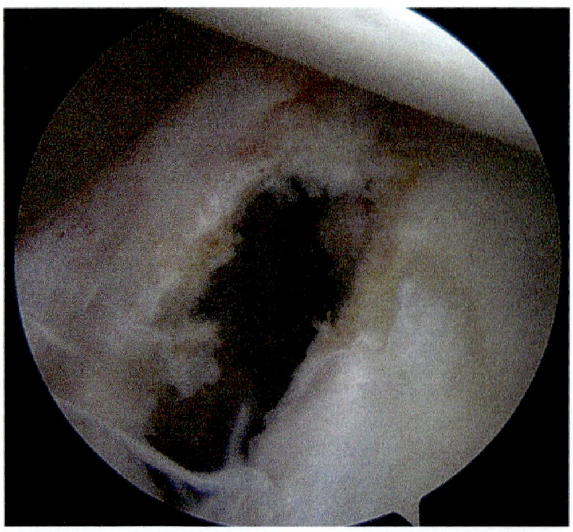

**Fig. 12.5** The subscapularis muscle belly can be observed following enough labrum release

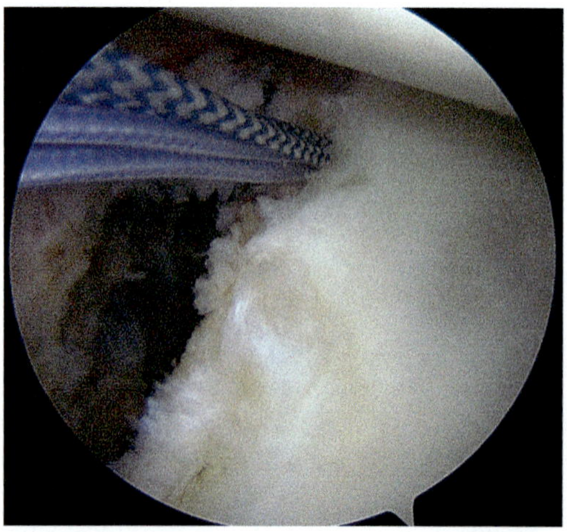

**Fig. 12.6** The first suture anchor was implanted at 5:30 o'clock

With viewing from anterolateral superior portal, the extent and location of the Hill- Sachs lesion is evaluated. The surface of the engaging Hill-Sachs lesion is gently freshened with a bur through the posterior portal (Fig. 12.8).

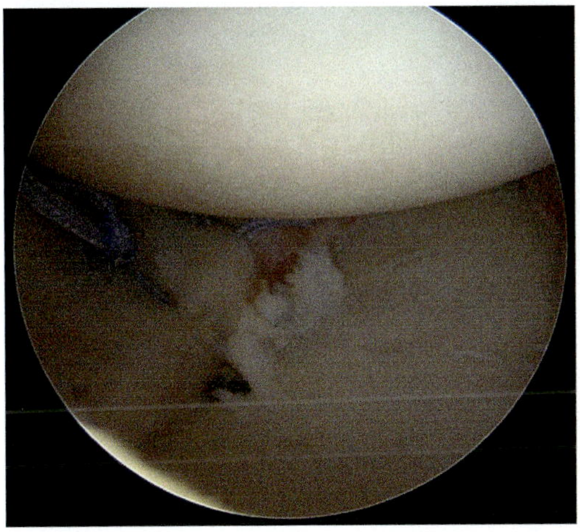

**Fig. 12.7** Bankart repair with suture anchors

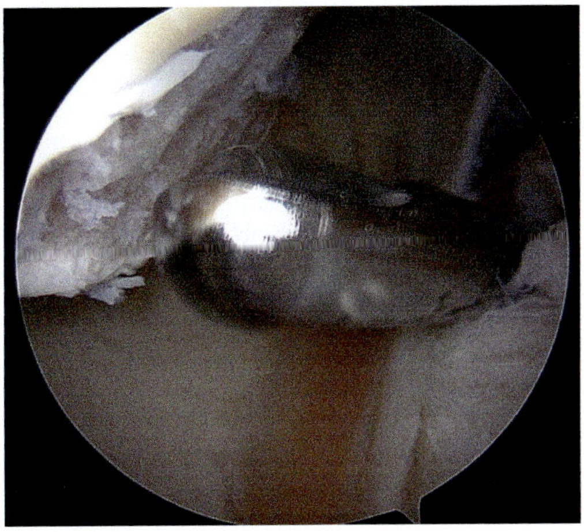

**Fig. 12.8** Debridement of Hill-Sachs lesion

Usually, two anchors are employed in remplissage technique and are placed in the most distal and superior aspects of the Hill-Sachs lesion in sequence. These anchors are placed in the inferior medial and superior medial margins of the defect (Fig. 12.9)

Following the sutures of two anchors being retrieved from anterior portal, the cannula in posterior portal is withdrawn outside the posterior capsule and infraspinatus tendon into the subdeltoid space.

A penetrating grasper is used to pass through the infraspinatus tendon and posterior casule, to retrieve the sutures individually through the posterior cannula, so that finally mattress knots could be tied extraarticular, in the subdeltoid space. If the visualization of knot tying is necessary, the arthroscope can be switched to the subacromial space to view the corresponding suture threads being tied in a mattress suture (Fig. 12.10a, b)

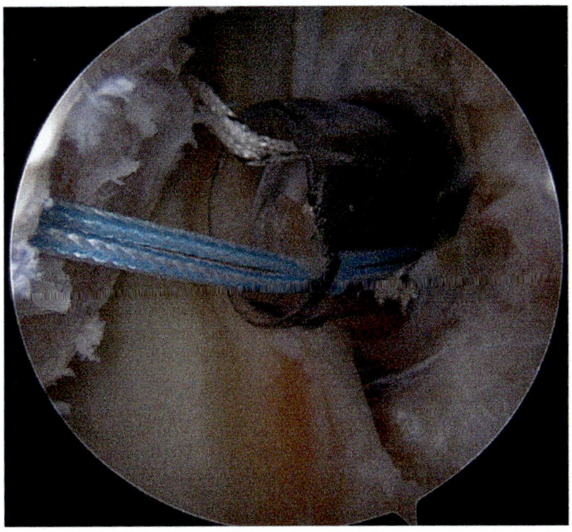

**Fig. 12.9** Two anchors were implanted inferior medial margin and superior medial margin of Hill-Sachs lesion respectively

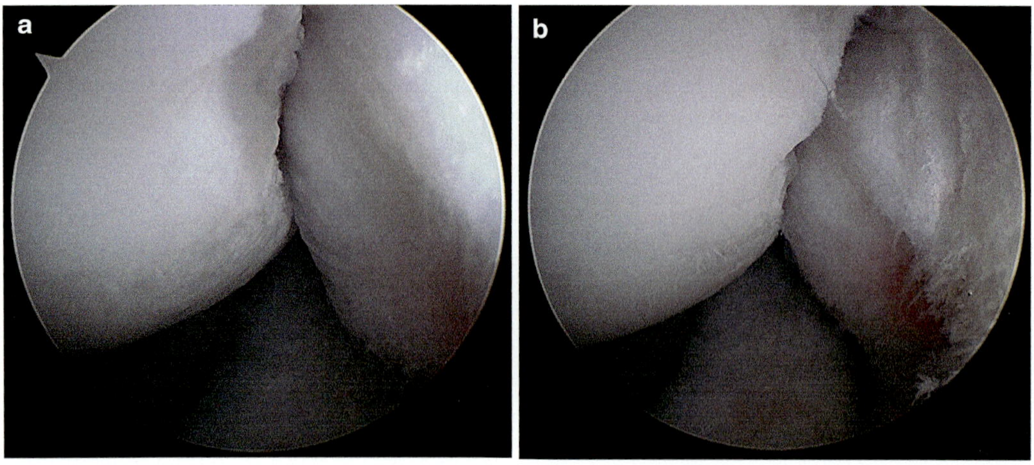


**Fig. 12.10** After remplissage technique. (**a**, **b**) the posterior capsule and posterior rotator cuff were filled into the Hill-Sachs lesion

**Conclusion**

Considering the high risk of failure of conservative management, the secondary lesions, and arthropathy following recurrent dislocation, surgical shoulder stabilization is recommended for traumatic anterior shoulder instability in the young athletes involved in shoulder demanding activities.

Bankart repair has satisfactory outcomes for the traumatic anterior shoulder instability with Bankart lesion, but without significant bone loss. If the engaging Hill-Sachs lesion is found at the same time, the additional remplissage technique will be a reliable supplemental procedure.

## References

1. Rowe CR. Prognosis in dislocations of the shoulder. J Bone Joint Surg Am. 1956;38-A(5):957–77.
2. McLaughlin HL, MacLellan DI. Recurrent anterior dislocation of the shoulder. II. A comparative study. J Trauma. 1967;7(2):191–201.
3. Rowe CR. Acute and recurrent anterior dislocations of the shoulder. Orthop Clin North Am. 1980;11(2):253–70.
4. Henry JH, Genung JA. Natural history of glenohumeral dislocation – revisited. Am J Sports Med. 1982;10(3):135–7.
5. Hoelen MA, Burgers AM, Rozing PM. Prognosis of primary anterior shoulder dislocation in young adults. Arch Orthop Trauma Surg. 1990;110(1):51–4.
6. Simonet WT, Cofield RH. Prognosis in anterior shoulder dislocation. Am J Sports Med. 1984;12(1):19–24.
7. Owens BD et al. The incidence and characteristics of shoulder instability at the United States Military Academy. Am J Sports Med. 2007;35(7):1168–73.
8. Amako M et al. Incidence and characteristics of traumatic shoulder instability in Japanese Military Cadets. Mil Med. 2016;181(6):577–81.
9. Godin J, Sekiya JK. Systematic review of rehabilitation versus operative stabilization for the treatment of first-time anterior shoulder dislocations. Sports Health. 2010;2(2):156–65.
10. Hovelius L, Rahme H. Primary anterior dislocation of the shoulder: long-term prognosis at the age of 40 years or younger. Knee Surg Sports Traumatol Arthrosc. 2016;24(2):330–42.
11. Habermeyer P, Gleyze P, Rickert M. Evolution of lesions of the labrum-ligament complex in posttraumatic anterior shoulder instability: a prospective study. J Shoulder Elb Surg. 1999;8(1):66–74.
12. Cetik O, Uslu M, Ozsar BK. The relationship between Hill-Sachs lesion and recurrent anterior shoulder dislocation. Acta Orthop Belg. 2007;73(2):175–8.
13. Yiannakopoulos CK, Mataragas E, Antonogiannakis E. A comparison of the spectrum of intra-articular lesions in acute and chronic anterior shoulder instability. Arthroscopy. 2007;23(9):985–90.
14. Kirkley A et al. Prospective randomized clinical trial comparing the effectiveness of immediate arthroscopic stabilization versus immobilization and rehabilitation in first traumatic anterior dislocations of the shoulder. Arthroscopy. 1999;15(5):507–14.
15. Bottoni CR et al. A prospective, randomized evaluation of arthroscopic stabilization versus nonoperative treatment in patients with acute, traumatic, first-time shoulder dislocations. Am J Sports Med. 2002;30(4):576–80.
16. Good CR, MacGillivray JD. Traumatic shoulder dislocation in the adolescent athlete: advances in surgical treatment. Curr Opin Pediatr. 2005;17(1):25–9.

17. Brophy RH, Marx RG. The treatment of traumatic anterior instability of the shoulder: nonoperative and surgical treatment. Arthroscopy. 2009;25(3):298–304.
18. Jakobsen BW et al. Primary repair versus conservative treatment of first-time traumatic anterior dislocation of the shoulder: a randomized study with 10-year follow-up. Arthroscopy. 2007;23(2):118–23.
19. Law BK et al. The surgical outcome of immediate arthroscopic Bankart repair for first time anterior shoulder dislocation in young active patients. Knee Surg Sports Traumatol Arthrosc. 2008;16(2):188–93.
20. Perthes Ü. Operationen bei habitueller Schulterluxation. Deutsche Zeitschrift für Chirurgie. 1906;85(1): 199–227.
21. Bankart AS. Recurrent or habitual dislocation of the shoulder-joint. Br Med J. 1923;2(3285):1132–3.
22. Taylor DC, Arciero RA. Pathologic changes associated with shoulder dislocations. Arthroscopic and physical examination findings in first-time, traumatic anterior dislocations. Am J Sports Med. 1997;25(3): 306–11.
23. Hintermann B, Gachter A. Arthroscopic findings after shoulder dislocation. Am J Sports Med. 1995;23(5):545–51.
24. Mazzocca AD et al. Arthroscopic anterior shoulder stabilization of collision and contact athletes. Am J Sports Med. 2005;33(1):52–60.
25. Franceschi F et al. Glenohumeral osteoarthritis after arthroscopic Bankart repair for anterior instability. Am J Sports Med. 2011;39(8):1653–9.
26. Castagna A et al. Arthroscopic bankart suture-anchor repair: radiological and clinical outcome at minimum 10 years of follow-up. Am J Sports Med. 2010;38(10):2012–6.
27. Ozturk BY et al. Return to sports after arthroscopic anterior stabilization in patients aged younger than 25 years. Arthroscopy. 2013;29(12):1922–31.
28. Hill HA, Sachs MD. The grooved defect of the humeral head. Radiology. 1940;35(6):690–700.
29. Calandra JJ, Baker CL, Uribe J. The incidence of Hill-Sachs lesions in initial anterior shoulder dislocations. Arthroscopy. 1989;5(4):254–7.
30. Spatschil A et al. Posttraumatic anterior-inferior instability of the shoulder: arthroscopic findings and clinical correlations. Arch Orthop Trauma Surg. 2006;126(4):217–22.
31. Longo UG et al. Shoulder injuries in soccer players. Clin Cases Miner Bone Metab. 2012;9(3):138–41.
32. Longo UG et al. Video analysis of the mechanisms of shoulder dislocation in four elite rugby players. J Orthop Sci. 2011;16(4):389–97.
33. Lynch JR et al. Treatment of osseous defects associated with anterior shoulder instability. J Shoulder Elb Surg. 2009;18(2):317–28.
34. Maffulli N et al. Sport injuries: a review of outcomes. Br Med Bull. 2011;97:47–80.
35. Boileau P et al. Risk factors for recurrence of shoulder instability after arthroscopic Bankart repair. J Bone Joint Surg Am. 2006;88(8):1755–63.
36. Rowe CR, Zarins B, Ciullo JV. Recurrent anterior dislocation of the shoulder after surgical repair. Apparent causes of failure and treatment. J Bone Joint Surg Am. 1984;66(2):159–68.
37. Burkhart SS, De Beer JF. Traumatic glenohumeral bone defects and their relationship to failure of arthroscopic Bankart repairs: significance of the inverted-pear glenoid and the humeral engaging Hill-Sachs lesion. Arthroscopy. 2000;16(7):677–94.
38. Armitage MS et al. Humeral head bone defects: remplissage, allograft, and arthroplasty. Orthop Clin North Am. 2010;41(3):417–25.
39. Longo UG et al. Management of primary acute anterior shoulder dislocation: systematic review and quantitative synthesis of the literature. Arthroscopy. 2014;30(4):506–22.
40. Yamamoto N et al. Contact between the glenoid and the humeral head in abduction, external rotation, and horizontal extension: a new concept of glenoid track. J Shoulder Elb Surg. 2007;16(5):649–56.
41. Di Giacomo G, Itoi E, Burkhart SS. Evolving concept of bipolar bone loss and the Hill-Sachs lesion: from "engaging/non-engaging" lesion to "on-track/off-track" lesion. Arthroscopy. 2014;30(1):90–8.
42. Metzger PD et al. Clinical application of the "glenoid track" concept for defining humeral head engagement in anterior shoulder instability: a preliminary report. Orthop J Sports Med. 2013;1(2):2325967113496213.
43. Neer 2nd CS, Foster CR. Inferior capsular shift for involuntary inferior and multidirectional instability of the shoulder. A preliminary report. J Bone Joint Surg Am. 1980;62(6):897–908.
44. Weber BG, Simpson LA, Hardegger F. Rotational humeral osteotomy for recurrent anterior dislocation of the shoulder associated with a large Hill-Sachs lesion. J Bone Joint Surg Am. 1984;66(9):1443–50.
45. Kazel MD et al. Percutaneous correction (humeroplasty) of humeral head defects (Hill-Sachs) associated with anterior shoulder instability: a cadaveric study. Arthroscopy. 2005;21(12):1473–8.
46. Kropf EJ, Sekiya JK. Osteoarticular allograft transplantation for large humeral head defects in glenohumeral instability. Arthroscopy. 2007;23(3):322 e1–5.
47. Sekiya JK et al. Hill-Sachs defects and repair using osteoarticular allograft transplantation: biomechanical analysis using a joint compression model. Am J Sports Med. 2009;37(12):2459–66.
48. Purchase RJ et al. Hill-sachs "remplissage": an arthroscopic solution for the engaging hill-sachs lesion. Arthroscopy. 2008;24(6):723–6.
49. Longo UG et al. Remplissage, humeral osteochondral grafts, weber osteotomy, and shoulder arthroplasty for the management of humeral bone defects in shoulder instability: systematic review and quantitative synthesis of the literature. Arthroscopy. 2014;30(12):1650–66.
50. Milchteim C et al. Outcomes of Bankart repairs using modern arthroscopic technique in an athletic population. Arthroscopy. 2016;32(7):1263–70.
51. Wolf EM, Arianjam A. Hill-Sachs remplissage, an arthroscopic solution for the engaging Hill-Sachs lesion: 2- to 10-year follow-up and incidence of recurrence. J Shoulder Elb Surg. 2014;23(6):814–20.

# Modified Open Bankart Repair and Capsular Shift for Recurrent Traumatic Anterior Shoulder Instability

13

Robert A. Arciero and Felix Dyrna

## Contents


| | | |
|---|---|---|
| 13.1 | **Introduction and Critical Literature Review** | 103 |
| 13.2 | **Indications** | 104 |
| 13.3 | **Description of the Technique** | 104 |
| 13.3.1 | Results After Open Bankart | 106 |
| 13.4 | **Rehab Program** | 107 |
| 13.5 | **Complications** | 107 |
| **References** | | 108 |



R.A. Arciero, MD (✉)
Orthopaedic Sports Medicine Division, University of Connecticut Health, 263 Farmington Avenue, Farmington, CT 06001, USA
e-mail: arciero@nso.uchc.edu

F. Dyrna, MD
Orthopaedic Sports Medicine Division, University of Connecticut Health, 263 Farmington Avenue, Farmington, CT 06001, USA

Department of Orthopaedic Sports Medicine, Technical University of Munich, Munich, Germany


## 13.1 Introduction and Critical Literature Review

The operative management of anterior shoulder instability is still controversial on the optimum method to prevent recurrent dislocations and restore stability without restriction of glenohumeral motion. Two possible options, arthroscopic or open surgery, for patients without significant bone loss (>20°) exist. Burkhart et al. [1] showed that glenoid bone loss greater than 25% correlates with an increased risk for recurrence after arthroscopic soft tissue stabilization to about 67%, whereas shoulders without significant bone defect demonstrated recurrence as only 4%, limiting our indication for soft tissue repairs alone. Each of those techniques has benefits and controversies, summarized in Table 13.1. A stable shoulder is fundamental not only for athlete's performance but also for daily living. Shoulder instability affects mainly young patients between the ages 15 and 35, resulting in a loss of life quality and activity level. Regardless of which intervention after a shoulder dislocation is performed, the ultimate goal is to prevent any recurrence. Open Bankart surgery has proven in multiple high-level evidence studies that with proper indications the results are excellent and the recurrence rate is as low as 0–5% [4, 6, 11]. Furthermore, in a direct comparison between arthroscopic and open Bankart, the favor clearly points in direction of the open procedure, revealing lower recurrence

© ISAKOS 2017
A.B. Imhoff, F.H. Savoie III (eds.), *Shoulder Instability Across the Life Span*,
DOI 10.1007/978-3-662-54077-0_13

**Table 13.1** Advantages and disadvantages to open and arthroscopic Bankart

| Open Bankart | Benefits | Arthroscopic Bankart |
|---|---|---|
| All knot will be tied extra-articularly in a mattress fashion | | Smaller incisions with minimal subscapularis trauma |
| Suture passage and amount in cooperated tissue can be controlled | | Detection of additional intra-articular pathologies |
| Lateral rotator interval closure possible | | Less postoperative pain |
| Higher percentage of labral footprint reconstruction | | Technically easier to perform |
| Freedom for anchor placement and repair construct configuration | | Lower chance of over-tensioning |
| Extension and degree of capsule shift; double-layer capsular repair | | Quicker rehabilitation |
| Capsule volume reduction and duplication especially if tissue quality is poor | | Shorter OR time |
| Separation of the capsule and subscapularis | | Cosmetically attractive |

rates [2, 3, 8, 9]. But no significant differences could be detected for return to sports rates, patient-specific outcome measures like the WOSI score or OA progression.

## 13.2 Indications

The open Bankart repair is a suitable option for a specific patient selection. In our hands this group includes mainly male collision athletes under the age of 20 years with limited glenoid bone loss (10–20%). Additional criteria for a preferred open procedure are multiple dislocations, greater than ten times, or intraoperatively presentation of unexpected poor capsulolabral tissue quality. We also think of it as a revision procedure of a failed but correct performed arthroscopic stabilization.

## 13.3 Description of the Technique

Patient is placed supine with a bolster supporting the medial border of the scapula to prevent scapular protraction. The head of the table is elevated modestly. Examination under anesthesia is performed to evaluate the glenohumeral joint regarding range of motion, laxity, and direction of instability. The arm is supported on a well-padded Mayo stand with the surgeon standing between the arm and thorax of the patient. Incision is marked as an anterior axillary incision along Langer's lines. A traditional deltopectoral approach is made mobilizing the cephalic vein laterally. While continuing the deeper exposure, the deltopectoral dissection should be extended proximally to the clavicle and distally to the level of the falciform ligament to create a better overview and avoid a keyhole field of view. A self-retaining retractor is used to maintain retraction of the deltoid and pectoralis major muscles. Next, the clavipectoral fascia is incised just lateral to the coracobrachialis muscle all the way up to the CA ligament. To retract the conjoins easier, a partial release of the Ca ligament superior and the falciform ligament inferior can be performed. One of the key parts to get access to the joint is now the subscapularis (SSC) tenotomy. We prefer a tenotomy. However, if the patient does not have a significant component of inferior laxity, a subscapularis split may be preferable. We secure the subscapularis with four non-resorbable sutures in a matrass fashion about 1.5 cm medial to its insertion site on the lesser tuberosity. Now incise the subscapularis in an L-shaped manner, from the superior edge vertically down toward the circumflex vessels and continue medial in fiber direction. Slowly and carefully separate the muscle from the underlying capsule, start inferior just above the circumflex vessels, and work superiorly; this way it is much easier to reflect them (Fig. 13.1). This will open up the rotator interval, which we like to close laterally right away to start out with a closed capsular structure prior to incision and shifting. The capsule will first be incised vertically on the lateral side, followed by a horizontal incision on the mid glenoid level creating a T-capsulotomy with superior and inferior leave (Fig. 13.2). This will expose the anterior glenoid rim and the Bankart lesion. The

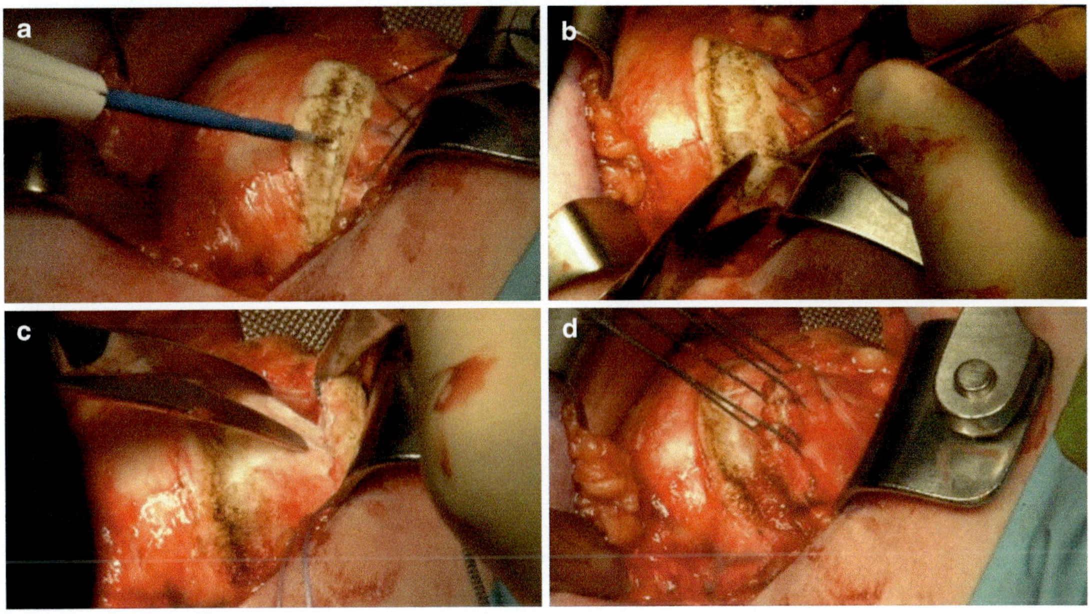

**Fig. 13.1** (**a**) Inital part of subscapualris tenotomy. (**b**) Using scissors to develop tissue plane between subscapualris tendon and capsule. (**c**) reflecting subscapualris tendon from anterior capsule. (**d**) subscapualris tendon released and tagged with permanent suture

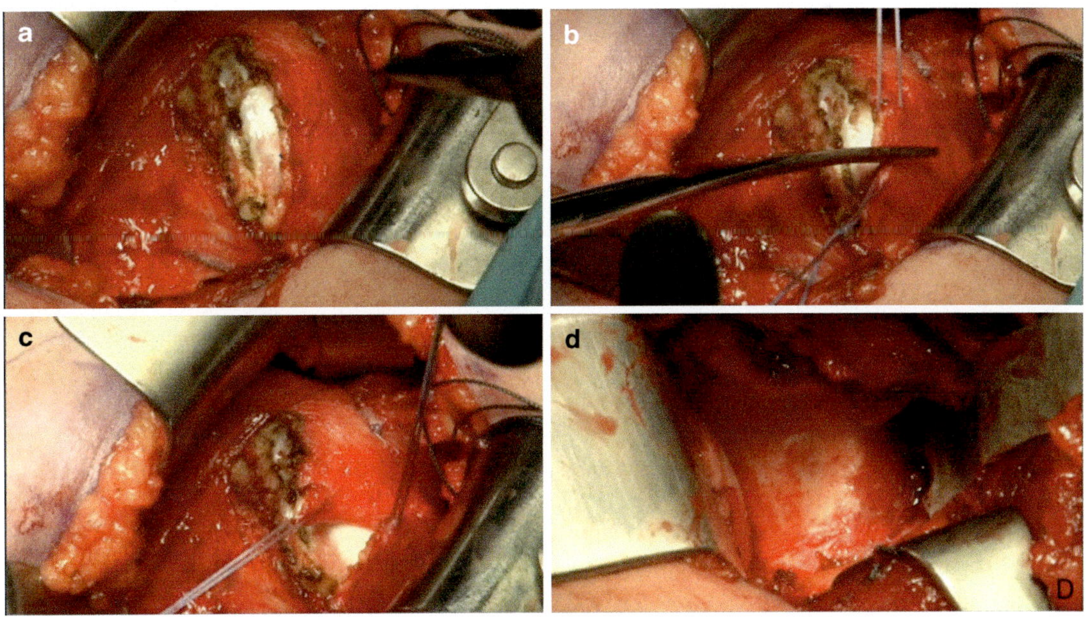

**Fig. 13.2** (**a**) Vertical capsulotomy after reflection of subscapualris tendon. (**b**) Horizontal capsulotomy creating two leaflets to the capsule. (**c**) demonstrating how leafs of capsule will be shifted. (**d**) scapular neck retractor placed exposing Bankart lesion

next step consists of mobilization of capsulolabral tissue and preparing the bony footprint on the glenoid neck. After that, suture anchors can be placed similar to arthroscopic techniques, starting inferior and extending along the rim depending on size of the Bankart lesion. Anchors can be placed in a single- or double-row configuration as the great exposure allows it. Sutures will be passed through

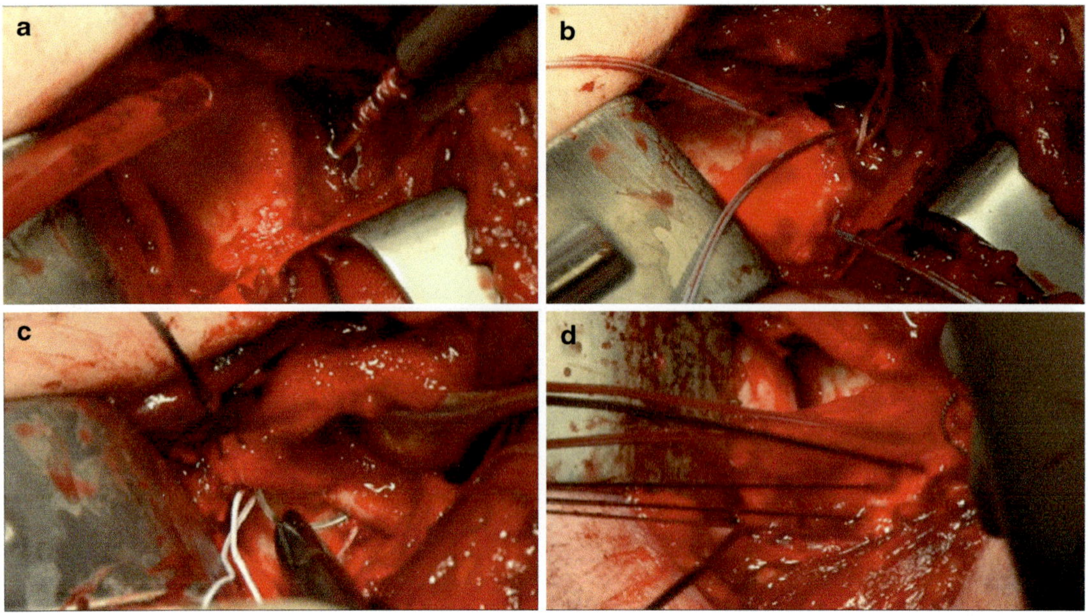


**Fig. 13.3** (**a**) Decortication of scapualr neck for healing. (**b**) double row of anchors placed for Bankart repair. (**c**) sutures being placed in a matress configuration. (**d**) mattress sutures tied through entire capsulolabral complex to repair Bankart lesion

the capsulolabral complex in a mattress fashion, being careful to avoid piercing the axillary nerve. Afterward, sutures can be tied, staring again inferiorly (Fig. 13.3). The Bankart repair is now completed at this stage, and the focus will be on the closure including the capsular shift and subscapularis reattachment. At this point we will put the arm in 30° of abduction and 30° of external rotation to avoid over-tensioning. We start out with the closure of the horizontal capsular incision by shifting the superior leave on top of the inferior leave medially but not tying this suture. In order to shift now the inferior capsule superiorly an adequate release has to be performed. The inferior capsule is dissected off the neck of the humerus and tagged with suture until superior shifting of the inferior leaf eliminates the inferior pouch. This is necessary to shift the inferior pouch of the capsule superiorly and laterally and reduce capsule volume. Optional suture anchors can be placed on the humeral neck to refix the superior and lateral shifted inferior capsule, which we would recommend. After shifting the inferior leaf superiorly, the superior leaf will be shifted inferiorly and tied on top (Fig. 13.4). We recommend checking range of motion to exclude the possibility of over-tensioning. The final step is the subscapularis reattachment; depending on your approach and takedown technique, this can be done by tendon to tendon suturing, doing a transosseous repair, or using suture anchors. Whichever technique is used ensures a meticulous and careful reattachment to avoid any subscapularis deficiency. Surgery ends with a wound closer and the arm in a shoulder immobilizer.

### 13.3.1 Results After Open Bankart

Recurrence as the most important outcome parameter after a shoulder stabilization procedure clearly demonstrates the value of open Bankart surgery with a low recurrence rate between 0% and 12.5% [4–6, 11, 12]. In direct comparison with arthroscopic procedures, the recurrence rates are lower and the need for revision surgeries is reduced [7, 12]. Additionally, limited bony lesion on the humeral head or the glenoid rim can be compensated with the

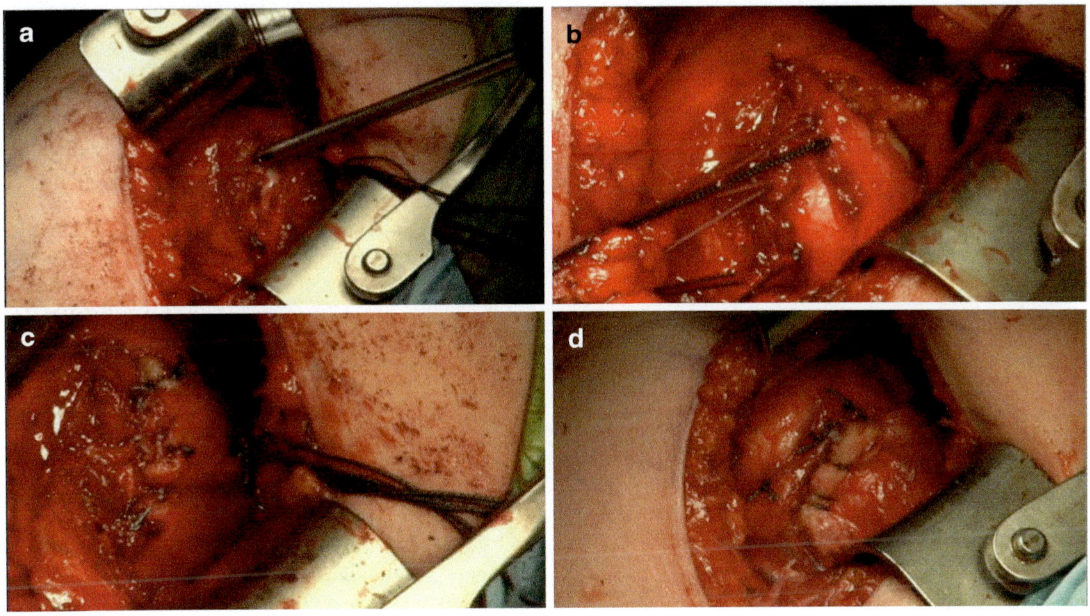


**Fig. 13.4** (**a**) Suture anchors placed on humeral neck for capsular shift. (**b**) inferior leaf of capsule shifted superolaterally to address capsular laxity. (**c**) completed shift after superior leaf of capsule shifted inferior lateral to give 2 layers to the repair. (**d**) subscapualris tendon re-attached

open procedure without increasing the risk for recurrence in contrast to the arthroscopic procedure [11]. The open stabilization appears to provide better results in a high-risk group of male collision athletes under the age of 25 [9]. Outcome scores like ASES, WOSI, VAS, SST, and Rowe do not differ in direct comparison between open and arthroscopic repair, both resulting in high functional and satisfying scores if the shoulder becomes stable [9, 10]. The range of motion after open repair is restricted more within the early postoperative period but did not reach significance at later follow-up time points when comparing both techniques [9]. Higher rates of return to contact sports and intense labor work are provided by the open Bankart procedure [7, 11], without a difference in complication rates and adverse events [9].

## 13.4 Rehab Program

We recommend shoulder immobilizer for 4 weeks, straight.

First 4 weeks we only allow passive mobilization with limited range of motion, external rotation up to 30°, and supine forward elevation up to 90°.

Start active ROM training after 4 weeks while protecting the subscapularis until week 6 with limited external rotation and no forced internal rotation.

Begin with strengthening at 6 weeks and return to sport in about 6 months.

## 13.5 Complications

Recurrent instability remains the primary complication. Postoperative hematoma and infection can occur but are very rare. The subscapularis reattachment has to be protected to avoid any kind of deficiency or rerupture. The risk for a complete retear is very low as shown in the published case series, but even without a complete rerupture, a postoperative atrophy of the upper portion and a noticeable insufficiency can be detected leading to lower outcome and satisfaction scores [13, 14]. Postoperative range of motion restriction can cause prorogated rehab or even the need of an arthroscopic release. Nerval structures such as the axillary nerve and musculocutaneus are in close relationship, but no complications have been reported.

## References


1. Burkhart SS, De Beer JF. Traumatic glenohumeral bone defects and their relationship to failure of arthroscopic Bankart repairs: significance of the inverted-pear glenoid and the humeral engaging Hill-Sachs lesion. Arthroscopy. 2000;16(7):677–94.
2. Cole BJ, Warner JJ. Arthroscopic versus open Bankart repair for traumatic anterior shoulder instability. Clin Sports Med. 2000;19(1):19–48.
3. Freedman KB, Smith AP, Romeo AA, Cole BJ, Bach BR. Open Bankart repair versus arthroscopic repair with transglenoid sutures or bioabsorbable tacks for Recurrent Anterior instability of the shoulder: a meta-analysis. Am J Sports Med. 2004;32(6):1520–7. doi:10.1177/0363546504265188.
4. Gill TJ, Zarins B. Open repairs for the treatment of anterior shoulder instability. Am J Sports Med. 2003;31(1):142–53.
5. Harris JD, Gupta AK, Mall NA, et al. Long-term outcomes after Bankart shoulder stabilization. Arthroscopy. 2013;29(5):920–33. doi:10.1016/j.arthro.2012.11.010.
6. Hubbell JD, Ahmad S, Bezenoff LS, Fond J, Pettrone FA. Comparison of shoulder stabilization using arthroscopic transglenoid sutures versus open capsulolabral repairs: a 5-year minimum follow-up. Am J Sports Med. 2004;32(3):650–4.
7. Lenters TR, Franta AK, Wolf FM, Leopold SS, Matsen FA. Arthroscopic compared with open repairs for recurrent anterior shoulder instability. A systematic review and meta-analysis of the literature. J Bone Joint Surg. 2007;89(2):244–54. doi:10.2106/JBJS.E.01139.
8. Mohtadi NGH, Bitar IJ, Sasyniuk TM, Hollinshead RM, Harper WP. Arthroscopic versus open repair for traumatic anterior shoulder instability: a meta-analysis. Arthroscopy. 2005;21(6):652–8. doi:10.1016/j.arthro.2005.02.021.
9. Mohtadi NGH, Chan DS, Hollinshead RM, et al. A randomized clinical trial comparing open and arthroscopic stabilization for recurrent traumatic anterior shoulder instability: two-year follow-up with disease-specific quality-of-life outcomes. J Bone Joint Surg Am. 2014;96(5):353–60. doi:10.2106/JBJS.L.01656.
10. Moroder P, Odorizzi M, Pizzinini S, Demetz E, Resch H, Moroder P. Open Bankart repair for the treatment of anterior shoulder instability without substantial osseous glenoid defects: results after a minimum follow-up of twenty years. J Bone Joint Surg Am. 2015;97(17):1398–405. doi:10.2106/JBJS.N.01214.
11. Pagnani MJ, Dome DC. Surgical treatment of traumatic anterior shoulder instability in american football players. J Bone Joint Surg. 2002;84-A(5):711–5.
12. Rhee YG, Ha JH, Cho NS. Anterior shoulder stabilization in collision athletes: arthroscopic versus open Bankart repair. Am J Sports Med. 2006;34(6):979–85. doi:10.1177/0363546505283267.
13. Sachs RA, Williams B, Stone ML, Paxton L, Kuney M. Open Bankart repair: correlation of results with postoperative subscapularis function. Am J Sports Med. 2005;33(10):1458–62. doi:10.1177/0363546505275350.
14. Scheibel M, Tsynman A, Magosch P, Schroeder RJ, Habermeyer P. Postoperative subscapularis muscle insufficiency after primary and revision open shoulder stabilization. Am J Sports Med. 2006;34(10):1586–93. doi:10.1177/0363546506288852.

# Humeral Avulsion of the Glenohumeral Ligaments (HAGL) in Shoulder Instability

14

Mark Ferguson

## Content

References .................................................................. 112

To prevent abnormal translation of the humeral head on the glenoid, the shoulder is stabilised by both static and dynamic mechanisms [1, 2]. The dynamic stabilisers include the rotator cuff and to a lesser degree the long head of the biceps and deltoid muscle. The static mechanisms include the bony configurations of the glenoid and humerus, the glenoid labrum, the joint capsule and the glenohumeral ligaments. The role of the capsular structures in preventing dislocation of the glenohumeral joint is well described [3–5]. Although the avulsion of the capsulolabral complex (Bankart lesion) accounts for more than 80% of instability cases, the humeral avulsion of the glenohumeral ligaments (HAGL) has only been reported in 1–9% of patients but may be even higher when looking at specific subgroups [6, 7]. Almost two-thirds of patients can have concurrent injury to the labrum or rotator cuff.

Nicola, in a short series of acute shoulder dislocations, was the first to describe the avulsion of the anterior inferior glenohumeral ligament (AIGHL) in 1942 [8]. Bach later described this injury in two patients with recurrent instability [9]. Wolf, in an arthroscopic study of 64 shoulders with shoulder instability, termed the acronym HAGL for humeral avulsion of glenohumeral ligaments [7].

The capsuloligamentous complex consists of the coracohumeral ligaments, superior glenohumeral ligament, middle glenohumeral ligament and inferior glenohumeral ligament (IGHL) [10].

M. Ferguson
Centre for Sports Medicine & Orthopaedics, University of Munich (TUM) Orthopaedic Sportsmedicine, Johannesburg, South Africa
e-mail: mferg@icon.co.za

© ISAKOS 2017
A.B. Imhoff, F.H. Savoie III (eds.), *Shoulder Instability Across the Life Span*,
DOI 10.1007/978-3-662-54077-0_14

The IGHL, which is attached medially to the glenoid labrum, is composed of the anterior band, posterior band and axillary pouch. The orientation of the pouch and bands creates a hammock-like structure on the anterior and posterior aspects of the glenoid. The anterior band of the IGHL therefore provides restraint to anterior and inferior translation with the arm in abduction and external rotation. With the arm in flexion and internal rotation, the posterior band of the IGHL spans the mid-portion of the joint providing posterior stability. The humeral insertion of the IGHL has been described as either a collar-like attachment close to the articular margin or as a V-shaped attachment with a base, anteriorly and posteriorly, close to the articular margin and the apex more distal on the humeral neck. Pouliart, in a large cadaveric and arthroscopic study, found on dissection from the outside that all had a capsular attachment in a V-form; however on visualisation this had a rounded collar-like appearance due to the presence of connecting synovial bands. Anteriorly, the most superior part of the IGHL joined the inferior fibres of the subscapularis tendon on the lesser tuberosity, while posteriorly it was attached to the distal part of the greater tuberosity adjacent to the superior fibres of the latissimus dorsi tendon [11].

The overwhelming majority of HAGL lesions are caused by traumatic injury. A small series of overhead athletes with IGHL avulsion due to repetitive microtrauma have been reported [12, 13]. Studies of arthroscopic findings in first-time dislocators have reported that traumatic shoulder dislocation or subluxation may result in (1) avulsion of the capsulolabral complex from the anterior glenoid rim (i.e. Bankart lesion), (2) avulsion of the IGHL from its humeral attachment (i.e. HAGL lesion) and (3) capsular tears or a combination of the above [14, 15]. These findings have been collaborated in cadaveric studies testing the tensile properties of the IGHL which demonstrated three possible locations of injury to occur: failure of the IGHL labral complex at the glenoid origin (40%), an intrasubstance tear (35%) and at the point of insertion on the humerus (25%) [4]. Gagey et al. however experimentally dislocated cadaver shoulders and noted capsular failure at the humeral side in as high as 63% of specimens [16].

Bui-Mansfield et al. developed the West Point classification system to organise the variety of concurrent injuries associated with the IGHL complex. The authors described six distinct forms of HAGL lesion based on anterior or posterior involvement, the presence or absence of bony avulsion and the presence of associated labral pathology: anterior HAGL, anterior bony HAGL (i.e. with associated bony avulsion), floating anterior IGHL (i.e. HAGL lesion with concurrent detachment of the anteroinferior labrum), posterior HAGL, posterior bony HAGL and floating posterior IGHL (i.e. HAGL lesion with concurrent detachment of the posterior inferior labrum). The anterior HAGL represents 93% of reported cases, whereas posterior HAGL represents only 7% of cases. This system does however not account for the finding of posterior HAGL with anterior labral pathology and vice versa as found in other studies on MR imaging of posterior HAGL lesions [17]. Furthermore, there is no evidence to suggest any correlation between the type of lesion and prognosis, and course of management using these classification systems.

In experimental sequential cutting studies evaluating the extent of humeral-based capsuloligamentous damage required for dislocation to occur, a high degree of correlation between the amount of cutting performed and the resulting degree of instability was found [18, 19]. The order in which the ligamentous cuts were made had no significant influence, but for dislocation to occur, at least three zones had to be cut.

Although large HAGL lesions can increase the passive motion of the glenohumeral joint in both neutral and external rotation, these differences are small and may be difficult to measure clinically [20]. That extensive lesions on the humeral side are required before dislocation can occur may be a factor explaining the relatively low incidence of HAGL lesions in clinical series.

From history, taking a traumatic shoulder injury event with or without subluxation or dislocation is described in 93% of the cases. It is important to ascertain the position of the arm at the time of injury, direction of instability and typically previous failed instability surgery. Although both traumatic Bankart and HAGL lesions occur with the arm in hyperabduction, HAGL lesions are more likely to occur with hyperabduction and external rotation. Bokor noted HAGL lesions in 14.6% of patients requiring revision of a previous failed procedure [21]. Occasionally, patients may present with non-specific symptoms like weakness, pain and poor function which may represent less extensive capsuloligamentous damage with subtle microinstability of the glenohumeral joint. All provocative tests to assess stability are similar to those for anterior and posterior capsulolabral pathology. Typically, the examiner should perform the apprehension, relocation, load-and-shift, posterior stress and posterior jerk tests. Examination for associated pathology of the rotator cuff should be performed including signs of subscapularis weakness.

Imaging studies should include a true AP with the shoulder in ER and IR, axillary view, Bernageau view and an outlet view. A small bony avulsion of the humeral neck is the only pathognomonic sign of inferior IGHL injury, but associated findings including humeral head impaction, glenoid rim fractures and glenohumeral malalignment must be excluded.

MRI, with or without intra-articular contrast, is the modality of choice for the assessment of a suspected HAGL lesion. The IGHL complex is best evaluated on coronal oblique or sagittal oblique T2-weighted fat-suppressed magnetic resonance images [22]. The normal IGHL anatomy appears as a U-shaped structure because of fluid distension of the axillary pouch. As a result of the loss of containment of contrast or joint fluid through the torn capsule and ligament, the presence of a HAGL lesion can cause the normally U-shaped axillary pouch to appear J-shaped.

Chronic HAGL lesions may be difficult to visualise on magnetic resonance images as the torn edge on the humeral side may scar down to the capsule with time. In a study of 42 patients with acute first-time dislocation, MRI was performed within 7 days of the injury and a follow-up MRI arthrogram after 30 days. Capsular ligament lesions were found in 22 patients (52.4%) in the acute stage and in 5 patients (11.9%) at follow-up. Nine patients (21.4%) had a humeral avulsion of the anterior glenohumeral ligament (HAGL lesion) on MRI. Three patients (7.1%) had this lesion at follow-up [23]. Understandably, only one study has determined the accuracy of standard MRI or magnetic resonance arthrography in detecting the presence of HAGL lesion. In 23 patients that underwent surgery for HAGL lesions, 16 lesions were seen on prospective MR reading [24].

In a retrospective study of 28 shoulders, posterior HAGL injuries were found to have complete tears (71%), partial tears (25%) and floating lesions (4%). There was concomitant bony HAGL avulsion in 7% of injuries. Associated traumatic glenohumeral disorders occurred in 93% of cases with the most common being reverse Hill-Sachs lesions (36%), anterior Bankart lesions (29%) and posterosuperior rotator cuff tears (25%). Of interest was the finding of concomitant anterior labral or capsular injury in 50% of patients, signifying bidirectional disruption of the capsule possibly due to the circle concept of injury [17].

HAGL lesions can be identified arthroscopically with a careful, thorough examination of the glenohumeral joint. In order to see the entire humeral attachment of the capsule, a 70° arthroscope and the use of accessory portals are employed.

Historically, the management of HAGL lesions has been conservative or surgical. George suggests incomplete lesions, and some detached lesions initially may be managed nonsurgically with physical therapy to rehabilitate the injured shoulder. The rate of recurrent instability for nonsurgical management of HAGL lesions in ten patients was reported as 90%. Surgery is indicated in young athletes, manual labourers, and recurrent instability and pain that do not improve with physical therapy and activity modification [25].

Both arthroscopic and open surgical repair techniques have been described. The arthroscopic techniques are technically challenging and require advanced portal placement and thorough knowledge of adjacent at-risk structures [26]. The lateral decubitus position does afford better access to the inferior capsule, particularly with advanced portal placement. The axillary pouch portal (i.e. Bhatia portal) is established using an outside-in technique and is marked with an 18-gauge spinal needle [27]. The anteroinferior (i.e. 5 o'clock) portal is established also using an outside-in technique with the shoulder placed in a neutral position to protect the musculocutaneous nerve and the axillary nerve [28].

The shoulder may also be placed in abduction and external rotation to improve the angle of approach necessary to reach the humeral insertion site [29]. Additionally a posteriorly directed force on the humeral head can open the anterior space and facillitate anchor placement. In floating lesions where there is concomitant labral pathology, it is advisable to first address the labral pathology first, going though the lateral capsule lesion to insert the anchors and then repair the humeral lesion, shifting the capsule as needed on the lateral side of the joint. This technique is equally applicable to posterior HAGL lesions.

Knotted or knotless suture anchors are routinely used and are placed at the anatomic insertion of the IGHL on the humeral neck. A repair using anchors placed in the humeral neck is more likely to restore the normal restraint to anterior translation than a juxtachondral repair [20]. Various suture-passing devices can be used to pass the sutures and secure the attachment usually tying the knots extracapsular.

Open anterior repair of the HAGL lesion is best performed in the beach chair position through a deltopectoral approach. In an effort to spare complete detachment of the subscapularis attachment with the standard approach, either a limited L-incision in the lower one-third of the subscapularis or by accessing the torn capsule from between the subscapularis and pectoralis major tendons can be used [30, 31].

Most reports on outcomes of HAGL lesions are limited to small series and case reports. In a recent systematic review, clinical outcomes, range of motion, rate of recurrence and complications following management of HAGL lesions were analysed [32]. There were 11 articles that met the inclusion criteria in which 42 shoulders were evaluated with a mean follow-up of 25.5 months. The overall rate of recurrence was 0% (0 of 25) in case of surgery with minimal reported loss of external rotation. The most frequently reported outcome score was the Rowe score with a mean postoperative value of 93.5 points.

Humeral avulsion of glenohumeral ligaments may occur in 9% of instability patients. A high index of suspicion is required in any traumatic episodes of shoulder instability. Careful clinical examination and early MRI investigation are necessary to make the diagnosis. Undiagnosed HAGL lesions may cause failed instability repair. Both arthroscopic and open surgical repair have a low recurrence of instability, but careful management of associated pathology is essential for successful outcomes.

## References

1. Abboud JA, Soslowsky LJ. Interplay of the static and dynamic restraints in glenohumeral instability. Clin Orthop Relat Res. 2002;(400):48–57.
2. Lippitt S, Matsen F. Mechanisms of glenohumeral joint stability. Clin Orthop Relat Res 1993;(291) 20–28.
3. Turkel SJ, Panio MW, Marshall JL, Gurgis FG. Stabilizing mechanisms preventing anterior dislocation of the glenohumeral joint. J Bone Joint Surg Am. 1981;63-A:1208–17.
4. Bigliani LU, Pollock RG, Soslowsky LJ, et al. Tensile properties of the inferior glenohumeral ligament. J Orthop Res. 1992;10:187–97.
5. Matsen FA. Glenohumeral instability. In: Rockwood CA, Matsen III FA, editors. The shoulder. Philadelphia: W. B. Saunders Co; 1990.
6. Tirman PF, Steinbach LS, Feller JF, Stauffer AE. Humeral avulsion of the anterior shoulder stabilizing structures after anterior shoulder dislocation: demonstration by MRI and MR arthrography. Skeletal Radiol. 1996;25:743–8.
7. Wolf EM, Cheng JC, Dickson K. Humeral avulsion of glenohumeral ligaments as a cause of anterior shoulder instability. Arthroscopy. 1995;11:600–7.
8. Nicola T. Anterior dislocation of the shoulder: the role of the articular capsule. J Bone Joint Surg. 1942;25:614–6.
9. Bach BR, Warren RF, Fronek J. Disruption of the lateral capsule of the shoulder: a cause of recurrent dislocation. J Bone Joint Surg (Br). 1988;70-B:274–6.
10. Brien SJ, Neves MC, Arnoczky SP, et al. The anatomy and histology of the inferior glenohumeral

ligament complex of the shoulder. Am J Sports Med. 1990;18:449–56.
11. Pouliart N, Gagey O. Reconciling arthroscopic and anatomic morphology of the humeral insertion of the inferior glenohumeral ligament. Arthroscopy. 2005;21(8):979–84. Elsevier.
12. Taljanovic MS, Nisbet JK, Hunter TB, Cohen RP, Rogers LF. Humeral avulsion of the inferior glenohumeral ligament in college female volleyball players caused by repetitive microtrauma. Am J Sports Med. 2011;39(5):1067–76.
13. Gehrmann RM, DeLuca PF, Bartolozzi AR. Humeral avulsion of the glenohumeral ligament caused by microtrauma to the anterior capsule in an overhand throwing athlete: a case report. Am J Sports Med. 2003;31(4):617–9.
14. Baker CL, Uribe JW, Whitman C. Arthroscopic evaluation of acute initial anterior shoulder dislocations. Am J Sports Med. 1990;18(1):25–8.
15. Taylor DC, Arciero RA. Pathologic changes associated with shoulder dislocations. Arthroscopic and physical examination findings in first-time, traumatic anterior dislocations. Am J Sports Med. 1997;25(3):306–11.
16. Gagey O, Gagey N, Boisrenoult P, Hue E, Mazas F. Etude expérimentale des luxations antéro-internes ou erecta de l'articulation scapulo-humérale. Rev Chir Orthop Reparatrice Appar Mot. 1993;79:13–21.
17. Rebolledo BJ, Nwachukwu BU, Konin GP, Coleman SH, Potter HG, Warren RF. Posterior humeral avulsion of the glenohumeral ligament and associated injuries: assessment using magnetic resonance imaging. Am J Sports Med. 2015;43(12):2913–7. American Orthopaedic Society for Sports Medicine.
18. Pouliart N, Gagey O. Simulated humeral avulsion of the glenohumeral ligaments: a new instability model. J Shoulder Elbow Surg. 2006;15(6):728–35. Elsevier.
19. Park KJ, Tamboli M, Nguyen LY, McGarry MH, Lee TQ. A large humeral avulsion of the glenohumeral ligaments decreases stability that can be restored with repair. Clin Orthop Relat Res. 2014;472(8): 2372–9.
20. Southgate DFL, Bokor DJ, Longo UG, Wallace AL, Bull AMJ. The effect of humeral avulsion of the glenohumeral ligaments and humeral repair site on joint laxity: a biomechanical study. Arthroscopy. 2013;29(6):990–7. Elsevier.
21. Bokor DJ, Conboy VB, Olson C. Anterior instability of the glenohumeral joint with humeral avulsion of the glenohumeral ligament. A review of 41 cases. J Bone Joint Surg Br. 1999;81(1):93–6.
22. Bui-Mansfield LT, Taylor DC, Uhorchak JM, Tenuta JJ. Humeral avulsions of the glenohumeral ligament: Imaging features and a review of the literature. AJR Am J Roentgenol. 2002;179(3):649–55.
23. Liavaag S, Stiris MG, Svenningsen S, Enger M, Pripp AH, Brox JI. Capsular lesions with glenohumeral ligament injuries in patients with primary shoulder dislocation: magnetic resonance imaging and magnetic resonance arthrography evaluation. Scand J Med Sci Sports. 2011;21(6):e291–7.
24. Magee T. Prevalence of HAGL lesions and associated abnormalities on shoulder MR examination Skeletal Radiol. 2014;43(3):307–13. Springer, Berlin, Heidelberg.
25. George MS, Khazzam M, Kuhn JE. Humeral avulsion of glenohumeral ligaments. J Am Acad Orthop Surg. 2011;19(3):127–33.
26. Lo IK, Lind CC, Burkhart SS. Glenohumeral arthroscopy portals established using an outside-in technique: Neurovascular anatomy at risk. Arthroscopy. 2004;20(6):596–602.
27. Bhatia DN, de Beer JF. The axillary pouch portal: a new posterior portal for visualization and instrumentation in the inferior glenohumeral recess. Arthroscopy. 2007;23(11):1241.
28. Davidson PA, Tibone JE. Anterior- inferior (5 o'clock) portal for shoulder arthroscopy. Arthroscopy. 1995;11(5):519–25.
29. Huberty D, Burkhart S. Arthroscopic repair of anterior humeral avulsion of the glenohumeral ligaments. Tech Should Elbow Surg. 2006;7(4):186–90.
30. Arciero RA, Mazzocca AD. Mini-open repair technique of HAGL (humeral avulsion of the glenohumeral ligament) lesion. Arthroscopy. 2005;21(9):1152.
31. Bhatia DN, DeBeer JF, van Rooyen KS. The "subscapularis-sparing" approach: a new mini-open technique to repair a humeral avulsion of the glenohumeral ligament lesion. Arthroscopy. 2009;25(6):686–90. Elsevier.
32. Longo UG, Rizello G, Ciuffreda M, Locher J, Berton A, et al. Humeral avulsion of the glenohumeral ligaments: a systematic review. Arthroscopy. 2016;32(9):1868–76.

# Open Coracoid Transfer: Indications, Technique, and Results

15

Giovanni Di Giacomo and Mark Ferguson

## Contents

15.1 **Indications**.................................................... 115
15.1.1 Open Coracoid Transfer.............................. 115

15.2 **Technique**.................................................... 119
15.2.1 Surgical Approach........................................ 119

15.3 **Alternative Techniques**............................. 122

15.4 **Results**........................................................ 123

**References**............................................................ 124

G. Di Giacomo, MD
Orthopaedic Department, Concordia Hospital for Special Surgery, Via delle Sette Chiese, 90, Rome, Italy
e-mail: concordia@iol.it

M. Ferguson, MB.ChB;FCS(SA)ortho
Centre for Sports Medicine & Orthopaedics, Johannesburg, South Africa
e-mail: mferg@icon.co.za

© ISAKOS 2017
A.B. Imhoff, F.H. Savoie III (eds.), *Shoulder Instability Across the Life Span*,
DOI 10.1007/978-3-662-54077-0_15

## 15.1 Indications

### 15.1.1 Open Coracoid Transfer

Transfer of the coracoid process to the anterior aspect of the glenoid was devised and described independently in three different centers, leading to different eponyms.

The technique as developed in the 1930s by Sir Rowley Bristow was described in 1958 by Arthur Helfet, one of Bristow's fellow [1].

The original Bristow procedure transfers distally through the subscapularis muscles only the tip of the coracoid process with its tendon attachments (short head of the biceps and coracobrachialis), such that the resected surface is in contact with the glenoid vault [2].

Fixation is achieved by means of the same sutures as those used for closure of the subscapularis muscle.

Helfet [2] modified the technique using a much larger fragment of the coracoid process which was secured to the scapular neck with a screw.

In 1954, a similar technique was reported in French literature; Latarjet [3] reported four cases of recurrent anterior shoulder dislocations by transferring the coracoid process to the anterior rim of the scapular neck through a horizontal split in the subscapularis, and screwed to the anterior glenoid, being orientated so that the tip was in line with the fibers of the conjoined tendon.

May (1970) [4] described a modification whereby the coracoid tip was secured by its cut cancellous surface to the anterior glenoid using a screw also placed through a split in the subscapularis muscle. He emphasized the importance of the tether created by the lower half of the subscapularis which acted to reinforce the deficient inferior glenohumeral ligament.

Bonnin (1973) [5] described further modification because he believed that the tethering of the lower half of the subscapularis caused excessive restriction of external rotation. He therefore divided the subscapularis muscle vertically before transfer and repaired it without shortening.

This also allowed a thorough inspection of the glenohumeral joint and more accurate placement of the screw.

The conjoined tendon of biceps and coracobrachialis was considered to act as a dynamic sling, preventing forward and downward movement of the humeral head when the arm was abducted.

Despite their frequent synonymous labeling as "Bristow-Latarjet" coracoid transfer, they represent distinct reconstructive procedures [6–9].

Latarjet coracoid transfer has a greater ability to restore glenohumeral joint stability. This restoration of stiffness will seemingly help normalize joint kinematics and kinetics by maintaining the joint in a well-reduced configuration, thus preventing excessive coracoid graft loading.

Latarjet procedure consistently outperformed the Bristow procedure in terms of restoring joint stiffness, and the stiffness of the Latarjet increases with the increasing anterior glenoid bone deficiency; this can be attributed to the progressively posterior positioning of the conjoined tendon origin on the coracoid tip as the graft is fixed to sequentially larger defect. This posterior translation of the tendon origin in turn can cause the tendon to wrap under the humeral head more completely, strengthening the dynamic sling effect. This progressive stiffening effect is not observed with the Bristow procedure.

When used for an isolated capsulolabral injury without glenoid bone loss, the Bristow procedure and the Latarjet procedure are equivalent in their ability to prevent dislocation.

However, when used for glenoid bone loss, the Latarjet reconstruction guarantees better stability [10].

The Latarjet procedure restores stability to the shoulder through a combination of bony and soft tissue mechanism. Augmentation of the anterior bony glenoid results in an increased glenoid surface area, thus preventing a Hill-Sachs lesion from engaging the anterior glenoid rim. More importantly, transfer of the coracobrachialis tendon with the coracoid through a split in the subscapularis creates a dynamic reinforcement to the deficient anteroinferior capsulolabral complex. This slinglike construct becomes taut with the shoulder in the abducted, externally rotated position typically associated with shoulder instability [1] (Fig. 15.1). The Latarjet procedure restores stability to the shoulder through a combination of bony and soft tissue mechanism. Augmentation of the anterior bony glenoid results in an increased glenoid surface area, thus preventing a Hill-Sachs lesion from engaging the anterior glenoid rim. More importantly, transfer of the coracobrachialis tendon with the coracoid through a split in the subscapularis creates a

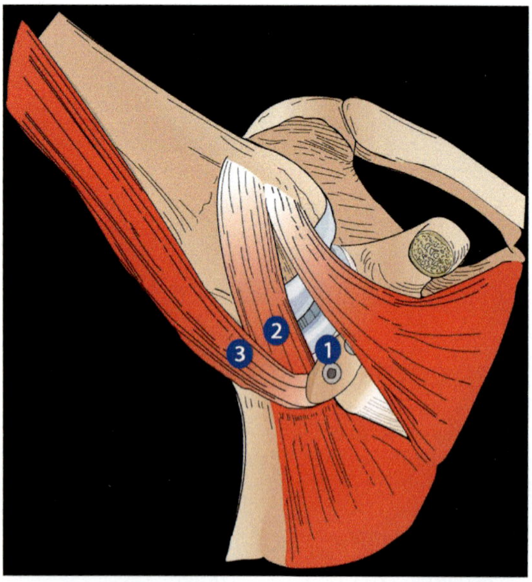


**Fig. 15.1** Effects of the Latarjet procedure: (*1*) increased glenoid surface area because the coracoid graft; (*2* e *3*) slinglike construct of subscapularis and common tendon that create a dynamic reinforcement to the deficient anteroinferior capsulolabral complex

dynamic reinforcement to the deficient anteroinferior capsulolabral complex. This slinglike construct becomes taut with the shoulder in the abducted, externally rotated position typically associated with shoulder instability [1]. According to this the main stabilizing mechanism of the Latarjet procedure is the sling effect produced by the subscapularis and conjoined tendons. The split subscapularis tendon provides muscle stability because the intersection of the transferred conjoined tendon adds tension to the inferior portion of the subscapularis; this principle works at both the end-range and midrange arm positions. The remaining stability is from suturing the coracoacromial ligament to the capsular flap at the end-range position (if performed) and from glenoid cavity reconstruction. The Latarjet procedure provides a superior stabilizing mechanism for the shoulder with anterior instability in the presence of the glenoid defect [11].

Since the Latarjet technique was developed well before recent arthroscopic capsuloplasty procedures, it follows that the indications for "coracoid transposition," although clearly considered a surgical procedure to treat inferior trauma-induced instability, may still differ slightly depending on the particular school of surgery, international scientific society, or geographical area.

It should be noted, however, that although the consensus is for "coracoid transposition" surgery (hereinafter called the "Latarjet technique") to be performed on patients with substantive glenoid bone loss, some surgical schools also include instability with minimum bone loss and poor quality soft tissue in their indications for surgery.

Many studies have evaluated the contributing factors for recurrent instability following nonoperative and operative treatment (arthroscopic capsulolabral repair/Bankart repair) of the anterior glenohumeral instability.

Risk factors for recurrent instability include young age [12, 13], anterior glenoid bone loss [14] or posterior humeral [15] bone loss (Hill-Sachs), underlying ligamentous laxity or multidirectional instability [16], prior ipsilateral anterior shoulder dislocation [16, 17], neurologic deficit or voluntary instability, prior or concurrent ipsilateral rotator cuff tear [18], and participation in contact or collision sports [13, 19–22].

In cases of anterior instability in which substantial glenoid bone deficiency is observed, an isolated Bankart repair is unlikely to result in a stable shoulder. Patients with glenoid bone loss measuring ≤15% can typically be treated with rehabilitation or soft tissue procedures alone [23]. For patients with an intermediate amount of bone loss (15–30% of the glenoid surface), it is important to consider the patient's demands on the shoulder when formulating a treatment plan. Low-demand patients may be treated successfully with either conservative methods or soft tissue procedures. However, high-demand patients will likely benefit from addressing the glenoid lesion to prevent recurrent instability [23]. For nearly all patients with bone loss measuring a ≥25% to 30% of the glenoid surface, a surgical procedure addressing the glenoid bone loss is necessary to prevent further instability [24].

Although these guidelines have been reflected in the literature, efforts should be made to reduce and fix displaced fracture of the glenoid rim in young, active patients to improve postoperative stability [25].

Burkhart and De Beer [14] recognized that one of the risk factors for failure of arthroscopic stabilization was based on the anatomic relation of the bone loss affecting the humeral head and the glenoid in critical positions. In fact, they introduced the concept of "significant bone loss." They defined a significant glenoid bone defect as in which the arthroscopic appearance of the glenoid, when viewed from a superior-to-inferior perspective, was an inverted pear. On the humeral side, they defined a significant bone defect to be an engaging Hill-Sachs lesion, oriented in such a way that it engaged the anterior glenoid in a position of athletic function (90° of abduction combined with external rotation of approximately 90°). They found that the instabilities associated with "engaging-type" Hill-Sachs lesions were at high risk of recurrence if treated with the classic arthroscopic capsuloligamentous repair, confirming that the restoration of the soft tissues alone would not be sufficient to contain the humeral head under stress.

However, this diagnostic technique could potentially cause an overdiagnosis of engaging

Hill-Sachs lesions because ligament insufficiency (Bankart lesion) might permit the humeral head to excessively translate anteriorly, thus facilitating engagement of the humeral defect with the glenoid rim [26].

The importance of bone loss on both the glenoid and humeral side has been increasingly studied; for the purpose of evaluating the size of the Hill-Sachs lesion together with the size of the glenoid, the "glenoid track" concept was introduced by Eiji Itoi [27].

The glenoid track is a contact zone of the glenoid on the humeral head with the arm at the end range of motion, e.g., in various degrees of elevation with the arm in maximum external rotation and maximum horizontal extension. This end range of motion is critical for anterior dislocation because the anterior soft tissue structures become tight and prevent the anterior translation of the humeral head in this position. It is this position that patients with recurrent anterior dislocation of the shoulder feel anterior apprehension. If the Hill-Sachs lesion is always covered by the glenoid at this end range of motion or, in other words, if the Hill-Sachs lesion stays within the glenoid track, the lesion does no harm, because it is always covered by the glenoid even at the end range of motion. On the other hand, if the lesion comes out of the glenoid coverage, it engages with the anterior rim of the glenoid and causes a dislocation. Clarifying the exact location of this contact zone or the glenoid track enables to evaluate any Hill-Sachs lesion for its risk of engagement [28].

A more recent evolution considers how both the glenoid and the humeral bone loss interact to determine whether their combination results in an "on-track" or "off-track" lesion, which may be more predictive of recurrent instability than looking at either side individually [29].

A method has been developed (both radiographic and arthroscopic) that uses the concept of the glenoid track to determine whether a Hill-Sachs lesion will engage the anterior glenoid rim, whether or not there is concomitant anterior glenoid bone loss. If the Hill-Sachs lesion engages, it is called an "off-track" Hill-Sachs lesion; if it does not engage, it is an "on-track" lesion. On the basis of this quantitative method, a treatment paradigm with specific surgical criteria for all patients with anterior instability, both with and without bipolar bone loss, can be applied.

Regardless of the degree of bipolar bone loss, anterior instability can be categorized as follows:

**Group 1**, glenoid defect of less than 25% plus on-track Hill-Sachs lesion – *treatment: arthroscopic Bankart repair*

**Group 2**, glenoid defect of less than 25% plus off-track Hill-Sachs lesion – *treatment: arthroscopic Bankart repair plus remplissage*

**Group 3**, glenoid defect of 25% or more plus on-track Hill-Sachs lesion – *treatment: Latarjet procedure*

**Group 4**, glenoid defect of 25% or more plus off-track Hill-Sachs lesion – treatment: *Latarjet procedure plus humeral-sided procedure (humeral bone graft or remplissage) if the Hill-Sachs lesion is engageable by surgeon on operating room table after Latarjet procedure or only Latarjet procedure if Hill-Sachs lesion is not engageable by surgeon after Latarjet procedure*

Numerous alternative sources of bone graft have been used to address the glenoid bone deficiency. Historically these have been osseous autografts from the iliac crest as described by Eden in 1918 and Hybbinette in 1932. They described the use of an L-shaped iliac crest bone block placed anterior to the glenoid under the periosteum, leaving the "L" arm of the graft extending lateral to the anterior glenoid. This was modified by Alvik who secured the graft into a preformed wedge-shaped groove on the anterior glenoid and later by De Palma who used screw fixation to secure the graft [30, 31]. Despite reports of positive outcomes, recurrent instability and a high incidence of moderate or severe arthritis developed with longer follow-up [32, 33].

More recently Warner reported on the anatomical fixation of autologous iliac crest using screws in 11 patients that had glenoid bone loss. Despite 9 of

11 cases having prior unsuccessful operative procedures at a mean follow-up of 33 months, all had improved ASES and Rowe scores with all patients returning to their pre-injury level of sport [34].

The Lyon group has recommended the use of the modified Eden-Hybbinette procedure for recurrent anterior dislocation after failed Latarjet with 79% good or excellent outcomes [35]. Arthroscopic-assisted procedures have recently been described using autologous iliac crest to restore the anterior bone loss using either screw fixation or a J-shaped press-fit technique [36, 37].

An alternative autologous option is the use of an ipsilateral distal clavicle resection which provides favorable osteochondral characteristics as a replacement for glenoid bone [38]. No clinical studies have yet been reported.

Current coracoid transfer procedures are non-anatomic, do have harvest morbidity, and are associated with an increasing number of complications. In a review of 45 level IV studies reporting outcomes following Bristow or Latarjet shoulder stabilization procedures, a total complication rate of 30% was reported [7].

Allograft reconstruction of glenoid bone loss represents a potential alternative to autologous coracoid use. There are numerous sources of allograft being used including glenoid, iliac crest, distal tibial plafond, femoral head, and humeral head. Some are osteochondral grafts and therefore theoretically provide both bone and hyaline cartilage surfaces. Data from studies using allograft for recurrent shoulder instability show excellent clinical outcomes, a low rate of recurrence, good graft union, and low rates of graft resorption [39]. All included studies were of level IV evidence, and the likelihood of methodological bias is increased. Unfortunately to this date, no comparative studies between the use of coracoid transfer and allograft for shoulder instability exist.

All of these alternative bone graft procedures restore stability by increasing the glenoid surface area alone and obviously do not have any sling effect from the conjoined tendon and inferior subscapularis.

## 15.2 Technique

### 15.2.1 Surgical Approach

The patient is instructed to shave the shoulder girdle and take a shower using antibacterial soap the night before surgery. Immediately before surgery, an interscalene block is placed for postoperative pain control. A general anesthetic is administered, and the patient is placed in the modified beach chair position with a 1-cm thick folded sheet placed under the scapula on the affected side, making the coracoid process readily palpable.

The deltopectoral approach is routinely used for the open treatment of anterior glenohumeral instability, regardless of the procedure that will be performed.

A 5-cm skin incision is made starting at the tip of the coracoid process and extending inferiorly.

The deltopectoral interval is located superiorly and medially by identifying the small triangular area devoid of muscle. The cephalic vein is identified in the deltopectoral interval and ligated with braided absorbable suture to prevent postoperative hematoma; the intermuscular plane is developed and retracted with right angle retractors, taking the cephalic vein laterally. Retraction of the vein medially carries the risk of injuring the large veins that drain the deltoid muscle.

A self-retaining retractor is then placed between the pectoralis major and the deltoid, completing the operative exposure (Fig. 15.2).

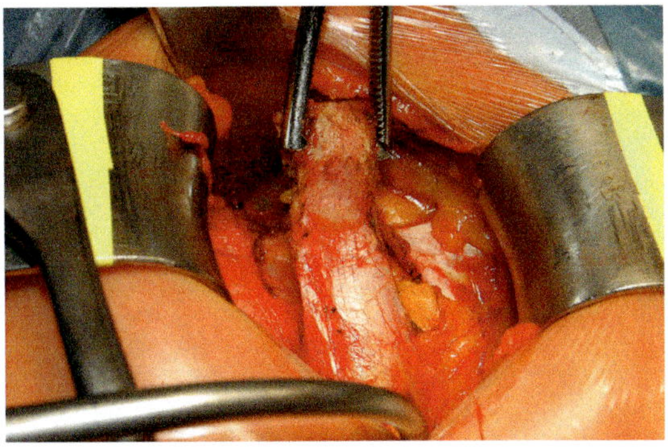

**Fig. 15.2** The *coracoid graft*

The arm is abducted and externally rotated. Mayo scissors are used to clear the superior aspect of the coracoid process, and a Hohmann retractor is placed over the top of the coracoid process. The conjoined tendon is identified, and the coracoacromial ligament and the coracohumeral ligament are completely transacted at its lateral coracoid insertion. The arm is placed in an internally rotated position, and the pectoralis minor tendon is identified and released from its coracoid insertion taking care not to disturb the blood supply to the coracoid process, which enters at the medial aspect of the coracoid insertion of the conjoined tendon (Fig. 15.3). After release of the pectoralis minor tendon, a periosteal elevator is used to expose the "knee" of the coracoid process by sliding it along its medial aspect. Cutting of the coracoid at the level of the "knee" is initiated with a microsagittal saw equipped with a 90° angled blade and completed with an osteotome. Grasping forceps are used to hold the coracoid process gripping the medial and lateral aspects; the arm is returned to the abducted and externally rotated position.

A gauze sponge is placed over the skin at the distal aspect of the incision, and the coracoid process is placed on the sponge by flipping it (the deep surface should be superficial and the superior aspect should be distal); any remaining soft tissue is removed from the deep surface of the coracoid process [40].

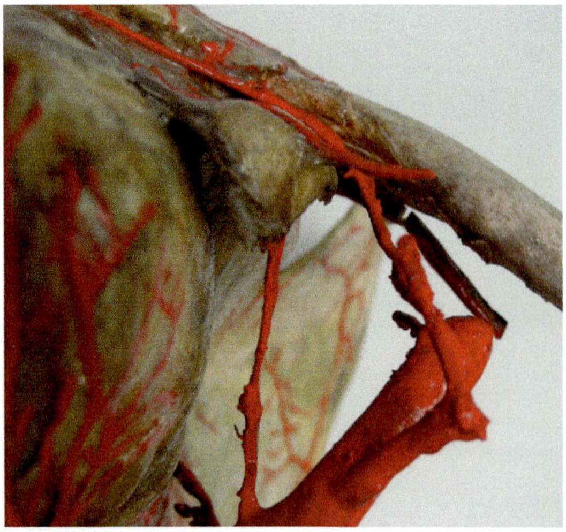

**Fig. 15.3** Pattern of the coracoid blood supply

The microsagittal saw and high-speed burr are then used to decorticate the deep surface of the coracoid bone graft; sterile saline solution is useful to reduce the heat caused by the saw during cutting. Exposing the cancellous bone will indicate that decortication has been performed correctly, and bleeding from cancellous bone will improve integration of the bone graft on the glenoid neck.

A drill guide allows the surgeon to create two dorsal-ventral holes in the coracoid graft using the 2.7-mm drill perpendicular to its long axis (if malleolar screws are intended to be used, the drill is 3.2 mm). The guide has a distance between centers equal to that of the wedged profile plate if intended to be used to improve bone-to-bone compression. The parallel positioning of the two wires guarantees that the two screws will be positioned perfectly parallel [41].

The lateral border of the conjoined tendon can be further released to additionally mobilize the coracoid process if necessary, and the coracoid process is placed beneath the arm of the self-retaining retractor holding the pectoralis major.

The subscapularis tendon and muscle is exposed with the arm by the side and externally rotated. The superior and inferior margins of the subscapularis should be identified.

The subscapularis muscle is divided in line with its fibers using Mayo scissors. Normally, the level of division is the junction of the middle and inferior thirds of the muscle; however, in the case of hyperlax patient, the junction of the superior and inferior half is selected to maximize the effect of the conjoined tendon sling and of the inferior sub-scap. The scissors are opened vertically, exposing the underlying capsule. To facilitate opening of the scissors and capsular exposure, it may be necessary to decrease the amount of external rotation of the arm. Taking down the subscapularis insertion (vertical tenotomy), whether partially or fully, requires protection of passive external rotation for at least 6 weeks in addition to graduated internal rotation strengthening program [42]. A subscapularis split may result in significantly less morbidity while also allowing the subscapularis to function as a "sling" component of the Latarjet reconstruction [42]. Once the capsula is well visualized, heavy forceps are used to develop the plane between the anterior surface of the scapula and the subscapularis muscle belly, allowing placement for a gauze sponge in the subscapularis fossa and elevating the subscapularis muscle off the capsule. A Hohmann-type retractor is placed on the anterior surface of the neck of the scapula as far medial as possible. The inferior portion of the subscapularis is retracted inferiorly, and using a scalpel, the lateral portion of the subscapularis is divided in line with its fibers to its insertion on the lesser tuberosity. The well-visualized underlying capsule allows vertical (close to the glenoid) or horizontal capsulotomy that will facilitate placement of a humeral head retractor into the glenohumeral joint. At this point, two retractors are used: a standard Fukuda retractor laterally for the humeral head and a forked glenoid-type retractor placed on the anterior scapular neck as medially as possible to improve visualization of the site of graft insertion. The superior portion of the subscapularis muscle is then retracted superiorly and held by a Steinmann pin driven into the surgical neck of the scapula (or by dedicated retractor). A small Hohmann retractor placed under the scapular neck could be useful.

The anteroinferior glenoid rim surface is cleared of soft tissue. With a high-speed burr, the anteroinferior glenoid neck is prepared for placement of the coracoid bone graft. The good exposure of the glenoid, obtained with the use of the specific retractors, makes it possible to obtain the best view of the surgical field. The anterior-inferior region of the glenoid neck is prepared to obtain bleeding from the bone and to attain correct leveling of the surface to aid the bone-to-bone contact between glenoid and coracoid graft.

At this point, the positioning of the coracoid is decided. Our criterion is biological and biomechanical [43]. Since the inferior part of the coracoid nearest the conjoined tendon is the most vascularized section, we tend to insert it where the greatest "bone loss" has occurred – usually at 3 and 5 o'clock – in order to allow optimal mechanical stimulation of the graft (mechanotransduction) (Fig. 15.4a, b).

The first guide wire (a 0.9-mm K-wire with threaded apical region) is inserted for subsequent drilling of the holes through the glenoid. The first wire to be inserted is the lower one in order to obtain correct positioning of the lower screw and therefore of the entire implant (wedge plate).

It is important to position this guide wire while precisely observing the lower glenoid margin to ensure that the distal screw will not be implanted too far down.

The coracoid graft offset is crucial; generally speaking, the coracoid has a lateromedial surface of approximately 2 cm; therefore, the first wire will be implanted approximately 1 cm medially

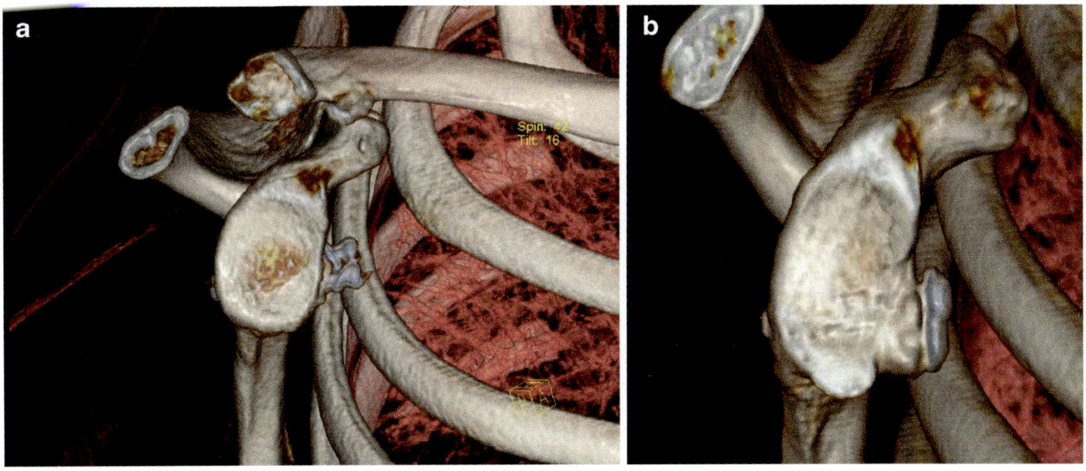


**Fig. 15.4** (**a**) CT en face view with subtraction of the humeral head is evident osteolysis of the coracoid graft when glenoid bone loss is mild. (**b**) CT en face view with subtraction of the humeral head is evident good integration of the most inferior part of the coracoid graft when glenoid bone loss is large

from the glenoid margin. The guide wire must be positioned parallel to the joint surface of the glenoid to avoid positioning the screws inside the joint in the following phase, which would cause serious damage to cartilage surfaces.

The second 0.9-mm K-wire with its guide is positioned, with indication of the offset if used.

To obtain better compression and load distribution between the coracoid graft and glenoid bone surface, a miniplate can be used (wedged profile plate; Arthrex Inc., Naples, FL, USA), the characteristics of which each correspond to a specific biomechanical function appropriate for the Latarjet procedure. The figure-of-eight configuration allows for better torsional orientation of the plate on the dorsal coracoid bone graft surface. This allows the plate to distribute the load evenly throughout the bone, avoiding stress risers that occur when screws only are used. When compressed during the screwing phase, the miniplate, positioned with the wedge profile oriented medially, will tilt the coracoid bone graft in that direction, aligning the bone contact surface between the coracoid graft and the steep glenoid neck. Four spikes on the plate are designed to hold the graft as a whole and to reduce traction forces from the conjoined tendon, at the same time improving plate and graft stability during surgical fixation: plate-coracoid-glenoid neck. The more the bone loss, the less steep is the glenoid neck. In this situation, the improved compression force effect from the plate is more important than the wedge effect; the wedge is useful in minor bone loss because of the steeper glenoid neck.

The coracoid graft is retrieved from under the pectoralis major and held with grasping forceps. The wedged profile plate, with its thickest margin placed medially, is centered with respect to the coracoid graft width and height and stabilized by the presence of the spikes on the plate. In this phase, it is advisable to be certain that the plate holes are centered over the bone graft holes to avoid a shift in the bone graft position when it is being screwed into place.

A cannulated temporary compression device (TCD) is used to stabilize the plate over the coracoid graft through the lower drilled. The TCD is used like a joystick. Positioning a guide wire in the upper bone hole helps keep the plate in place on the bone graft while the TCD is being screwed onto the coracoid graft.

Incorrect positioning of the wedge of the plate – pulling with the grasper punch or with the TCD positioning the graft too far cranially – could damage the musculocutaneous nerve that crosses through the short head of the biceps and coracobrachialis muscles.

A partially threaded 3.75-mm screw (length usually between 34 and 36 mm) is inserted first through the upper coracoid screw hole. The TCD is then removed, leaving the K-wire as a guide for a 3.75-mm cannulated screw through the lower coracoid screw hole. It is again important to have an optimal view of the glenoid region to align the bone graft with the glenoid surface.

Because of the medial wedge of the plate, the slight medial tilt will improve contact between screw head and plate. Both screws must engage the posterior cortex of the scapula. The Fukuda retractor is removed, and the arm is placed in abduction and external rotation. The capsule and subscapularis muscle are sutured in lateral to medial fashion with the arm at 20° of external rotation. As the Latarjet procedure is effective, we do not stress the need for capsular repair on the glenoid or capsular reinforcement. We perform a capsular repair only for patients with associated hyperlaxity. The triple effect of the Latarjet procedure is thus achieved, with the coracoid bone graft positioned in the anterior portion of the glenoid, the subscapularis muscle split, and the conjoined tendon positioned astride the lower portion of the subscapularis [41].

## 15.3 Alternative Techniques

To achieve the graft compression to the glenoid, different techniques can be used:

- One or two screws: 3.5-mm, 4.5-mm, 6.5-mm unicortical, bicortical, ± washer.
- The conventional fixation described in the literature uses either a 3.5-mm diameter bicortical screw or a 4.5-mm diameter malleolar screw. Several problems have been described

in the literature about this mode of fixation. For Huguet et al. [44], Walch et al. [45], and Vander Maren et al. [46], fixation with a 3.5-mm screw can be held responsible for a large number of complete lyses. As regards the 4.5-mm screws, they may be the source of fractures because of their size. Therefore, a compromise should be found between a bulky screw showing strong fixation and a smaller-diameter screw which does not weaken the bone block.

- Hovelius et al. [8] report recurrences decreased and subjective results improved when a horizontal capsular shift was added to the coracoid transfer: two or three suture anchors should be placed in the native glenoid to assist with capsular repair after Latarjet coracoid transfer. In right shoulders, these anchors should be positioned at the 4 and 5 o'clock positions relative to the glenoid face. In left shoulders, they should be positioned at the 7 and 8 o'clock positions [8].
- The anterior capsula can be reinforced closing it to the coracoacromial ligament stamp remaining on the medial aspect of the coracoid graft if previously grafted with the coracoid process [47].

## 15.4 Results

Bhatia et al. [48] performed a systematic review of outcomes after the Latarjet procedure. Eight studies reported recurrence rates of 0–8% with follow-up between 6 months and 14 years. Bessiere et al. [49] compared arthroscopic Bankart repair versus open Latarjet procedure and found the rate of recurrent instability at 5 years of follow-up to be 24% after arthroscopic Bankart repair and 12% after Latarjet procedure. Hovelius et al. [50] in a long-term follow-up study exceeding 10 years after a Bristow-Latarjet procedure reported recurrence to be 3.4% and 13.4% if subluxation were included. The rate of significant recurrence of instability with the need for further surgery was lower than 1%. Of the patients, 98% were very satisfied or satisfied at follow-up.

Latarjet procedure provides excellent long-term clinical results. The prevalence of postoperative development of arthritis and progression of preoperative arthritis is only 23.5%, which is mild arthritis (stage 1 or 2) in 14.7% or severe arthritis (stage 3) in 8.8% [47].

Singer et al. [51] reported on 14 Bristow-Latarjet procedures with a mean follow-up of 20.5 years. They demonstrated an excellent or good Rowe score in 93% despite a 71% rate of glenohumeral arthritis in the involved shoulders. Allain et al. [52] reported on 58 Latarjet procedures with a mean follow-up of 14.3 years, good or excellent results in 88% according to the Rowe score. Sixty-two percent of the patients had postoperative arthritis, and severe arthritis was seen in 36%. Hovelius et al. [14, 50] reported on the outcomes of 118 Bristow-Latarjet reconstructions at a mean follow-up of 15.2 years; they reported 98% good or excellent Rowe scores and a 13.8% recurrence of instability (including subluxations). Forty-nine percent of their patients had arthritis at final follow-up.

The surgical technique has a substantial influence on the long-term development of arthritis after coracoid transfer.

In the studies by Singer et al. and Allain et al. [51, 52], patients underwent a tenotomy of the subscapularis muscle, which was reattached after coracoid grafting. This approach may lead to an external rotation deficit after the subscapularis is repaired, which may lead to arthritis in the long term because of change in glenohumeral joint contact forces. Allain et al. [52] described a mean 20° loss of external rotation postoperatively overall and a mean 29° loss of external rotation in 18 patients in whom they repaired the subscapularis with an overlapping technique. Singer et al. [51] described that 86% of patients had an external rotation deficit, and their mean external rotation was only 19° in the patients with grade 3 arthropathy. We recommend a horizontal subscapularis splitting technique that does not require reattachment of the tendon. Maynou et al. [53] recently described improved functional outcomes and greater preservation in external rotation in patients who underwent a subscapularis split compared with a tenotomy during the Latarjet procedure.

Therefore, the subscapularis split approach may contribute to our lower rate of long-term arthritis.

Reported risk factors for arthritis have included age at initial dislocation and at the time of surgery, number of preoperative dislocations, excessive anterior tissue tightening, intra-articular hardware, lateral overhang of the bone block, and longer follow-up [16, 52, 54–66].

This suggests that postoperative arthritis is caused not only by the Latarjet procedure but also by the natural history of the glenohumeral joint.

Coracoid reabsorption is, in our view, erroneously considered a complication by several authors in the literature. In our experience, if the surgical procedure is correctly performed carefully following the steps described above, reabsorption is simply the physical phenomenon known as "Wolff's law", i.e., coracoid graft reabsorption that is inversely proportional to the original glenoid bone loss. The greater the glenoid deficit, the greater will be the mechanotransduction stimulating transplant integration, with recreation of the concavity and arch of the glenoid bone, both of which ensure anteroinferior glenohumeral joint stability.

Warner [67] reported 6% of superficial infection most in workers' compensation claim and smokers.

Literature reports rate of neurologic injuries 10%, involving musculocutaneous nerve, radial nerve, and axillary nerve. Neurologic injury following stabilization procedures is thought to be caused by traction, patient malpositioning, and inadvertent suturing. Transient nerve injuries usually do not affect long-term outcomes.

## References


1. Matton D, Van Looy F, Geens S. Recurrent anterior dislocations of the shoulder joint treated by the Bristow-Latarjet procedure. Historical review, operative technique and results. Acta Orthop Belg. 1992;58(1):16–22.
2. Helfet AJ. Coracoid transplantation for recurring dislocation of the shoulder. J Bone Joint Surg Br. 1958;40(2):198–202.
3. Latarjet M. Treatment of recurrent dislocation of the shoulder. Lyon Chir. 1954;49(8):994–7.
4. May Jr VR. A modified Bristow operation for anterior recurrent dislocation of the shoulder. J Bone Joint Surg Am. 1970;52(5):1010–6.
5. Bonnin JG. Transplantation of the coracoid tip: a definitive operation for recurrent anterior dislocation of the shoulder. Proc R Soc Med. 1973;66(8):755–8.
6. Paladini P, Merolla G, De Santis E, Campi F, Porcellini G. Long-term subscapularis strength assessment after Bristow-Latarjet procedure: isometric study. J Shoulder Elb Surg. 2012;21(1):42–7.
7. Griesser MJ, Harris JD, McCoy BW, Hussain WM, Jones MH, Bishop JY, Miniaci A. Complications and re-operations after Bristow-Latarjet shoulder stabilization: a systematic review. J Shoulder Elb Surg. 2013;22(2):286–92.
8. Hovelius L, Sandström B, Olofsson A, Svensson O, Rahme H. The effect of capsular repair, bone block healing, and position on the results of the Bristow-Latarjet procedure (study III): long-term follow-up in 319 shoulders. J Shoulder Elb Surg. 2012;21(5):647–60.
9. Boileau P, Mercier N, Roussanne Y, Th'elu CE, Old J. Arthroscopic Bankart-Bristow-Latarjet procedure: the development and early results of a safe and reproducible technique. Arthroscopy. 2010;26(11):1434–50.
10. Doursounian L, Debet-Mejean A, Chetboun A, Nourissat G. Bristow-Latarjet procedure with specific instrumentation: study of 34 cases. Int Orthop. 2009;33(4):1031–6.
11. Yamamoto N, Muraki T, An KN, Sperling JW, Cofield RH, Itoi E, Walch G, Steinmann SP. The stabilizing mechanism of the Latarjet procedure: a cadaveric study. J Bone Joint Surg Am. 2013;95(15):1390–7.
12. Arciero RA, Wheeler JH, Ryan JB, McBride JT. Arthroscopic Bankart repair versus nonoperative treatment for acute, initial anterior shoulder dislocations. Am J Sports Med. 1994;22(5):589–94.
13. Hovelius L, Augustini BG, Fredin H, Johansson O, Norlin R, Thorling J. Primary anterior dislocation of the shoulder in young patients. A ten-year prospective study. J Bone Joint Surg Am. 1996;78(11):1677–84.
14. Burkhart SS, De Beer JF. Traumatic glenohumeral bone defects and their relationship to failure of arthroscopic Bankart repairs: significance of the inverted-pear glenoid and the humeral engaging Hill-Sachs lesion. Arthroscopy. 2000;16(7):677–94.
15. Weber BG, Simpson LA, Hardegger F. Rotational humeral osteotomy for recurrent anterior dislocation of the shoulder associated with a large Hill-Sachs lesion. J Bone Joint Surg Am. 1984;66(9):1443–50.
16. Hawkins RH, Hawkins RJ. Failed anterior reconstruction for shoulder instability. J Bone Joint Surg Br. 1985;67(5):709–14.
17. Rowe CR, Pierce DS, Clark JG. Voluntary dislocation of the shoulder. A preliminary report on a clinical, electromyographic, and psychiatric study of twenty-six patients. J Bone Joint Surg Am. 1973;55(3):445–60.
18. Robinson CM, Kelly M, Wakefield AE. Redislocation of the shoulder during the first six weeks after a pri-

mary anterior dislocation: risk factors and results of treatment. J Bone Joint Surg Am. 2002;84(9):1552–9.
19. Bacilla P, Field LD, Savoie 3rd FH. Arthroscopic Bankart repair in a high demand patient population. Arthroscopy. 1997;13(1):51–60.
20. O'Neill DB. Arthroscopic Bankart repair of anterior detachments of the glenoid labrum. A prospective study. J Bone Joint Surg Am. 1999;81(10):1357–66.
21. Pagnani MJ, Dome DC. Surgical treatment of traumatic anterior shoulder instability in American football players. J Bone Joint Surg Am. 2002;84(5): 711–5.
22. Zaffagnini S, Marcheggiani Muccioli GM, Giordano G, Bonanzinga T, Grassi A, Nitri M, Bruni D, Ravazzolo G, Marcacci M. Long-term outcomes after repair of recurrent post-traumatic anterior shoulder instability: comparison of arthroscopic transglenoid suture and open Bankart reconstruction. Knee Surg Sports Traumatol Arthrosc. 2012;20(5):816–21.
23. Piasecki DP, Verma NN, Romeo AA, Levine WN, Bach Jr BR, Provencher MT. Glenoid bone deficiency in recurrent anterior shoulder instability: diagnosis and management. J Am Acad Orthop Surg. 2009;17(8):482–93.
24. Mologne TS, Provencher MT, Menzel KA, Vachon TA, Dewing CB. Arthroscopic stabilization in patients with an inverted pear glenoid: results in patients with bone loss of the anterior glenoid. Am J Sports Med. 2007;35(8):1276–83.
25. Bigliani LU, Newton PM, Steinmann SP, Connor PM, McIlveen SJ. Glenoid rim lesions associated with recurrent anterior dislocation of the shoulder. Am J Sports Med. 1998;26(1):41–5.
26. Kelkar R, Wang VM, Flatow EL, et al. Glenohumeral mechanics. A study of articular geometry, contact, and kinematics. J Shoulder Elb Surg. 2001;10:73–84.
27. Yamamoto N, Itoi E, Abe H, Minagawa H, Seki N, Shimada Y, Okada K. Contact between the glenoid and the humeral head in abduction, external rotation, and horizontal extension: a new concept of glenoid track. J Shoulder Elb Surg. 2007;16(5):649–56.
28. Schrumpf MA, Maak TG, Delos D, Jones KJ, Dines DM, Walch G, Dines JS. The management of anterior glenohumeral instability with and without bone loss: AAOS exhibit selection. J Bone Joint Surg Am. 2014;1596(2):e12.
29. Di Giacomo G, Itoi E, Burkhart SS. Evolving concept of bipolar bone loss and the Hill-Sachs lesion: from "engaging/non-engaging" lesion to "on-track/off-track" lesion. Arthroscopy. 2014;30(1):90–8.
30. Schrøder HA, Fristed PB. Recurrent dislocation of the shoulder: the Alvik modification of the Eden-Hybinette operation. Acta Orthop Scand. 2009;56(5):396–9.
31. De Palma AF. Surgery of the shoulder. Philadelphia: JB Lippincott Co; 1950.
32. Rahme H, Wikblad L, Nowak J, Larson S. Long-term clinical and radiological results after Eden-Hybbinette operation for anterior instability of the shoulder. J Shoulder Elbow Surg. 2003;(12):15–9.
33. Hindmarsh J, Lindberg A. Eden-Hybbinette's operation for recurrent dislocation of the humeroscapular joint. Acta Orthop Scan. 1967;(38):459–78.
34. Warner JJP. Anatomical glenoid reconstruction for recurrent anterior glenohumeral instability with glenoid deficiency using an autogenous tricortical iliac crest bone graft. Am J Sports Med. 2006;34(2):205–12.
35. Lunn JV, Castellano-Rosa J, Walch G. Recurrent anterior dislocation after the Latarjet procedure: outcome after revision using a modified Eden-Hybinette operation. J Shoulder Elb Surg. 2008;17(5):744–50.
36. Giannakos A, Vezeridis P, Schwartz D, Jany R, Lafosse L. All-Arthroscopic Revision Eden-Hybinette Procedure for Failed Instability Surgery: Technique and Preliminary Results. Arthroscopy. 2017;33(1):39–48. doi: 10.1016/j.arthro.2016.05.021. Epub 2016 Jul 16. Arthroscopy Association of North America.
37. Anderl W, Pauzenberger L, Laky B, Kriegleder B, Heuberer PR. Arthroscopic implant-free bone grafting for shoulder instability with glenoid bone loss: clinical and radiological outcome at a minimum 2-year follow-up. Am J Sports Med. 2016;44(5):1137–45.
38. Tokish J, Fitzpatrick K, Cook J, Mallon W. Arthroscopic distal clavicular autograft for treating shoulder instability with glenoid bone loss. Arthrosc Tech. 2014;3(4):e475–81. Elseiver.
39. Sayegh E, Mascarenhas R, Chalmers P, Cole B, et al. Allograft reconstruction for glenoid bone loss in glenohumeral instability: a systematic review. Arthroscopy. 2014;30(12):1642–9. Arthroscopy Association of North America.
40. Edwards TB, Walch G. The Latarjet procedure for recurrent anterior shoulder instability: rationale and technique. Operative Tech Sports Med. 2012;20(1):57–64.
41. Di Giacomo G et al. Shoulder instability – alternative surgical techniques. Milan: Springer; 2011.
42. Schroder DT, Provencher MT, Mologne TS, Muldoon MP, Cox JS. The modified Bristow procedure for anterior shoulder instability: 26-year outcomes in Naval Academy midshipmen. Am J Sports Med. 2006;34:778–86.
43. Di Giacomo G, de Gasperis N, Costantini A, De Vita A, Beccaglia MA, Pouliart N. Does the presence of glenoid bone loss influence coracoid bone graft osteolysis after the Latarjet procedure? A computed tomography scan study in 2 groups of patients with and without glenoid bone loss. J Shoulder Elb Surg. 2014;23(4):514–8.
44. Huguet D, Pietu G, Bresson C, Potaux F, Letenneur J. Anterior instability of the shoulder in athletes: apropos of 51 cases of stabilization using the Latarjet-Patte intervention. Acta Orthop Belg. 1996;62(4):200–6.
45. Walch G, the "Duplay" group. Plaidoyer pour l'utilisation d'une fiche de cotation commune dans les instabilités de l'épaule. Paris: Communication au premier congrès pour la chirurgie de l'épaule et du coude; 1987.
46. Vander Maren C, Geulette B, Lewalle J, Mullier J, Autrique JC, Thiery J, Deneufbourg J. Coracoid process abutment according to Latarjet versus the

Bankart operation. A comparative study of the results in 50 cases. Acta Orthop Belg. 1993;59(2):147–55.
47. Mizuno N, Denard PJ, Raiss P, Melis B, Walch G. Long-term results of the Latarjet procedure for anterior instability of the shoulder. J Shoulder Elbow Surg. 2014;23(11):1691–9.
48. Bhatia S, Frank RM, Ghodadra NS, et al. The outcomes and surgical techniques of the Latarjet procedure. Arthroscopy. 2014;30(2):227–35.
49. Bessiere C, Trojani C, Pelegri C, Carles M, Boileau P. Coracoid bone block versus arthroscopic Bankart repair: a comparative paired study with 5-year follow-up. Orthop Traumatol Surg Res. 2013;99(2):123–30.
50. Hovelius L, Sandström B, Sundgren K, Saebö M. One hundred eighteen Bristow-Latarjet repairs for recurrent anterior dislocation of the shoulder prospectively followed for fifteen years: study I – clinical results. J Shoulder Elb Surg. 2004;13:509–16.
51. Singer GC, Kirkland PM, Emery RJ. Coracoid transposition for recurrent anterior instability of the shoulder. J Bone Joint Surg Br. 1995;77:73–6.
52. Allain J, Goutallier D, Glorion C. Long-term results of the Latarjet procedure for the treatment of anterior instability of the shoulder. J Bone Joint Surg Am. 1998;80:841–52.
53. Maynou C, Cassagnaud X, Mestdagh H. Function of subscapularis after surgical treatment for recurrent instability of the shoulder using a bone-block procedure. J Bone Joint Surg Br. 2005;87:1096–101.
54. Bigliani LU, Weinstein DM, Glasgow MT, Pollock RG, Flatow EL. Glenohumeral arthroplasty for arthritis after instability surgery. J Shoulder Elb Surg. 1995;2:87–94.
55. Buscayret F, Edwards TB, Szabo I, Adeleine P, Coudane H, Walch G. Glenohumeral arthrosis in anterior instability before and after surgical treatment: incidence and contributing factors. Am J Sports Med. 2004;32:1165–72.
56. Chapnikoff D, Besson A, Chantelot C, Fontaine C, Migaud H, Duquennoy A. Bankart procedure: clinical and radiological long-term outcome. Rev Chir Orthop Reparatrice Appar Mot. 2000;86:558–65.
57. Fabre T, Abi-Chahla ML, Billaud A, Geneste M, Durandeau A. Longterm results with Bankart procedure: a 26-year follow-up study of 50 cases. J Shoulder Elb Surg. 2010;19:318–23.
58. Hawkins RJ, Angelo RL. Glenohumeral osteoarthrosis: a late complication of the Putti-Platt repair. J Bone Joint Surg Am. 1990;72:1193–7.
59. Hovelius L, Sandström B, Saebö M. One hundred eighteen Bristow-Latarjet repairs for recurrent anterior dislocation of the shoulder prospectively followed for fifteen years: study IIdthe evolution of dislocation arthropathy. J Shoulder Elb Surg. 2006;15:279–89.
60. O'Driscoll SW, Evans DC. Long-term results of staple capsulorrhaphy for anterior instability of the shoulder. J Bone Joint Surg Am. 1993;75:249–58.
61. Ogawa K, Yoshida A, Matsumoto H, Takeda T. Outcome of the open Bankart procedure for shoulder instability and development of osteoarthritis: a 5- to 20-year follow-up study. Am J Sports Med. 2010;38:1549–57.
62. Pelet S, Jolles BM, Farron A. Bankart repair for recurrent anterior glenohumeral instability: results at twenty-nine years' follow-up. J Shoulder Elb Surg. 2006;15:203–7.
63. Privitera DM, Bisson LJ, Marzo JM. Minimum 10-year follow-up of arthroscopic intra-articular Bankart repair using bioabsorbable tacks. Am J Sports Med. 2012;40:100–7.
64. Rosenberg BN, Richmond JC, Levine WN. Long-term followup of Bankart reconstruction: incidence of late degenerative glenohumeral arthrosis. Am J Sports Med. 1995;23:538–44.
65. Zuckerman JD, Matsen FA. Complications about the glenohumeral joint related to the use of screws and staples. J Bone Joint Surg Am. 1984;66:175–80.
66. Zwaag HVD, Brand R, Obermann WR, Rozing PM. Glenohumeral osteoarthrosis after Putti-Platt repair. J Shoulder Elb Surg. 1999;8:252–8.
67. Shah AA, Butler RB, Romanowski J, Goel D, Karadagli D, Warner JJ. Short-term complications of the Latarjet procedure. J Bone Joint Surg Am. 2012;94(6):495–501.

# Arthroscopic Latarjet: Technique and Results

# 16

Emilio Calvo and María Valencia-Mora

## Contents


16.1 **Rationale and Indications of Arthroscopic Latarjet** ........ 127

16.2 **Surgical Technique of the Arthroscopic Latarjet Procedure** ........ 129

16.2.1 Joint Evaluation and Capsulolabral Complex Dissection ........ 130

16.2.2 Coracoid Process and Conjoint Tendon Dissection, Preparation, and Harvesting ........ 130

16.2.3 Subscapularis Preparation and Split ........ 131

16.2.4 Coracoid Transfer and Fixation ........ 131

16.2.5 Capsulolabral Reattachment ........ 132

16.3 **Results of Arthroscopic Latarjet** ........ 132

**Conclusion** ........ 135

**References** ........ 135



E. Calvo, MD, PhD, MBA (✉)
M. Valencia-Mora, MD, PhD
Shoulder and Elbow Reconstructive Surgery Unit, Department of Orthopaedic Surgery and Traumatology, IIS-Fundación Jiménez Díaz, Universidad Autónoma, Madrid, Spain
e-mail: ecalvo@fjd.es



© ISAKOS 2017



A.B. Imhoff, F.H. Savoie III (eds.), *Shoulder Instability Across the Life Span*,
DOI 10.1007/978-3-662-54077-0_16


The best operative procedure to address anterior recurrent instability in both the index and revision setting remains a subject of orthopedic surgical debate, and Latarjet has been considered the ideal choice in certain circumstances. This chapter briefly describes the rationale for arthroscopic Latarjet procedure, presents indications and future trends for the procedure and the personal technique of the senior author, and summarizes the state of the current results of arthroscopic Latarjet procedure literature.

## 16.1 Rationale and Indications of Arthroscopic Latarjet

When addressing anterior recurrent instability of the shoulder, multiple treatment options have been described, including nonoperative management, open or arthroscopic soft tissue stabilization techniques, or bone block transfer procedures. Arthroscopic Bankart is still considered the gold standard treatment for anterior instability that addresses the most common lesion associated with a shoulder dislocation: a capsulolabral avulsion from the glenoid rim [1]. However, it has been made clear that there are certain situations in which the risk of failure after Bankart repair is so high that other alternatives should be considered, especially in young active athletes involved in overhead or collision sports, in cases of poor soft tissue quality, or bony glenoid or humeral defects or revision surgery [2].

The Latarjet procedure involves the detachment of the pectoralis minor from the coracoid process, the incision of the coracoacromial ligament leaving a stump of the ligament attached to the coracoid, and the completion of an osteotomy at the base of the coracoid so that it could be mobilized and placed as a bone block against the anterior glenoid neck. The coracoid process is passed through a horizontal split performed between the subscapularis muscle fibers, and positioned vertically adjacent to the articular surface on the inferior equator of the anterior glenoid neck, where it is secured with two screws. The stabilizing effect of the technique is obtained by four mechanisms: first, the increase of the articular surface by the bone graft; second, the sling effect provided by the conjoint tendon when it is tensioned in abduction and external rotation; third, the tensioning of the lower subscapularis by means of the conjoint tendon in its new position; and fourth, the reinforcement of the anterior ligament structures by suturing the stump of the coracoacromial ligament on the anterior capsule.

Coracoid transfer techniques have a long history in Europe, where they have been regarded as the procedure of choice in anterior shoulder instability by certain surgeons [3, 4]. However, the most frequent accepted indication for coracoid transfer techniques is anterior shoulder instability encompassing a bony Bankart lesion or a true fracture of the anterior or inferior glenoid rim. The rationale for this indication is to reconstruct the glenoid surface with the coracoid. There is not clear consensus on the minimum size of the bony lesion to indicate the procedure, but we found that glenoid loss of more than 15% of the inferior glenoid diameter represents a superior risk of postoperative recurrence after shoulder stabilization with arthroscopic Bankart [2].

The presence of a large engaging Hill–Sachs lesion is considered an indication to perform the capsulotenodesis of the posterior capsule and the infraspinatus tendon to the humeral bone defect (remplissage) or a bone graft to the humeral head. The Latarjet technique will lengthen the arc of the anterior glenoid, thereby increasing the degree of external rotation that can be achieved before the lesion approaches the glenoid rim in these cases. Furthermore, a large Hill–Sachs lesion frequently occurs in combination with glenoid bone loss. In this way, the Latarjet operation effectively addresses both lesions without the need for additional procedure on the humeral head.

Another potential indication for coracoid transfer techniques is in the patient with severe soft tissue loss involving the anterior labroligamentous structures. Such deficient soft tissues can be found in patients with intrinsic poor tissue quality or after multiple failed soft tissue procedures for instability or thermal capsular necrosis. The "sling effect" of the conjoint tendon provided by the coracoid transfer resists the anterior translation of the humeral head in the position of abduction and external rotation, but also the lengthening of the anterior glenoid arc effectively prevents glenohumeral dislocation. Although some authors have recommended using soft tissue allografts, this especial setting can also be amenable of coracoid transfer techniques based on the intraoperative observation in revision cases that a new anterior pseudocapsular tissue is formed after the Latarjet technique. Concerning other soft tissue abnormalities, Lafosse and Boyle [5] also consider the presence of a HAGL lesion an indication for shoulder stabilization using the arthroscopic Latarjet technique based on their disappointing experience of a higher risk of shoulder stiffness after soft tissue repair technique with anchors. The group Lyonnais conducted by Gilles Walch reported also satisfactory results of open Latarjet in cases of recurrent shoulder instability associated with rotator cuff tears [6].

Gerber and coworkers have recently shown that coracoid transfer as described by Latarjet can effectively restore anterior glenohumeral shoulder stability if previous operation(s) have failed to do so [7]. Patients engaged in high-risk sports (climbing, rugby, football) or occupations needing a safe and stable shoulder, or who have a high risk of recurrence due to the intensity and action of their activity, are also ideal candidates for these procedures [8, 9]. It is well known that epilepsy can be devastating for shoulder stability [10]. Shoulder instability in epileptic patients is frequently associated with large bone defects and poor outcome. Coracoid transfer techniques may offer a stronger reconstruction than soft tissue procedures in these patients.

## 16.2 Surgical Technique of the Arthroscopic Latarjet Procedure

Although several techniques on arthroscopic bone block procedures have been published, Lafosse et al. first [11] and Boileau et al. later [12] have described an arthroscopic Latarjet procedure. This technique affords the benefits of a bone block procedure in a less invasive manner than the open procedure. Additionally, the procedure offers the potential for more precise bone block positioning; concomitant joint abnormalities can be treated at the same procedure, reduce scar tissue, improve cosmesis, decrease post-op pain, and provide greater subjective patient satisfaction. The arthroscopic Latarjet technique presented in this report is the procedure followed by the authors and corresponds to a modification of that described by Lafosse et al. [13]. It requires the Latarjet kit manufactured by DePuy Synthes Mitek (Raynham, MA, USA).

The arthroscopic Latarjet is performed with the patient anesthetized under a combination of single-shot interscalene regional block and general anesthesia and is placed in the beach chair position with the arm free to allow movement of the arm. The shoulder is draped wide including a major portion of the hemithorax to permit access through the more medial portals. Arterial blood pressure is controlled and arthroscopic pump is mandatory to prevent bleeding during the extra-articular procedure, and it is recommended to monitor cerebral blood flow using near infrared spectroscopy for optimal patient safety. Seven portals are used for this technique of arthroscopic Latarjet (Fig. 16.1). The A portal is the conventional posterior soft spot portal and is used for

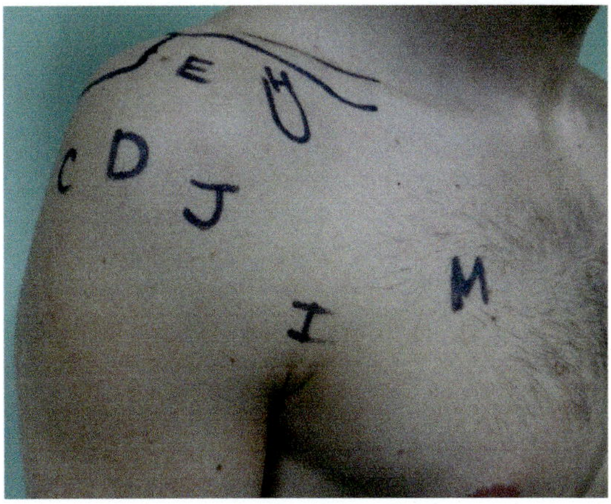


**Fig. 16.1** Portals for arthroscopic Latarjet

visualization. The D portal is the anterolateral portal positioned 1 cm lateral and anterior to the anterolateral acromial angle. It is aligned with the superior border of the subscapularis and is used for visualization and also for instrumentation during coracoid process preparation. The E portal is the classic anterior working portal for soft tissue stabilization and is used mostly for capsulolabral dissection and later reattachment at the end of the bony procedure. The H portal is located just anterior to the clavicle and superior to the coracoid and is used for coracoid preparation and osteotomy. The I portal is an axillary portal created at the most inferior part of the deltopectoral crease. It is used mostly for visualization during coracoid preparation and for subscapularis split. The J portal is in the midway between the D and I portals and is used for visualization along the major part of the extra-articular procedure as well as instrumentation during various stages. The M (medial) portal is initially used for preparation of the medial coracoid, to perform the subscapularis split and to introduce the transparent double-barrel cannula from the Latarjet kit, which is used for coracoid handling and final fixation. It is created at the intersection between a transverse horizontal line at the level of the most inferior deltopectoral crease and a parasagittal vertical line at the level of the glenohumeral joint, and it is located approximately 8–10 cm medial to the I portal. The technique is described in five surgical steps.

### 16.2.1 Joint Evaluation and Capsulolabral Complex Dissection

After a thorough diagnostic shoulder arthroscopic evaluation is performed with the arthroscope inserted through the A portal, the E portal is created, and the rotator interval is completely removed to gain access to the capsulolabral complex, coracoid process, and conjoint tendon. Care should be taken to preserve the biceps pulley. The coracoacromial ligament is detached from the lateral aspect of the coracoid process. Should any intra-articular abnormality is found, it should be corrected before proceeding with the Latarjet procedure, with the exception of anterior capsulolabral or glenoid injuries. Engagement of the Hill–Sachs lesion with the anterior glenoid is assessed by abduction and external rotation of the shoulder. The extent and characteristics of bony anterior glenoid injuries are much better evaluated later visualizing from anterior D to E portals.

The labrum is carefully peeled off from the anterior glenoid with a radiofrequency probe, and a cleavage plane between the anterior capsule and the posterior articular aspect of the subscapularis developed until the capsule is completely independent of the subscapularis from two to six o'clock positions. Then the labrum is transected at the two o'clock position and the capsulolabral complex fully retracted inferiorly and hidden into the axillary pouch to allow free passage of the graft through the subscapularis at a later stage.

With the rotator interval widely open, a needle is inserted just above and parallel to the superior edge of the subscapularis to orient the D portal. The lateral and inferior aspects of the coracoid can be skeletonized using a radiofrequency probe or a shaver inserted through the D portal.

### 16.2.2 Coracoid Process and Conjoint Tendon Dissection, Preparation, and Harvesting

After glenohumeral joint preparation, the arthroscope is moved into the D portal, allowing the inferolateral J portal to be created under direct visualization. A shaver or a radiofrequency probe is inserted through the J portal to remove any soft tissue remaining in the lateral and inferior aspect of the coracoid. It is also used to dissect the lateral border and anterior aspect of conjoint tendon as well as the superior aspect of the coracoid making sure that any soft tissue is cleared to the origin of the coracoclavicular ligaments. It is recommended to release the lateral border of the conjoint tendon as inferiorly as possible reaching the insertion of the pectoralis major tendon to facilitate later coracoid graft mobilization. The mobility of the coracoid process should be tested while it is released. This is especially important in revision cases where scar tissue might preclude soft tissue mobilization. The arthroscope is then moved to this J portal and the M portal created to begin with the coracoid harvesting process. During all the process of coracoid dissection and harvesting, we found it very useful to use switching sticks inserted through the D and E portals to elevate the deltoid and pectoralis major in order to create additional working space and improve visualization in the anterior extra-articular region of the shoulder.

The coracoid harvesting process is performed visualizing from the I portal, which allows a frontal view of the tip of the coracoid. The pectoralis minor is resected from the coracoid using a radiofrequency probe inserted through the M portal. While performing this step, the brachial plexus and the musculocutaneous nerve may be at risk. To prevent any inadvertent damage of nerves, it is recommended to use the probe always facing superiorly. Once the coracoid is completely exposed, an additional portal (H) is created above the coracoid in order to gain access for pre-drilling the coracoid osteotomy. Coagulation of a branch of the cephalic vein can help avoid potential bleeding when creating this superior portal. A commercially available cannulated $\alpha\beta$ drill guide has been developed to aid in the coracoid harvest process. The guide is inserted through the H portal and should be accommodated between the middle and medial third of the width of the coracoid process (two-thirds lateral and one-third medial) and at minimum of 7 mm posterior to the coracoid tip to avoid lateral or anterior screw placement. The drill guide aids in the insertion of two ($\alpha$ and $\beta$) K-wires that perforate the coracoid process superiorly to inferiorly (Fig. 16.2). Once the coracoid is drilled, the guide

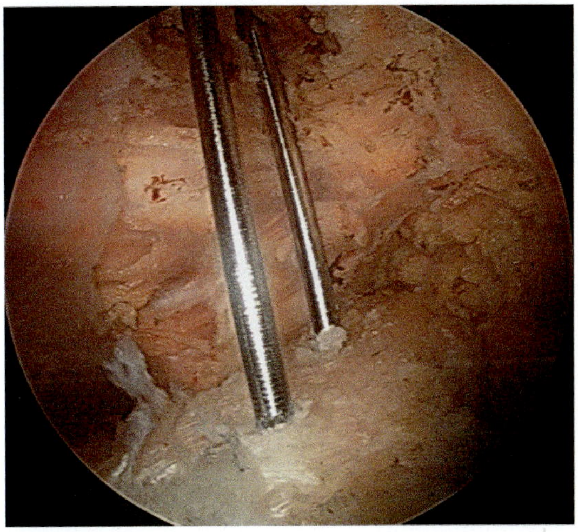

**Fig. 16.2** Anterior view of the coracoid process from the I portal. Two K-wires perforating the coracoid process superiorly to inferiorly have been inserted with the aid of the αß drill guide. The K-wires will be used to drive the cannulated drill that will perforate the holes for the top-hat washers and the screws

is removed and the position of the wires evaluated on the superior and inferior aspects of the coracoid. The holes are then drilled using the cannulated coracoid step drill bit and then tapped. A "top-hat" washer is inserted into each hole with the K-wire still in place as a guide.

Attention is now turned toward coracoid osteotomy. The osteotomy is started on the superior, lateral, and medial surfaces of the coracoid process creating a through with a forefoot cutting drill bit power tool inserted through the superior H portal. A minimal 4 mm security distance between the osteotomy line and the posterior is recommended to avoid fracture of the graft. Once the coracoid base is osteotomized at the superior, medial, and lateral cortical bone, the osteotomy is performed from the H portal using the curved osteotome. The coracoid is then retracted medially and inferiorly to expose completely the anterior aspect of the subscapularis.

### 16.2.3 Subscapularis Preparation and Split

Before starting the split of the subscapularis, the connective tissue covering the anterior aspect of the subscapularis tendon and muscle is fully

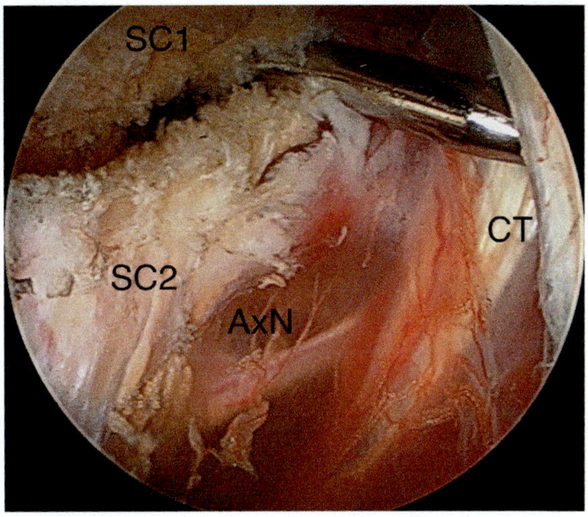


**Fig. 16.3** Image of the subscapularis split. A Wissinger rod has pierced the muscle to establish the level and the subscapularis divided medial to lateral in superior (SC1) and inferior (SC2) portions. The axillary nerve (AxN) determines the medial limit. *CT* conjoint tendon

resected using a shaver. The ideal level of the split should be established between the middle third and inferior third of the tendon. To define this level, it is helpful to insert a Wissinger rod through the posterior portal that will pierce the subscapularis at the four o'clock level of the glenoid. After verification of correct level through various portals, a split in the subscapularis is created using radiofrequency probe inserted either through the M or I portals. It is advised to extend the subscapularis split as wide as possible to facilitate the passage of the graft into the joint. The lesser tuberosity and the axillary nerve delineate the lateral and medial limits of the split, respectively. The axillary nerve should be visualized with caution (Fig. 16.3). Placing the dull large trocar through the muscle and onto the glenoid can complete the split and externally rotating the shoulder with the arm adducted.

### 16.2.4 Coracoid Transfer and Fixation

For coracoid transfer, the subscapularis split is opened by retracting the superior two-thirds of the tendon with the Wissinger rod inserted through the joint and the inferior third with an additional rod inserted thorough the I portal. The coracoid is fixed to a transparent double-barrel cannula inserted through the medial M portal that will be used to drive the graft. Two long coracoid-holding screws are passed through the bores of this cannula and the top hats into the bone. The coracoid can now be fully mobilized with the remainder of soft tissue attachments released. Before transferring the coracoid to the glenoid, the undersurface of the coracoid and the anterior glenoid rim are decorticated using a motorized arthroscopic burr without suction. This burr can be inserted either through the lateral D or superior H portals for the coracoid and through the J or I portals for the glenoid.

To facilitate the mobilization of the coracoid graft toward the glenoid, the scapula is retracted posteriorly, and the arm placed in internal rotation and forward flexion, thereby releasing the conjoint tendon and opening the subscapularis split. The double-barrel cannula is now used to joystick the coracoid graft into proper position on the glenoid, while usually visualizing from a J portal. Optimal positioning is about 1–2 mm medially to the cartilage in the axial plane and inferiorly to the glenoid equator in the sagittal plane surface ensuring bony congruence. Once the graft is satisfactorily positioned, two long K-wires are used to drill through the graft, glenoid, and finally through the posterior shoulder skin. We recommend drilling first the inferior wire to ensure bony contact. Once the graft is stabilized on the glenoid surface with these two long K-wires, the long screws that fixed the graft to the double-barrel cannula are removed and two holes drilled with a 3.2 mm cannulated drill driven by the K-wires starting with the inferior hole. Screw length measurement is carried out using the laser marks on the drill bit when the posterior glenoid cortex is perforated (usually 28–34 mm). The inferior screw is then inserted and the process repeated for the superior screw. Care must be taken to alternately tighten the screws to provide adequate compression without fracturing the graft. The final graft position is checked through J, D, and posterior A portals and any prominences gently abraded with a burr. Once it is confirmed that the coracoid position is adequate, the K-wires are removed posteriorly and the cannula retrieved anteriorly. It is also important to check that the subscapularis muscle is completely anterior to the coracoid graft permitting full excursion in external rotation. In addition, the head of the screws should not interfere with the humeral head during internal rotation.

### 16.2.5 Capsulolabral Reattachment

Glenohumeral osteoarthritis at long-term follow-up has been reported as complication of the Latarjet procedure. Bouju et al. have recently reported a lower incidence of osteoarthritis (8.5%) compared to previously published series with a minimum 10-year follow-up [14]. In this investigation, the strictly extracapsular situation of the bone block appeared as an important factor in limiting long-term osteoarthritis, and capsule reinsertion seemed to alleviate the radiologic complications. Based on these findings, we consider that the capsulolabral complex should be reconstructed unless the capsular tissue is in a poor condition.

In this last step of the procedure, a forceps is inserted through the E portal to grasp the capsulolabral complex from the inferior axillary pouch and reduce it back to the anterior glenoid rim visualizing the joint from the conventional posterior A portal. The labrum is reattached to the anterior glenoid rim using conventional anchors, and in this manner, the graft is left outside the joint. The anchor located at two o'clock position should be inserted first and the upper part of the labrum reattached to stabilize the labrum in its anatomic position. Then the labrum is sutured superiorly to inferiorly to the six o'clock position. All suture anchors are recommended to avoid impaction of the anchors with the coracoid screws.

## 16.3 Results of Arthroscopic Latarjet

Long-term studies of the open Latarjet procedure have confirmed its efficacy in terms of safety for the patient and stability of the joint. It provides excellent results and patient satisfaction with an overall recurrence rate of 0–8% [4, 15–17]. However, literature regarding the long-term results of all-arthroscopic Latarjet is still scarce. As mentioned before, the rationale for arthroscopic Latarjet is that it would combine the excellent results obtained by means of the open technique with the advantages that arthroscopy provides. The main concern about the arthroscopic procedure is the learning curve with the neurovascular risk that it implies [18]. Arthroscopic Latarjet offers potential advantages: firstly, the avoidance of a diagnostic previous shoulder arthroscopy in order to evaluate the soft tissue quality and bony defect and need to reconversion to an open surgery; secondly, the visual control of the joint during coracoid placement that could avoid malpositioning of the graft and screw prominence [19, 20]; thirdly, the possibility to detect and treat other intra-articular lesions such as superior or posterior tears as well as cartilage defects; and lastly, a faster recovery based on diminished postoperative pain, scar tissue, and stiffness [21].

In 2010, Lafosse et al. published their earlier results of the first 100 shoulders undergoing all-arthroscopic Latarjet shoulder stabilization [5]. At a mean follow-up of 26 months, patient-reported outcomes revealed 91% excellent scores and 9% good, with quick return to work and sports, satisfactory graft position in 78% of the cases, and low complication rate. However, they reported a mean external rotation loss of 18°. In 2014, Dumont et al. published the results from the same group at 5-year follow-up [22]. This series was constituted by 62 patients (64 shoulders) with a mean age at the time of the surgery of 29.4 years. Of them, 20% had undergone a previous arthroscopic Bankart repair at a mean of approximately 4 years earlier. None of them reported dislocations at final follow-up; just one of them complained of subluxations. The reoperation rate was 15.6%. One patient returned for a displaced coracoid graft and eight patients because of hardware impingement, and one patient required a total shoulder arthroplasty for glenohumeral arthrosis.

Boileau et al. published also their earlier results in 2010, with excellent clinical outcomes in terms of increase in Rowe and WOSI scores [12]. They reported a need for open conversion in 12% of the cases, but no neurological complications were recorded. With regard to the position of the bone block, it was deemed to be subequatorial in 98% of the cases and flush with glenoid surface in 92% of the cases. There was one block fracture and seven migrations.

More recently, Metais et al. have published the longest series of Latarjet surgery comparing the open technique with two different arthroscopic techniques (fixation with screws or cortical button) [19]. They included 390 patients and did not find differences in mean increase in functional outcome, apprehension, recurrence rate, nerve injury, or incidence of infection. However, all of the cases of neurological complications occurred in the screw fixation arthroscopic group. Motion range restriction was minimal with all three techniques, but external rotation at 90° of abduction and internal rotation in neutral were better after open surgery. Marion et al. have published the early results of a comparative prospective study comparing open and arthroscopic procedures and have not found differences in any of the parameters studied but the less degree of postoperative pain in the arthroscopic group [20].

The importance of the learning curve has been outlined and studied by many authors. All of them advise of the difficulty of the technique and the need for a dedicated experience in both open and arthroscopic shoulder surgery. Calvo et al. found that surgical time decreases significantly after the first ten cases, and the subscapularis split and coracoid passage and fixation into the glenohumeral joint were the most difficult steps of the procedure [23]. Cunningham et al. compared the learning curve of arthroscopic Latarjet to the open procedure and found that ten cases were needed to overcome the need for conversion and 20 cases to achieve equal operating time [24]. Although they did not find differences in final outcome or patient satisfaction, there was a higher incidence of complications (screw placement inaccuracy, persistent apprehension, and recurrence rate) with the arthroscopic technique. Kany et al. also published their learning curve results with the focus on screw positioning [25].

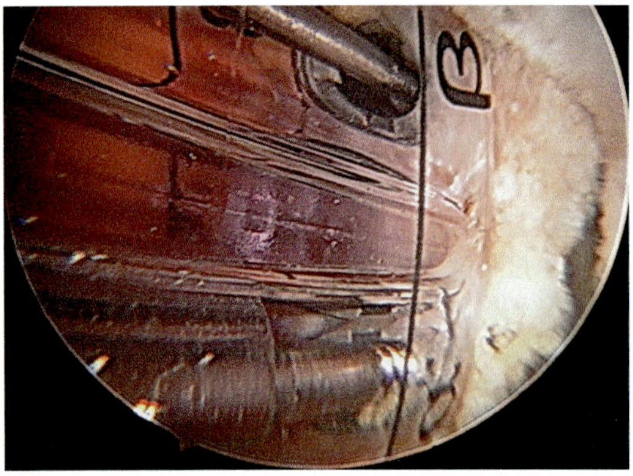

**Fig. 16.4** Anterior view of the coracoid process. The graft has been transported using the double-barrel transparent cannula and stabilized on the anterior glenoid rim with two long K-wires. The coracoid tunnels have been drilled and the inferior screw is being inserted

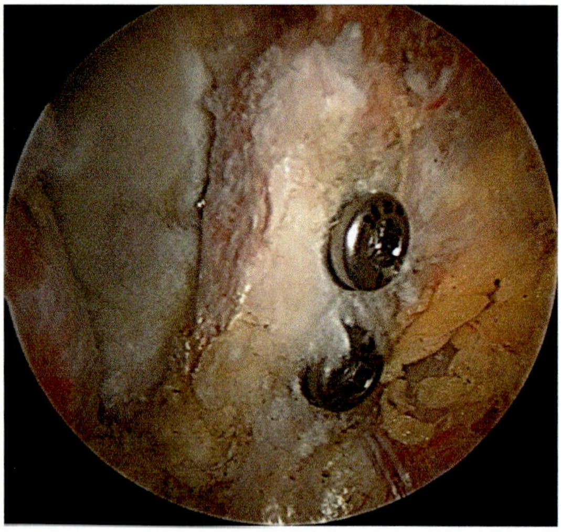

**Fig. 16.5** Imaging of a right shoulder with the coracoid graft in place. Note that the lateral aspect of the coracoid has been abraded to correct any lateral protrusion

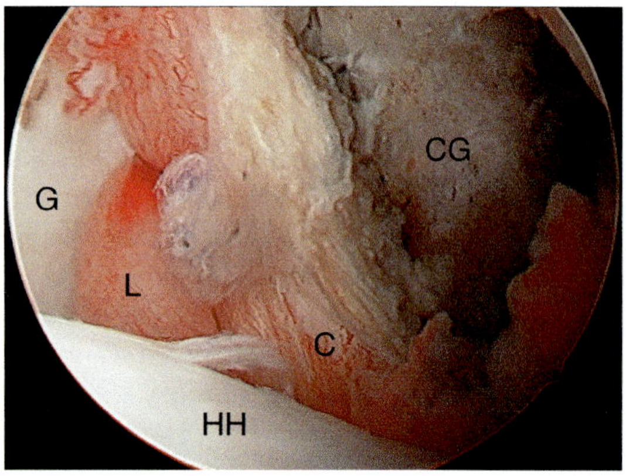


**Fig. 16.6** Latarjet finalized. The capsulolabral complex has been reattached and the coracoid graft remains extra-articular. *G* glenoid, *HH* humeral head, *L* labrum, *C* capsule, *CG* coracoid graft

In their series, the coracoid graft was accurately positioned in the sagittal plane in 91.5% of the cases and 81% in the axial plane. When comparing cases performed in the initial period with those performed in the last period, they found a significant decrease in surgical time and also in the risk of graft malpositioning. The position of the bone graft has been traditionally considered a key factor determining the long-term clinical and radiological outcome of bone block procedures [26]. The risk of osteoarthritis is higher when there is an overhanging position of the bone block, and, conversely, when the bone block is too medial or above the equator, it can result in recurrent instability [14, 26, 27] (Figs. 16.4, 16.5, and 16.6).

Early complication rate (intraoperative and immediate postoperative) has been one of the main concerns of most surgeons when thinking of changing from an open technique to the arthroscopic procedure. However, recent reports did not find any statistically significant differences between open and arthroscopic procedures in American or European perspective [19, 23, 28]. Fracture of the coracoid graft is the most frequent complication, with an incidence of 0–7% [19, 23]. Neurological complications have been also reported infrequently but in general, they are transient palsies that resolve with time (0.8%). Axillary [25, 28], musculocutaneous [29], and more rarely suprascapular nerves can be involved [30]. In order to make the arthroscopic Latarjet safer and to reduce hardware-related and neurological complications related to anteroposterior drilling, Boileau has described a new fixation method involving a guided surgical approach for graft positioning and the use of specific suture buttons for fixation [31]. The reported initial results at 2-year follow-up of this technique are promising with a 96% satisfactory graft positioning, excellent clinical results, and no need for reintervention in any of the patients. There were no neurological complications, graft fracture, or migration. The consolidation rate was 91% at 6 months. Regarding late complications, re-dislocation, apprehension, or late instability-related arthrosis development, similar rates than with open procedures have been reported [19]. In order to avoid the risk of osteoarthritis and make the graft extra-articular, Boileau et al. also promoted the combined Bankart–Latarjet procedures. This author also reported low recurrence rate when both techniques were performed together [12, 19].

### Conclusion

The arthroscopic Latarjet offers a minimally invasive and effective surgical option for recurrent anterior shoulder instability. The experience of the senior author and that reported by others shows that arthroscopic Latarjet constitutes a reliable and safe technique. However, the procedure is technically demanding, and it is recommended to be performed by surgeons with sound anatomic knowledge, advanced arthroscopic skills, and familiarity with the specialized instrumentation.

## References


1. Hintermann B, Gachter A. Arthroscopic findings after shoulder dislocation. Am J Sports Med. 1995;23(5):545–51.
2. Calvo E, Granizo JJ, Fernández-Yruegas D. Criteria for arthroscopic treatment of anterior instability of the shoulder. J Bone Joint Surg Br. 2005;87:677–83.
3. Hovelius L, Körner L, Lundberg B, et al. The coracoid transfer for recurrent dislocation of the shoulder. Technical aspects of the Bristow-Latarjet procedure. J Bone Joint Surg Am. 1983;65(7):926–34.
4. Allain J, Goutallier D, Glorion C. Long-term results of the Latarjet procedure for the treatment of anterior instability of the shoulder. J Bone Joint Surg Am. 1998;80(6):841–52.
5. Lafosse L, Boyle S. Arthroscopic Latarjet procedure. J Shoulder Elbow Surg. 2010;19:2–12.
6. Jouve F, Graveleau N, Nové-Josserand L, et al. Recurrent anterior instability of the shoulder associated with full thickness rotator cuff tear: results of surgical treatment. Rev Chir Orthop Reparatrice Appar Mot. 2008;94(7):659–69.
7. Schmid SL, Farshad M, Catanzaro S, et al. The Latarjet procedure for the treatment of recurrence of anterior instability of the shoulder after operative repair: a retrospective case series of forty-nine consecutive patients. J Bone Joint Surg Am. 2012;94:e75(1-7).
8. Neyton L, Young A, Dawidziak B, et al. Surgical treatment of anterior instability in rugby union players: clinical and radiographic results of the Latarjet-Patte procedure with minimum 5-year follow-up. J Shoulder Elbow Surg. 2012;21(12):1721–7.
9. Cerciello S, Edwards TB, Walch G. Chronic anterior glenohumeral instability in soccer players: results for a series of 28 shoulders treated with the Latarjet procedure. J Orthop Traumatol. 2012;13(4):197–202.
10. Goudie EB, Murray IR, Robinson CM. Instability of the shoulder following epilepsy. J Bone Joint Surg Br. 2012;94(6):721–8.
11. Lafosse L, Lejeune E, Bouchard A, et al. The arthroscopic Latarjet procedure for the treatment of anterior shoulder instability. Arthroscopy. 2007;23(11):e1241–5.
12. Boileau P, Mercier N, Roussanne Y, et al. Arthroscopic Bankart-Bristow-Latarjet procedure: the development and early results of a safe and reproducible technique. Arthroscopy. 2010;26(11):1434–50.
13. Rosso C, Bongiorno V, Samitier G, et al. Technical guide and tips on the all-arthroscopic Latarjet procedure. Knee Surg Sports Traumatol Arthrosc. 2016;24:564–72.
14. Bouju Y, Gadéa J, Stanovici J, et al. Shoulder stabilization by modified Latarjet-Patte procedure: Results at a minimum 10 years' follow-up, and role in the prevention of osteoarthritis. Orthop Traumatol Surg Res. 2014;100:S213–8.
15. Hovelius L, Sandström B, Sundgren K, et al. One hundred eighteen bristow-latarjet repairs for recurrent anterior dislocation of the shoulder prospectively followed for fifteen years (study I): clinical results. J Shoulder Elbow Surg. 2004;13(5):509–16.
16. Hovelius L, Vikerfors O, Olofsson A, et al. Bristow-Latarjet and Bankart: a comparative study of shoulder stabilization 185 shoulders during a seventeen-year follow-up. J Shoulder Elbow Surg. 2011;20(7):1095–101.
17. Bhatia S, Frank RM, Ghodadra NS, et al. The outcomes and surgical techniques of the Latarjet procedure. Arthroscopy. 2014;30(2):227–35.
18. Shah AA, Butler RB, Romanowski J, et al. Short-term complications of the Latarjet procedure. J Bone Joint Surg Am. 2012;94(6):495–501.
19. Metais P, Clavert P, Barth J, et al. Preliminary clinical outcomes of Latarjet-Patte coracoid transfer by arthroscopy vs. open surgery: Prospective multicentre study of 390 cases. Orthop Traumatol Surg Res. 2016;102(8S):S271–6. pii: S1877-0568(16)30113-X.
20. Marion B, Klouche S, Deranlot J, et al. A prospective comparative study of arthroscopic versus mini-open latarjet procedure with a minimum 2-year follow-up. Arthroscopy. 2016;pii: S0749-8063(16)30455–8.

21. Nourissat G, Neyton L, Metais P, et al. Functional outcomes after open versus arthroscopic Latarjet procedure: a prospective comparative study. Orthop Traumatol Surg Res 2016;pii: S1877-0568(16)30114–1.
22. Dumont GD, Fogerty S, Rosso C, et al. The arthroscopic latarjet procedure for anterior shoulder instability 5-year minimum follow-up. Am J Sports Med. 2014;42(11):2560–6.
23. Calvo E, Avila C, Morcillo D. Arthroscopic Latarjet: my learning curve. In: Boileau P, editor. Shoulder concepts, arthroscopy, arthroplasty and fractures, vol. 2014. Montpellier: Sauramps Medical; 2014. p. 165–70.
24. Cunningham G, Benchouk S, Kherad O, et al. Comparison of arthroscopic and open Latarjet with a learning curve analysis. Knee Surg Sports Traumatol Arthrosc. 2016;24(2):540–5.
25. Kany J, Flamand O, Grimberg J, et al. Arthroscopic latarjet procedure: is optimal positioning of the bone block and screws possible? A prospective computed tomography scan analysis. J Shoulder Elbow Surg. 2016;25(1):69–77.
26. Hovelius LK, Sandström BC, Rösmark DL, et al. Long-term results with the Bankart and Bristow-Latarjet procedures: recurrent shoulder instability and arthropathy. J Shoulder Elbow Surg. 2001;10(1):445–52.
27. Gordins V, Hovelius L, Sandström B, et al. Risk of arthropathy after the Bristow-Latarjet repair: a radiologic and clinical thirty-three to thirty-five years of follow-up of thirty-one shoulders. J Shoulder Elbow Surg. 2015;24(5):691–9.
28. Athwal GS, Meislin R, Getz C, et al. Short-term complications of the arthroscopic Latarjet procedure: a North American experience. Arthroscopy. 2016;32(10):1965–70.
29. Boileau P, Thélu CÉ, Mercier N, Ohl X, et al. Arthroscopic Bristow-Latarjet combined with Bankart repair restores shoulder stability in patients with glenoid bone loss. Clin Orthop Relat Res. 2014;472(8):2413–24.
30. Sastre S, Peidro L, Méndez A, Calvo E. Suprascapular nerve palsy after arthroscopic Latarjet procedure: a case report and review of literature. Knee Surg Sports Traumatol Arthrosc. 2016;24(2):601–3.
31. Boileau P, Gendre P, Baba M, et al. A guided surgical approach and novel fixation method for arthroscopic Latarjet. J Shoulder Elbow Surg. 2016;25(1):78–89.

# Prevention of Complications of Bone Block Procedures: Latarjet

# 17

Kevin D. Plancher, Allison M. Green, Margaret A. Harvey, and Stephanie C. Petterson

## Contents


| | | |
|---|---|---|
| **17.1** | **Introduction** | 137 |
| **17.2** | **Intraoperative Complications** | 138 |
| 17.2.1 | Graft Malpositioning | 138 |
| 17.2.2 | Neurovascular Injury | 138 |
| 17.2.3 | Graft Fracture | 138 |
| **17.3** | **Postoperative Complications** | 139 |
| 17.3.1 | Loss of External Rotation | 139 |
| 17.3.2 | Nonunion or Fibrous Union | 139 |
| 17.3.3 | Recurrent Glenohumeral Instability | 139 |
| 17.3.4 | Graft Osteolysis | 140 |
| 17.3.5 | Shoulder Arthritis/Cartilage Damage | 140 |
| 17.3.6 | Infections | 140 |
| **Conclusions** | | 141 |
| **References** | | 141 |



K.D. Plancher, MD (✉)
Plancher Orthopaedics and Sports Medicine, 1160 Park Avenue, New York 10128, NY, USA

Department of Orthopaedics, Albert Einstein College of Medicine, New York, NY, USA

Orthopaedic Foundation, Stamford, CT, USA
e-mail: kplancher@plancherortho.com

A.M. Green, PhD • S.C. Petterson, MPT, PhD
Plancher Orthopaedics and Sports Medicine, 1160 Park Avenue, New York 10128, NY, USA

M.A. Harvey, DO
Department of Orthopaedics, Albert Einstein College of Medicine, New York, NY, USA


## 17.1 Introduction

First described by Michel Latarjet in 1954, the Latarjet procedure involves the transfer of the coracoid process and the conjoined tendon to the anterior glenoid rim and has become the gold-standard treatment for the management of recurrent anterior shoulder instability in the setting of glenoid bone loss [1]. This procedure enhances the stability of the shoulder in three ways: 1) the increased bony surface area increases the congruent arc of motion, 2) the conjoined tendon provides a dynamic sling effect in abduction and external rotation, and 3) the capsular repair increases stability [2]. The Latarjet procedure has been reported to produce relatively low recurrent instability rates of less than 10% in the majority of series [3, 4]; however, complication rates as high as 30% have been reported [2, 5]. While the arthroscopic Latarjet as first described by Lafosse in 2007 has become popularized, available long-term evidence on the effectiveness of arthroscopic techniques are limited [28]. This chapter will review intraoperative and postoperative complications associated with the Latarjet procedure and provides tips on how to avoid these complications.


© ISAKOS 2017


A.B. Imhoff, F.H. Savoie III (eds.), *Shoulder Instability Across the Life Span*,
DOI 10.1007/978-3-662-54077-0_17

## 17.2 Intraoperative Complications

### 17.2.1 Graft Malpositioning

Graft positioning is a critical aspect of the Latarjet procedure. Due to limited visualization of the anterior-inferior glenoid during an open Latarjet procedure, accurate positioning of the graft can be challenging. The consensus is that the graft should be positioned between 2 o'clock and 5 o'clock on the glenoid face of a right shoulder and between 10 o'clock and 7 o'clock on the glenoid face of a left shoulder, just medial to the chondral surface of the glenoid [2]. Placement of the graft too high on the glenoid can result in recurrent instability as it will not provide a bony restraint for the humeral head. Iatrogenic suprascapular nerve injury from a superior malpositioned screw can also occur [6–10]. Placement of the graft too low can make it difficult for the inferior screw to gain adequate purchase in the glenoid for stable fixation, possibly resulting in a fibrous nonunion [11]. Medial placement can result in recurrent instability through insufficient bone blocking, whereas lateral placement creates lateral overhang, a known risk factor for osteoarthritis (OA) [6, 12]. It has been suggested that visualization is improved with the arthroscopic Latarjet procedure, possibly decreasing the incidence of graft malpositioning. Commercially available guides can also aid in the proper positioning of the graft.

### 17.2.2 Neurovascular Injury

Transient and permanent neurovascular injuries to the musculocutaneous nerve, axillary nerve, radial nerve, brachial plexus, suprascapular nerve, and axillary artery have been reported in the literature [5]. While Shah et al. reported a 10% incidence of neurologic injury in their series of 48 shoulders [27], a 2013 systematic review reported an average 1.4% rate of neurovascular injuries across open and arthroscopic procedures, including 11 musculocutaneous, 6 axillary, and 4 trunk level brachial plexus nerve injuries [5].

A good understanding of the local shoulder anatomy is necessary to avoid these complications. In a cadaveric study, Lo et al. reported the anteromedial portion of the coracoid tip was closest to neurovascular structures [30]. The average distance from the anteromedial portion of the coracoid to the axillary nerve, the musculocutaneous nerve, the lateral cord, and the axillary artery was 30.3 ± 3.9 mm, 33.0 ± 6.2 mm, 28.5 ± 4.4 mm, and 36.8 ± 6.1 mm, respectively.

During the open Latarjet procedure, the high-risk stages for nerve injury are glenoid exposure and coracoid graft placement [13]. Recommendations to avoid iatrogenic injury include maintaining excellent visualization of the glenohumeral anatomy throughout the procedure and meticulous surgical technique around the coracoid, specifically the medial aspect. When removing structures from the coracoid, care must be taken to peel them directly from the bone to avoid inadvertent neurovascular injury. To avoid a traction injury to the musculocutaneous nerve, the coracoid must also be dissected free of soft tissue prior to its placement on the glenoid. Retraction around the glenoid should be kept to a minimum as a long operative time is a risk factor for axillary nerve injury [13].

If a nerve injury occurs, a computerized tomography (CT) scan of the shoulder should be obtained to evaluate screw placement and graft positioning [2]. If no abnormalities are noted, up to 3 months of observation are recommended to see whether the patient's symptoms resolve spontaneously. If symptoms do not resolve, management options include nerve transfers and muscle flaps. While rare, if a vascular injury occurs, consultation with vascular surgery is recommended.

### 17.2.3 Graft Fracture

The coracoid process measures 21 ± 2 to 26 ± 2.9 mm in length and averages 9.3 ± 1.3 mm in thickness; therefore, extreme care must be taken during graft harvest and preparation to avoid fracture [14, 15]. A 2.5–3.0 cm graft is desirable to allow careful size for drill hole placement. The risk of graft fracture can be minimized through careful screw placement. While the optimal distance between screws is still debated, mean distances of 7.8–9 mm have produced good results [15, 16]. The use of commercially available guides, as stated previously, can aid in avoiding aberrant hole placement that can lead to graft fracture. Additionally, cancellous bone from drilling should be cleared before screw insertion, and excessive tightening should be avoided to prevent penetration or fracture of the graft. A washer or plate can be used to reinforce osteoporotic or otherwise poor-quality bone before drilling to minimize this complication.

If graft fracture occurs, the remaining bone quantity and quality as well as the direction of the fracture will influence management decisions [2]. For a longitudinal fracture or poor-quality bone, a modified Eden-Hybinette procedure can be utilized. In this procedure, a wedge-shaped, bicortical, or tricortical graft is harvested from the ipsilateral iliac crest and secured to the anterior glenoid rim [17]. For transverse fractures with adequate quality and quantity of bone, a bioabsorbable anchor can be used to supplement the hold of a single screw with good purchase. Alternatively, or in the case of a screw hole blowout, a buttress plate can be used to provide compression.

## 17.3 Postoperative Complications

### 17.3.1 Loss of External Rotation

Loss of external rotation range of motion is common following the Latarjet procedure, with average losses of 13° reported in a recent systematic review [5]. This potential complication is not surprising, as the method by which the glenoid bone graft prevents engagement of a Hill-Sachs lesion is by extending the glenoid arc so that the shoulder cannot externally rotate far enough to engage the lesion over the front of the graft. Additionally, the tethering effect of the transferred conjoined tendon further restricts external rotation [18]. It has been reported that the arthroscopic Latarjet procedure results in larger losses in external rotation [5]. While a definitive reason for this discrepancy is unknown, the relatively longer length of time needed to perform the arthroscopic procedure has been hypothesized [5]. Furthermore, a subscapularis split has demonstrated less loss of external rotation than subscapularis tenotomy with subsequent reattachment [19]. Repairing the capsule to the coracoclavicular stump with the arm in external rotation may decrease the loss of postoperative external rotation [31]. Immediate postoperative physical therapy may also help to regain external rotation and limit loss of motion [31].

### 17.3.2 Nonunion or Fibrous Union

The incidence of nonunion or fibrous union has been reported up to 9% after a Latarjet procedure [5]. They are commonly incidental findings and are unlikely to lead to recurrence of instability or require reoperation. These patients often report good to excellent functional outcomes following surgery [2, 5, 20]. To obtain good compression and better healing potential, the anterior-inferior glenoid rim and underside of the coracoid graft should be decorticated to flat surfaces. Placement of screws parallel to the glenoid face will also reduce the incidence of graft nonunion [2].

### 17.3.3 Recurrent Glenohumeral Instability

While recurrence of instability after the Latarjet procedure is low, it is usually the result of surgical errors, patient characteristics such as ligamentous hyperlaxity or seizure disorder, or a subsequent trauma [3, 4]. Correct graft placement is key as demonstrated by Hovelius et al. who reported recurrence of instability in 83% of patients when the graft was placed 1 cm or more medial to the anterior glenoid edge [21]. In addition to correct graft placement, a capsular shift can be added to reinforce stability and minimize recurrence as demonstrated by their 4% recurrence rate of instability with the addition of a horizontal capsular shift procedure [21].

In the rare instances when recurrent glenohumeral instability occurs following Latarjet procedure, revision surgery is often technically difficult due to scar tissue from the previous surgery and the revision nature of the procedure [2]. The open or arthroscopic modified Eden-Hybinette procedure using an iliac crest bone graft is the most common salvage procedure used to restore stability following a failed Latarjet procedure. The Eden-Hybinette procedure, when utilized as a revision procedure in patients with recurrent instability following Latarjet procedure, has a reported failure rate of 12% and good overall results in a large published series [17]. Arthroscopic capsuloplasty and/or remplissage are alternative considerations to restore glenohumeral stability [22].

### 17.3.4 Graft Osteolysis

Graft osteolysis is a common complication following the Latarjet procedure, with rates of up to 65% reported in the literature [23]. Osteolysis is most commonly seen in the superficial portion of the proximal coracoid and least commonly seen in the distal portion of the graft which exhibits the best rate of bone healing [2, 23]. Despite its prevalence, osteolysis has been demonstrated to be a largely radiographic phenomenon with no associated increase in recurrent instability or detrimental effect on functional outcomes [2]. Graft osteolysis may be decreased by avoiding significant devascularization of the coracoid graft. Limiting the release of the pectoralis minor to the tip of the coracoid may decrease the risk of devascularization. In the rare instance of osteolysis resulting in recurrent instability, revision with allograft reconstruction or the modified Eden-Hybinette procedure is the best management option.

### 17.3.5 Shoulder Arthritis/Cartilage Damage

OA is a common long-term consequence of the Latarjet procedure with reported incidence rates of 20% at 20 years and over 60% at 35 years following surgery [19, 20, 24]. It is currently unclear whether patients who undergo a Latarjet procedure are at an increased risk of OA development compared to patients who undergo Bankart surgery as it is difficult to distinguish between OA occurring as a result of traumatic dislocation and OA caused by the surgical procedure [2]. Risk factors for development of OA include an age of 23 years or older at first dislocation, participation in high demand sports, and lateral overhang of the coracoid graft [19, 20, 24]. As a result, correct graft positioning, specifically avoiding excessive lateral placement, may reduce the risk of OA development later in life. If lateral overhang of the graft is noted intraoperatively, it should be addressed either by removal of excess graft or by changing the position of the graft. Additionally, external rotation deficits should be minimized as they may lead to arthritis in the long term because of associated changes in glenohumeral joint contact forces [25, 26]. As previously stated, tenotomy of the subscapularis muscle with subsequent reattachment following coracoid grafting should be avoided in favor of a horizontal subscapularis splitting technique to minimize external rotation loss and lower incidence rates of glenohumeral OA [19].

### 17.3.6 Infections

Infections, while rare, do occur following open and arthroscopic Latarjet which could lead to coracoid graft failure and recurrence of instability. Griesser et al. in their systematic review reported a <0.1% infection rate; however, rates as high as 6% for superficial wounds have been reported by Warner et al. [5, 27]. Superficial infections typically respond to antibiotic treatment in conjunction with irrigation and debridement, if needed. An infectious disease consultation may be required when managing deep infections which may also necessitate prolonged intravenous antibiotics and screw and graft removal. In the event of graft failure, the infection must be definitively resolved before considering revision procedures such as the Eden-Hybinette. An antiseptic skin wash should be used for 1 week preoperatively in conjunction with shorter operating room times to decrease the risk of postoperative infection [29, 30].

## Conclusions

The Latarjet is a well-established procedure for the management of anterior shoulder instability in the setting of glenoid bone loss but is not without disadvantages. The overall complication rate associated with the Latarjet procedure remains high and is commonly the result of positioning the bone block and utilization of screws. The best way to avoid complications during and following the Latarjet procedure is by maintaining impeccable surgical technique during graft preparation and placement. Through careful transfer of the coracoid process, complications can be minimized and patients can return to high levels of activity without fear of recurrent shoulder instability. Furthermore, as described by Boileau et al. in 2016, an arthroscopic Latarjet with a guide system and suture button fixation appears to have the potential to improve positioning and eliminate neurovascular complications associated with screw fixation, yielding good healing of coracoid in 91% of cases [32].

## References


1. Latarjet M. Treatment of recurrent dislocation of the shoulder. Lyon Chir. 1954;49(8):994–7.
2. Gupta A, Delaney R, Petkin K, Lafosse L. Complications of the Latarjet procedure. Curr Rev Musculoskelet Med. 2015;8:59–66.
3. Longo UG, Loppini M, Rizzello G, Ciuffreda M, Maffulli N, Denaro V. Latarjet, Bristow, and Eden-Hybinette procedures for anterior shoulder dislocation: systematic review and quantitative synthesis of the literature. Arthroscopy. 2014;30(9):1184–211.
4. Butt U, Charalambous CP. Complications associated with open coracoid transfer procedures for shoulder instability. J Shoulder Elbow Surg. 2012;21(8):1110–9.
5. Griesser MJ, Harris JD, McCoy BW, Hussain WM, Jones MH, Bishop JY, et al. Complications and reoperations after Bristow-Latarjet shoulder stabilization: a systematic review. J Shoulder Elbow Surg. 2013;22:286–92.
6. Hovelius L, Korner L, Lundberg B, Akermark C, Herberts P, Wredmark T, et al. The coracoid transfer for recurrent dislocation of the shoulder. Technical aspects of the Bristow-Latarjet procedure. J Bone Joint Surg Am. 1983;65(7):926–34.
7. Huguet D, Pietu G, Bresson C, Potaux F, Letenneur J. Anterior instability of the shoulder in athletes: apropos of 51 cases of stabilization using the Latarjet-Patte intervention. Acta Orthop Belg. 1996;62(4):200–6.
8. Willemot LB, Eby SF, Thoreson AR, Debeer P, Victor J, An KN, et al. Iliac bone grafting of the intact glenoid improves shoulder stability with optimal graft positioning. J Shoulder Elbow Surg. 2015;24(4):533–40.
9. Ladermann A, Denard PJ, Burkhart SS. Injury of the suprascapular nerve during latarjet procedure: an anatomic study. Arthroscopy. 2012;28(3):316–21.
10. Shishido H, Kikuchi S. Injury of the suprascapular nerve in shoulder surgery: an anatomic study. J Shoulder Elbow Surg. 2001;10(4):372–6.
11. Weppe F, Magnussen RA, Lustig S, Demey G, Neyret P, Servien E. A biomechanical evaluation of bicortical metal screw fixation versus absorbable interference screw fixation after coracoid transfer for anterior shoulder instability. Arthroscopy. 2011;27(10):1358–63.
12. Torg JS, Balduini FC, Bonci C, Lehman RC, Gregg JR, Esterhai JL, et al. A modified Bristow-Helfet-May procedure for recurrent dislocation and subluxation of the shoulder. Report of two hundred and twelve cases. J Bone Joint Surg Am. 1987;69(6):904–13.
13. Delaney RA, Freehill MT, Janfaza DR, Vlassakov KV, Higgins LD, Warner JJ. 2014 Neer Award Paper: neuromonitoring the Latarjet procedure. J Shoulder Elbow Surg. 2014;23(10):1473–80.
14. Bachy M, Lapner PL, Goutallier D, Allain J, Hernigou P, Benichou J, et al. Coracoid process x-ray investigation before Latarjet procedure: a radioanatomic study. J Shoulder Elbow Surg. 2013;22(12):e10–4.
15. Young AA, Baba M, Neyton L, Godeneche A, Walch G. Coracoid graft dimensions after harvesting for the open Latarjet procedure. J Shoulder Elbow Surg. 2013;22(4):485–8.
16. Rosso C, Bongiorno V, Samitier G, Dumont GD, Szollosy G, Lafosse L. Technical guide and tips on the all-arthroscopic Latarjet procedure. Knee Surg Sports Traumatol Arthrosc. 2016;24(2):564–72.
17. Lunn JV, Castellano-Rosa J, Walch G. Recurrent anterior dislocation after the Latarjet procedure: outcome after revision using a modified Eden-Hybinette operation. J Shoulder Elbow Surg. 2008;17(5):744–50.
18. Burkhart SS, DeBeer JF, Barth JR, Cresswell T, Roberts C, Richards DP. Results of modified Latarjet reconstruction in patients with anteroinferior instability and significant bone loss. Arthroscopy. 2007;23(10):1033–41.
19. Mizuno N, Denard PJ, Raiss P, Melis B, Walch G. Long-term results of the Latarjet procedure for anterior instability of the shoulder. J Shoulder Elbow Surg. 2014;23(11):1691–9.
20. Leroux T, Wasserstein D, Veillette C, Khoshbin A, Henry P, Chahal J, et al. Epidemiology of primary anterior shoulder dislocation requiring closed reduction in Ontario, Canada. Am J Sports Med. 2014;42(2):442–50.
21. Hovelius L, Sandstrom B, Olofsson A, Svensson O, Rahme H. The effect of capsular repair, bone

block healing, and position on the results of the Bristow-Latarjet procedure (study III): long-term follow-up in 319 shoulders. J Shoulder Elbow Surg. 2000;1(4):256–61.
22. Poberaj B, Marjanovic B. Outcomes and failures after open Latarjet stabilization. Med Fluminensis. 2015;51(1):191–4.
23. Di Giacomo G, Costantini A, de Gasperis N, de Vita A, Lin BKH, Francone M, et al. Coracoid graft osteolysis after the Latarjet procedure for anteroinferior shoulder instability: a computed tomography scan study of twenty-six patients. J Shoulder Elbow Surg. 2011;20(6):989–95.
24. Gordins V, Hovelius L, Sandstrom B, Rahme H, Bergstrom U. Risk of arthropathy after the Bristow-Latarjet repair: a radiologic and clinical thirty-three to thirty-five years of follow-up of thirty-one shoulders. J Shoulder Elbow Surg. 2015;24(5):691–9.
25. Allain J, Goutallier D, Glorion C. Long-term results of the Latarjet procedure for the treatment of anterior instability of the shoulder. J Bone Joint Surg Am. 1998;80:841–52.
26. Singer GC, Kirkland PM, Emery RJ. Coracoid transposition for recurrent anterior instability of the shoulder. J Bone Joint Surg Br. 1995;77:73–6.
27. Shah AA, Butler RB, Romanowski J, Goel D, Karadagli D, Warner JJ. Short-term complications of the Latarjet procedure. J Bone Joint Surg Am. 2012;94(6):495–501.
28. Lafosse L, Lejeune E, Bouchard A, Kakuda C, Gobezie R, Kochhar T. The arthroscopic Latarjet procedure for the treatment of anterior shoulder instability. Arthroscopy. 2007;23(11):1242.e1-5.
29. Saltzman MD, Nuber GW, Gryzlo SM, Marecek GS, Koh JL. Efficacy of surgical preparation solutions in shoulder surgery. J Bone Joint Surg Am. 2009;91(8):1949–53.
30. Lo IK, Burkhart SS, Parten PM. Surgery about the coracoid: neurovascular structures at risk. Arthroscopy. 2004;20(6):591–5.
31. Plancher KD, Petterson SC. Arthroscopic bankart repair with suture anchors: tips for Success. Oper Tech Sports Med. 2013;21(4):192–200.
32. Boileau P, Gendre P, Baba M, Thélu CÉ, Baring T, Gonzalez JF, Trojani C. A guided surgical approach and novel fixation method for arthroscopic Latarjet. J Shoulder Elbow Surg. 2016;25(1):78–89.

# Posterior Instability of the Shoulder

# 18

Blandine Marion, André Thès, and Philippe Hardy

## Contents


18.1 **Introduction** 143

18.2 **Anatomy and Pathogenesis of Posterior Instability of the Shoulder** 144
18.2.1 Traumatic Posterior Dislocation 144
18.2.2 Recurrent Posterior Instability (Posterior Subluxations) 144

18.3 **Pathogenesis and Anatomy** 145
18.3.1 Soft Tissue Defects 147
18.3.2 What to Remember 147

18.4 **Clinical Evaluation** 149

18.5 **Radiological Examination** 150

18.6 **Treatment** 151
18.6.1 Surgical Treatment: What Are the Available Surgical Treatments? 151

18.7 **Treatment of Traumatic Posterior Dislocations** 151
18.7.1 Reduction 152
18.7.2 Anterior Deltopectoral Approach 152
18.7.3 Posterior Approach 153
18.7.4 Stabilization 153
18.7.5 McLaughlin Technique 154
18.7.6 Filling the Humeral Impression Defect with a Bone Graft 155
18.7.7 Rotational Osteotomy of the Humerus 156
18.7.8 Posterior Iliac Bone Block 157
18.7.9 Total Shoulder Arthroplasty 157

18.8 **Treatment of Recurrent Posterior Instability** 158
18.8.1 General Information 158
18.8.2 Surgical Bone Repair Techniques 159
18.8.3 Repair of the Labrum Associated with Capsular Plication 166
18.8.4 Isolated Posterior Capsular Plication 166
18.8.5 Rotator Interval Closure 166
18.8.6 Postoperative Follow-Up and Physical Therapy 167

**Conclusion** 167

**References** 167

**Suggested Reading** 167



B. Marion, MD • A. Thès, MD
P. Hardy, MD, PhD (✉)
Hopital Ambroise Pare Universite Paris Ile de France Ouest, 9, Avenue Charles de Gaulle, 92100 Boulogne, France
e-mail: ph.hardy@aphp.fr;
http://www.paris-ouest-orthopedie.com


## 18.1 Introduction

Posterior shoulder instability is rare, representing less than 5% of all shoulder dislocations, and its diagnosis is often delayed. There is very little consensus on the classification and terminology for this entity which is characterized by several factors that may be present in different degrees. The clinical presentation of posterior instability is not as clear as anterior instability, and numerous patients presenting with posterior instability may not be diagnosed or may be treated for other conditions. Thus, the presence of trauma, the association of constitutional laxity, the uni- or multidirectional features of the instability, the ability to voluntarily reproduce posterior instability, and the psychological context of the patient are all factors that may be more or less involved. Recent progress in the understanding of posterior


© ISAKOS 2017


A.B. Imhoff, F.H. Savoie III (eds.), *Shoulder Instability Across the Life Span*,
DOI 10.1007/978-3-662-54077-0_18

instability has helped more clearly define the possible treatment options by taking into account the disease, the pathogenesis, as well as the diagnostic and therapeutic means available.

To establish a therapeutic strategy, three fundamental questions must be asked:

What is the main cause of the posterior instability? In other words, traumatic lesions must be differentiated from recurrent instability (subluxation, multidirectional hyperlaxity).

When is surgical treatment necessary?

Which surgical technique should be used (soft tissue repair, bone surgery)?

A full medical history and physical examination associated with specific imaging tests are necessary to determine the exact pathogenesis and the appropriate treatment options in these cases.

Several variables should be taken into account during patient assessment, including the mechanism of injury (true traumatic posterior dislocation, posterior subluxation, cumulative microtraumas), the direction of instability (posterior, posteroinferior, or multidirectional), and the model of instability (voluntary or involuntary). These factors will help define a treatment strategy that is adapted to each type of posterior instability.

## 18.2 Anatomy and Pathogenesis of Posterior Instability of the Shoulder

Successful treatment of posterior instability of the shoulder should begin by identifying all structural anomalies in the involved shoulder including a combination of several possible lesions in the labrum, the capsule, the ligaments, and the rotator cuffs.

Traumatic posterior dislocations must be clearly differentiated from posterior subluxations (or recurrent posterior instability) because the anatomical lesions and therapeutic options of the two differ markedly.

### 18.2.1 Traumatic Posterior Dislocation

Traumatic posterior dislocation is secondary to a traumatic episode and is usually associated with an impression defect of the humeral head. This may occur following direct trauma in young athletes or after a fall (road or domestic accident) onto a flexed, adducted, internally rotated arm, as well as from a violent contraction of the internal rotator muscles during a seizure or electric shock.

Treatment is determined by the size of the cartilage defect and the delay in diagnosis, which is frequently observed in so-called chronic dislocations (locked dislocations).

The limit between acute and chronic dislocation is 3–6 weeks depending on the authors. This notion is important because it determines the treatment strategy.

Posterior dislocation can be associated with a fracture of the tuberosity of the surgical neck of the humerus resulting in two-, three-, or four-fragment dislocation fractures which are outside the scope of this chapter and which may be treated with standard internal fixation.

### 18.2.2 Recurrent Posterior Instability (Posterior Subluxations)

This is a distinct entity that is not necessarily associated with trauma and whose management is specific, including conservative treatment (physical therapy) or surgical posterior reconstruction techniques of the shoulder. The patient presents with pain and/or instability which usually occurs during anterior elevation, internal rotation, and adduction.

Posterior subluxations are considered to be *traumatic* if there has been an identifiable injury or *atraumatic* even if they are secondary to cumulative microtraumas.

*Atraumatic posterior subluxations* are divided into *voluntary or involuntary* instability:

- Atraumatic voluntary subluxations are considered to be recurrent and intentional or non-intentional.
- Atraumatic involuntary subluxations are positional and demonstrable by the patient or non-positional and not demonstrable by the patient.

Although they may seem complicated, these classifications are essential because they determine whether surgical treatment is needed. Thus, voluntary intentional atraumatic subluxations suggest a psychiatric context which excludes surgical treatment, while surgery may be indicated in certain voluntary unintentional subluxations if physical therapy fails.

Recurrent posterior instability can be *unidirectional* or one element of *multidirectional* laxity. Although the posterior component may play a role in true symptomatic multidirectional instability (different degrees of anterior, posterior, and inferior instability together), this is rare. Generally, multidirectional laxity includes symptomatic posterior instability, frequently associated with inferior laxity.

Thus, certain authors consider posterior instability associated with inferior laxity, whose symptoms may be difficult to identify, to be bidirectional instability to distinguish it from real multidirectional instability (on all three planes) or pure recurrent unidirectional posterior instability where inferior involvement frequently goes unrecognized.

## 18.3 Pathogenesis and Anatomy

Anatomical posterior lesions may present as isolated labral lesions or be associated with true avulsion of the posterior capsular periosteum (reverse/posterior Bankart lesions), capsular laxity which is frequently posteroinferior, bone lesions such as posterior glenoid fractures or defects, or an anterior humeral head impression defect (McLaughlin lesion) (Fig. 18.1). These lesions may be encountered depending on the type of instability.

The pathogenesis of atraumatic posterior instability is a subject of debate, and several anatomical structures are involved (bone or soft tissue defects).

**Bone Defects** Bone abnormalities include excessive humeral and glenoid retroversion and glenoid dysplasia. Anatomical studies have revealed that normal bone retroversion is approximately −4°. Weishaupt et al. have shown that all patients with recurrent posterior instability of the shoulder had glenoid retroversion (mean 7.8° (3–21.4°)).

Kim et al. showed that loss of chondrolabral containment was always present in shoulders with symptoms of posterior instability (Fig. 18.2).

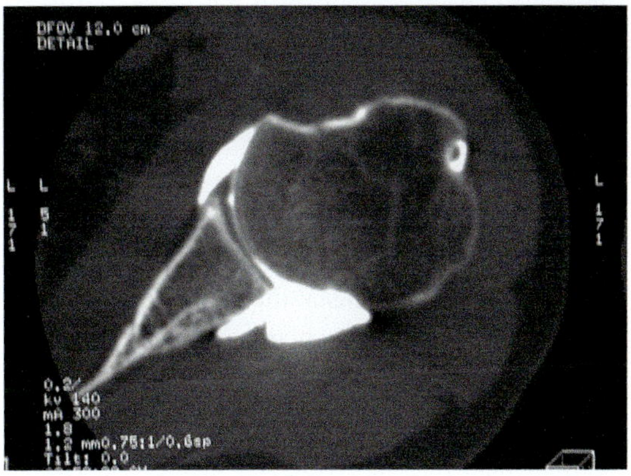

Fig. 18.1 Arthro-CT showing an anterior Hill-Sachs lesion and a posterior Bankart lesion

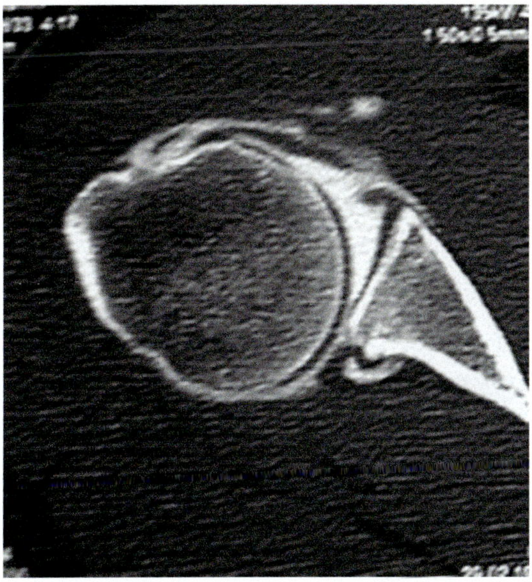

Fig. 18.2 Arthro-CT showing a typical Kim lesion

They evaluated four measurements to determine bony containment of the scapulohumeral articulation (bony and chondrolabral version of the glenoid, height of the labrum, and glenoid depth) measured on T2-weighted MR arthrography in 33 shoulders presenting with atraumatic posterior instability (subluxation). The measurements were compared to 33 age-matched control patients with no glenohumeral abnormalities. The angles of version of the bony and chondrolabral portions of the glenoid were measured on three consecutive planes (superior 25%, middle 50%, and inferior 75% in relation to the superior glenoid labrum) perpendicular to the long axis of the glenoid. Although the posterior instability group had greater retroversion of both the bony and chondrolabral portion of the glenoid on the middle and inferior planes, the chondrolabral portion of the glenoid had more retroversion than the bony portion on the inferior plane. The height of the posterior portion of the labrum was decreased on the inferior plane in the group with shoulder instability. Glenoid depth in the middle and inferior planes was significantly shallower in the group with instability.

Thus, the loss of containment in the chondrolabral portion of the glenoid in the middle and inferior planes is consistently found in shoulders with atraumatic posterior instability, and it is mainly due to a loss of posterior labral height (Fig. 18.3).

According to Kim et al., the loss of chondrolabral containment is due to cumulative microtraumas on the posterior glenoid labrum, which is initially a normal size until retroversion gradually develops by a mechanism of "rim loading" (Fig. 18.4). With the loss of chondrolabral height,

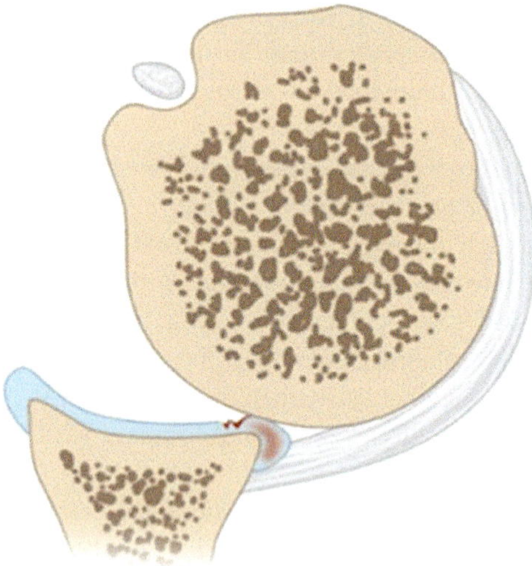

**Fig. 18.4** "Rim loading": A labral lesion develops from cumulative subluxations of the humeral head on the posterior glenoid labrum. This stress on the posterior labrum first produces retroversion of the labrum and then a stress fracture and finally posterior labral detachment

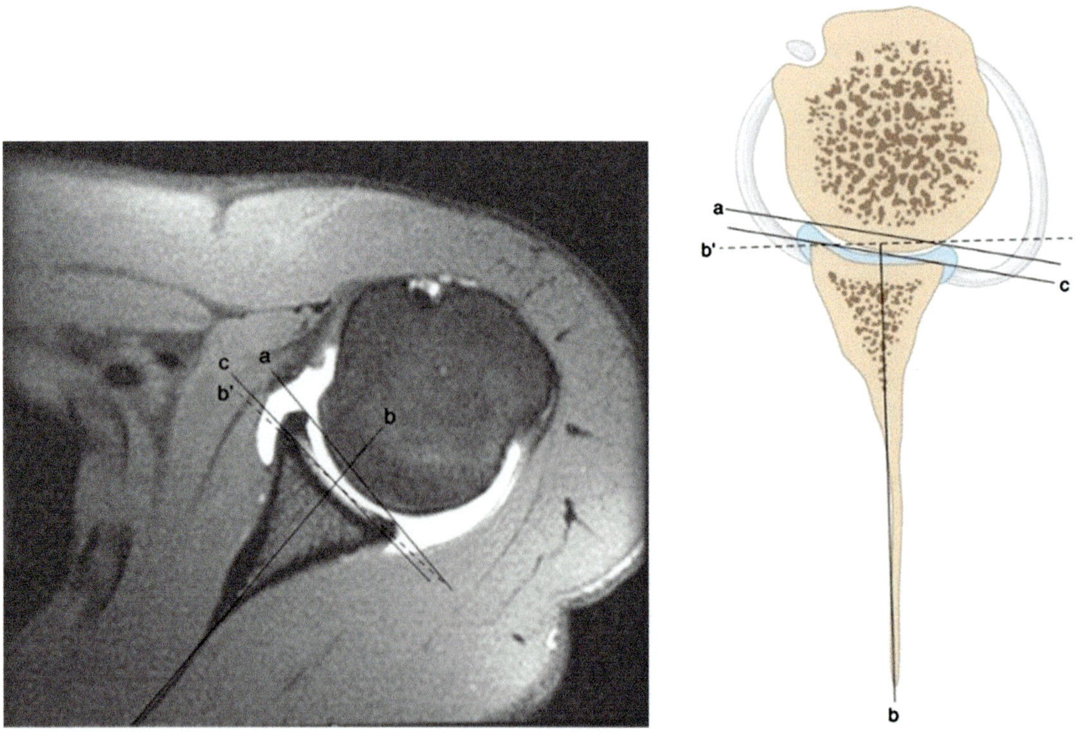


**Fig. 18.3** Figure showing measurement of glenoid chondrolabral and bony version. (Seung-Ho Kim et al. [1]) (**a**) Chondrolabral glenoid plane, (**b**) plane of the body of the scapula (*b'*) plane perpendicular to *b*, (**c**) plane of the bony glenoid. The angle between *a* and *b'* (perpendicular to *b*) represents chondrolabral glenoid version. The angle between *c* and *b'* represents bony glenoid version

the labrum loses its function as a dynamic stabilizer of the shoulder and less effectively preserves centering of the scapulohumeral joint.

### 18.3.1 Soft Tissue Defects

Soft tissue defects include incompetent rotator interval structures such as the coracohumeral and superior and inferior glenohumeral ligaments.

In general, the consensus on the pathogenesis of posterior atraumatic instability is excessive capsular laxity.

A lesion of the glenoid labrum reinforces scapulohumeral congruence by doubling the depth of the glenoid. Any change in chondrolabral integrity can disturb scapulohumeral rhythm and favor the development of posterior instability.

*Kim et al.* reported that all patients who underwent arthroscopic surgery for posterior instability had various degrees of damage to the posterior and inferior glenoid labrum.

Labral lesions were classified into four types:

*Type I:* Incomplete detachment, the posterior labrum is separated from the glenoid but is not medially displaced. This type is more frequent in traumatic posterior instability than in multidirectional instability.

*Type II:* A posterior marginal crack, which is frequently called a "Kim lesion" and which is an incomplete and unidentified avulsion of the posterior labrum.

*Type III:* Chondrolabral erosion.

*Type IV:* Labral flap tear (Fig. 18.5).

The "Kim lesion" corresponds to a superficial tear between the posterior labrum and the glenoid cartilage, without complete detachment of the labrum. The posterior labrum has lost its normal height and become flattened, resulting in glenoid chondrolabral retroversion. Arthroscopic palpation identifies fluctuation of the posterior labrum revealing defective attachment of the deep portion of this structure.

The hypothesis of the pathogenesis of the Kim lesion is based on a theory of repetitive "rim loading." Because the posterior capsule is attached to the inferior portion of the posterior labrum, posterior and inferior loading first affects the inferior portion of the posterior labrum and the insertions of the deep portion of the labrum. Moreover, loading on the posterior-inferior portion of the labrum during posterior subluxation is less than that in anterior instability, which explains why the labral tear only involves the deep portion of the labral insertion and does not extend to the superficial portion. "Rim loading" of the humeral head on the posterior labrum during repetitive subluxation creates a shear force between the bony glenoid and the labrum, resulting in the development of a marginal crack in the chondrolabral junction. Thus the triad of indications for a Kim lesion includes a marginal crack or erosion, chondrolabral retroversion, and incomplete unidentified avulsion. A Kim lesion is fairly similar to an intratendinous tear of the cuff tendon, which is frequently overlooked or not identified during an initial arthroscopic examination.

The four types of labral lesions represent different degrees of severity. Over time a "Kim lesion" can develop into a *type IV* lesion due to complete detachment when a marginal crack extends to the deep part of the tear.

The marginal crack present in posterior instability is different from similar lesions which are often found under other conditions, such as degenerative lesions. Thus, the marginal crack itself is not a sign of posterior instability. Symptomatic inferior and posterior subluxations with a positive Jerk Test (painful clunk) confirm a diagnosis of true posterior instability.

### 18.3.2 What to Remember

Capsular laxity alone cannot explain the symptoms associated with atraumatic posterior instability. Loss of chondrolabral containment is always found in shoulders with posterior instability and is the result of cumulative microtraumas to the posterior labrum. With the loss of chondrolabral containment, the static stabilizer of the shoulder loses its function, and the dynamic stabilizers of the shoulder are less effective in centering the humeral head in the glenohumeral joint.

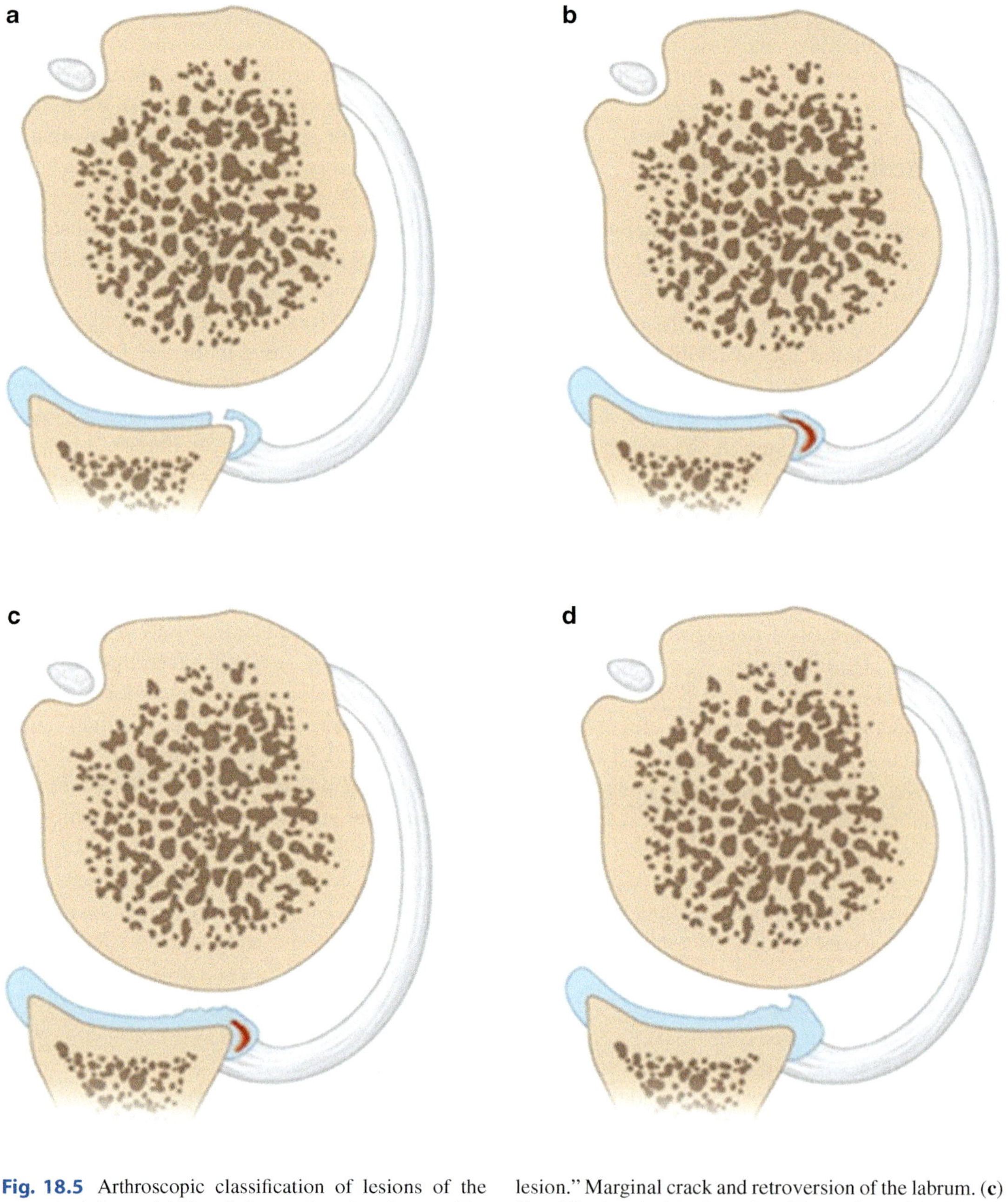


**Fig. 18.5** Arthroscopic classification of lesions of the posterior labrum. (**a**) Type I: incomplete detachment. The posterior labrum is detached from the glenoid but there is no displacement. (**b**) Type II: marginal crack or "Kim lesion." Marginal crack and retroversion of the labrum. (**c**) Type III: chondrolabral erosion. The surface of the labrum is frayed and its deep portion is loose. (**d**) Type IV: mobile labral tear, "flap tear"

Different types of labral lesions may be found in patients with posterior instability of the shoulder and have been classified by Kim.

The Kim lesion corresponds to a tear between the posterior labrum and the glenoid cartilage without complete detachment of the labrum.

The posterior labrum loses its normal height and becomes flat, with progressive retroversion of the chondrolabral glenoid.

Palpation of the lesion identifies fluctuation of the posterior labrum and reveals a loose attachment of the deep portion of this structure.

## 18.4 Clinical Evaluation

Careful investigation of the patient's medical history can provide information on the direction, the mechanism, and the severity of instability. The patient's limitation of daily sports activities or the symptoms at presentation help determine the therapeutic strategy.

Slight discomfort of the shoulder during daily activities such as pain or weakness when carrying something heavy or slight pain following intense physical activity can be managed by conservative medical treatment alone, such as physical therapy.

An in-depth bilateral and comparative examination is indispensable. Examination of the asymptomatic shoulder is performed first, to identify laxity and mobility including examination of range of motion, strength, and scapulohumeral rhythm.

More specific tests for instability include:

The anterior-posterior ("drawer test") is performed with the patient in the sitting position, the shoulder relaxed, and elbow flexed with the forearm resting on the thigh. The examiner, placed behind the patient, seizes the humeral head with one hand while the other hand stabilizes the acromioclavicular portion of the shoulder, as she/he moves the humeral head in an anterior and posterior direction, to evaluate humeral head displacement, patient apprehension, and blocking or cracking suggesting a possible labral lesion.

The "sulcus sign" is an examination with the patient in the same position. The examiner applies downward traction to the lower part of the arm; a visible, more or less marked sulcus or step-off deformity on the inferior rim of the acromion is a sign of inferior laxity of the shoulder.

Two sensitive and specific physical tests, the "*Jerk Test*" and "*Kim Test*," are based on provoking pain by compression of the labral lesion.

The Jerk Test (Fig. 18.6) is performed with the patient in the seated position by stabilizing the scapula of the patient with one hand, with the arm in 90° abduction and neutral rotation. The examiner takes the elbow and presses the humerus in a proximal and axial direction. Then

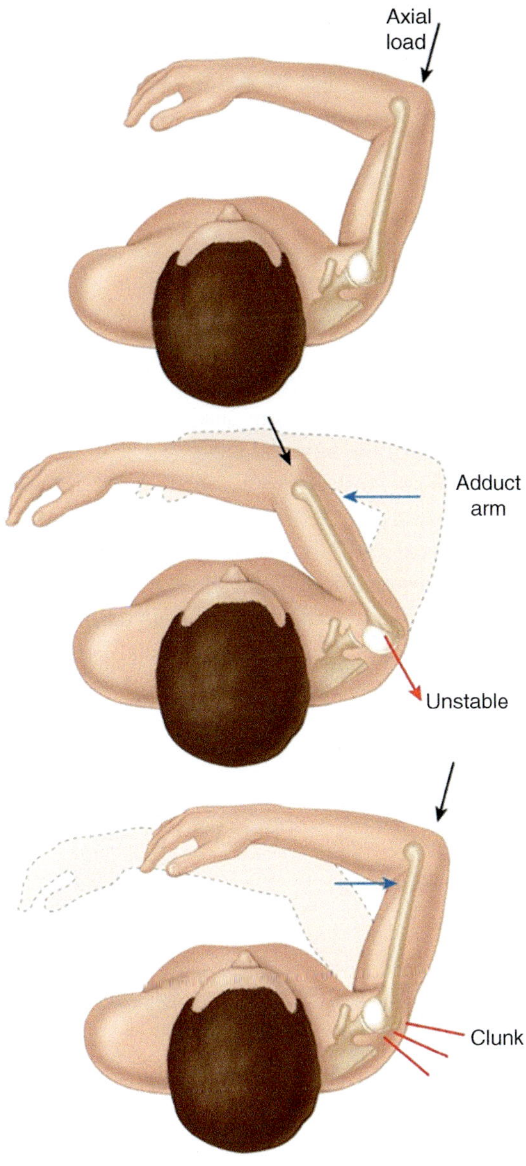


**Fig. 18.6** The Jerk Test. (Matsen et al. [3])

in the same position, the examiner moves the arm into horizontal adduction and internal rotation with one hand as she/he pushes it backward while the other hand stabilizes the scapula. In the presence of posterior instability, a sudden "jerk" may occur when the humeral head springs backward out of its socket and then returns to its original place when it is returned to its original position.

The test is positive when there is a sudden "clunk" of the humeral head. Painful and non-painful positive Jerk Tests are differentiated. A painful and positive Jerk Test is always associated with a posterior labral lesion.

The *Kim Test* (Fig. 18.7) is performed with the patient in the seated position and the arm in 90° abduction. The examiner holds the elbow and the lateral aspect of the proximal arm and then applies a strong axial loading force while elevating the arm diagonally to 45° and applying downward and backward force. Sudden posterior pain indicates a positive test regardless of any associated clunk of the humeral head.

The Kim Test is more sensitive for inferior labral lesions, while the Jerk Test is more sensitive for posterior labral lesions.

The Kim and Jerk Tests should be interpreted in relation to two components: pain and "clunk" response. A pain without the "clunk" sign suggests that there is a posterior labral lesion, while pain with the clunk sign indicates posterior instability with a labral lesion.

## 18.5 Radiological Examination

A radiographic examination includes standard X-rays: AP and axillary lateral views and a comparative Bernageau glenoid profile view to evaluate any bony anomalies suggesting anterior instability.

MR arthrography (MRA) is the most sensitive test to identify lesions of the posterior labrum and obtain a precise assessment of congruence of the humeral head and the posterior glenoid. It is used to identify any loss of labral height or of the posterior cartilage and a labral tear. MRA or CT arthrography improves visualization of labral lesions, as well as visualization of the articular capsule, humeral avulsion glenohumeral ligament (HAGL) injury, associated posterior labrum periosteal sleeve avulsions (POLPSA), and lesions of the subscapularis tendon. These techniques can also be used to evaluate capsule volume which may be increased in the posterior and axillary portions.

Lesions of the posterior labrum may be classified using the classification by Kim et al. (Fig. 18.8).

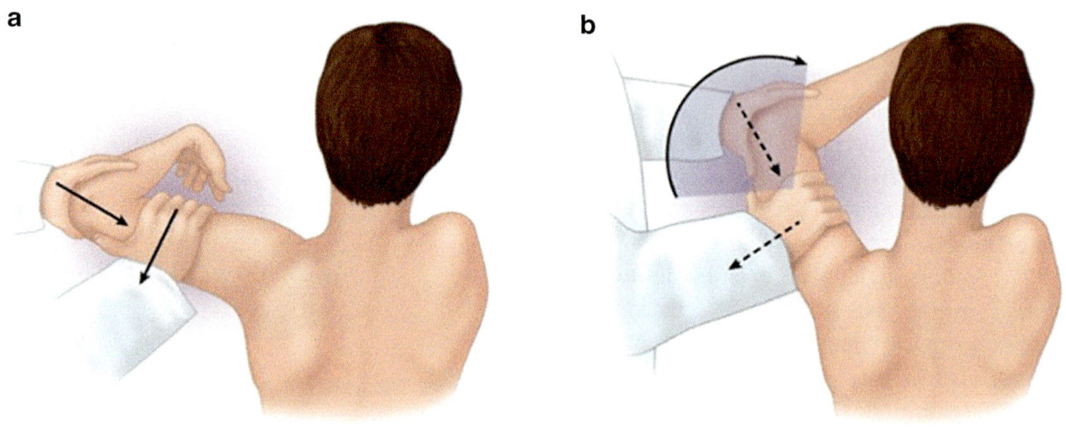


**Fig. 18.7** Kim Test (Kim et al. [2])

**Fig. 18.8** Kim classification

| Arthroscopic classification | | MR Classification | |
|---|---|---|---|
| I | Incomplete stripping | I | Separation without displacement |
| II | Marginal crack | II | Incomplete avulsion |
| III | Chondrolabral erosion | III | Loss of contour |
| IV | Flap tear | | |

The use of CT is limited to cases in which severe bony glenoid lesions are suspected and when precise measurements are needed to plan surgery of the bony portions of the glenoid.

## 18.6 Treatment

### 18.6.1 Surgical Treatment: What Are the Available Surgical Treatments?

Treatment of posterior instability may include osseous surgical procedures (glenoid osteotomy and bone block (Scott technique), rotational osteotomy of the proximal humerus, posterior bone block, bone graft of anterior humeral defects, arthroscopic or open surgical treatment, etc.) and isolated or associated capsuloligamentary procedures (posterior capsulolabral repair (reverse Bankart procedure), posterior capsulorrhaphy alone or associated with bicipital tendon transfer (Boyd), or posterior capsular plicature (posterior Putti-Platt procedure)).

These techniques have been described for isolated posterior instability or for multidirectional laxity. Thus, posterior capsulorrhaphies may be described in a chapter on posterior instability or predominantly posterior multidirectional instabilities.

A comparative analysis of the results in the literature is difficult because of the frequently small size of the study populations which include different types of posterior instability. The combination of surgical techniques, the inclusion of patients who have undergone multiple surgeries, and the frequent association of multidirectional laxity make it difficult to evaluate the different techniques. Depending on the series, the results of open posterior surgical stabilization techniques are satisfactory in 50–95% of cases.

More recently, advances in arthroscopic techniques have provided better understanding of the pathogenic mechanisms of these lesions and allowed the development of diverse capsulolabral repair techniques (Wolff, Mac Intyre, etc.).

## 18.7 Treatment of Traumatic Posterior Dislocations

Humeral displacement is posterosuperior subacromial in most cases, while displacement below the scapular spine is rare.

Osseous lesions mainly involve the humeral head with an impression fracture of the anteromedial aspect of the humeral head called a McLaughlin lesion ("reverse Hill-Sachs lesion" by Anglo-Saxon authors) whose size and depth partly determine the treatment indications, especially if chronic locked dislocation is present.

Osseous posterior glenoid lesions are rare and always limited.

Posterior capsular lesions are probably always present in the form of detachment of the posteroinferior labrum with avulsion of the posterior capsular periosteum (reverse Bankart lesion):

- Posterior cuff tears have rarely been reported in the literature, while supraspinatus lesions have been described, mainly in the form of partial-thickness tears of the deep portion of this structure.
- Anterior soft tissue lesions (joint capsule and subscapularis) have been described by Vichard and Samilson. An anterior joint capsule tear associated with a subscapularis tear favors intra-articular dislocation of the long head of the biceps and irreducible dislocation (Velghe).
- A fracture of the lesser tuberosity can be associated with posterior dislocation, and when this feature is identified on radiography, this diagnosis should be looked for.

It is essential to determine how old the dislocation is to avoid performing closed reduction in a chronic dislocation because the risk of epiphyseal fracture is high. Neviaser and Moseley established 3 weeks as the limit between acute/recent and chronic/old undiagnosed dislocations.

The main criteria to determine the therapeutic strategy are the time since the injury, the size of the bone defect, the age and activity of the patient, and the physician's usual practices. Most of the surgical techniques described here have been used for treatment of traumatic posterior dislocations (locked or not) or for recurrent posterior instability.

The therapeutic options have been gradually updated in the past few decades, and they will be described in relation to their optimal indications; certain techniques are indicated for various types of posterior instability.

### 18.7.1 Reduction

Several parameters must be evaluated before reduction:

- The patient's general condition and functional status
- An absence of associated fractures on preoperative X-rays
- Dislocation has been formally identified as chronic
- Precise evaluation of active range of motion deficit
- The presence of osteoporosis on X-rays
- The patient's ability to follow a functional physical therapy protocol

The possibility of excluding this option in elderly patients with limited functional needs or medical problems that could make physical therapy difficult should be considered. Posterior dislocation may be amazingly well tolerated in elderly patients who have very little pain and who have sufficient elevation of the shoulder for their daily activities.

Nevertheless, the external rotation deficit must be tolerable and allow bringing the hand to the mouth and if possible to the forehead. Excluding this treatment option in these patients has been reported in a study by Hawkins in seven cases who received conservative functional treatment and who were followed up for 5.5 years, with no clinical worsening.

Closed reduction can be attempted if the deficit is <25% of the articular surface, if the injury is less than 3 weeks old, and in the absence of associated fractures.

The techniques are the same for chronic locked dislocations as for recent dislocations, but reduction is more difficult, is less frequently successful, and is more frequently complicated by fractures.

Performed under general anesthesia with the patient in the supine position and the muscles relaxed, reduction is obtained by axial traction on the limb which is slightly flexed, in internal rotation and adduction, aided by direct pressure on the posterior portion of the shoulder.

If the humeral head is locked in the posterior glenoid rim, gentle medial rotation should free the cuff and the posterior capsule, lateral traction should remove the humeral head from the glenoid rim, and then careful lateral rotation should achieve reduction.

Stability of the shoulder is tested and if it is stable during internal rotation, the arm is immobilized for 3 weeks in neutral rotation. The patient is not allowed to put the hand behind the body during this time. If the humeral head defect is minimal or slight, reduction is often easy and stability is satisfactory even in internal rotation. Recurrence is rare, normal function is usually recovered, and the bone deficit tends to fill in spontaneously.

In the presence of residual instability or a significant bone deficit (but <25%), the arm is immobilized in slight external rotation (20°) at 20° abduction and 10–15° extension for 6 weeks. Immobilization can be shorter in patients over the age of 60.

Open reduction should be performed:

- If closed reduction is unsuccessful
- If dislocation occurred more than 3 weeks before
- In the presence of open dislocation
- For dislocation with a humeral head impression defect of > 30%
- For dislocation with a fracture of the neck or the lesser tuberosity

The anterior and posterior surgical approaches have both advantages and disadvantages.

### 18.7.2 Anterior Deltopectoral Approach

The patient is installed in the beach-chair position, and the arm should be mobile during the operation. Deltopectoral incision: because the upper limb is in internal rotation, the long head of the biceps tendon is the correct reference to identify the rotator interval that is open to reach the joint. In locked forms of dislocation, mobilization of the humeral head is often difficult, and sectioning of the coracohumeral and superior glenohumeral ligaments, which are frequently retracted, greatly facilitates humeral head reduction.

Sometimes a tenotomy of the upper part of the subscapularis muscle can improve articular exposure. The dislocation is reduced under visual control by unblocking the humeral head from the posterior glenoid rim with a movement of internal rotation followed by lateral traction and external rotation of the limb while sometimes placing posterior pressure directly on the humeral head.

If the reduction is stable (small bone defects), the rotator interval is closed and the shoulder is immobilized. In case of instability, Cicak transfers the superior third of the subscapularis to the defect with transosseous sutures knotted behind the intertubercular sulcus. The shoulder is then immobilized in slight lateral rotation for 3 weeks.

The use of the deltopectoral approach may be indicated if a subscapularis transfer is planned because of a large humeral head defect. Articular exposure is obtained by a subscapularis tenotomy or an osteotomy of the lesser tuberosity (cf McLaughlin technique).

The anterior approach makes it possible to release any existing interposition of the long head of the biceps which may make reduction difficult.

### 18.7.3 Posterior Approach

This approach is recommended by certain authors (Dubousset) who feel that the anterior approach does not allow reconstruction on the posterior capsuloligamentary plane, which could favor the development of recurrent posterior instability.

The patient is installed in the lateral decubitus position, and the cutaneous incision follows the inferior border of the scapular spine and then curves laterally along the posterior border of the deltoid. The posterior deltoid is detached and reflected downward and outward. The emergence of the axillary nerve from the quadrangular space is identified. The teres minor and the infraspinatus are vertically sectioned, and then the joint capsule is opened to expose the posteromedial articular surface of the humeral head that is dislocated behind the glenoid. The arm is medially rotated to expose the glenoid and the anterior defect of the humeral head. Reduction of old dislocations can be difficult because of capsuloligamentary and anterior muscle retractions, and this anterior release is the most difficult part of these posterior approaches.

For the author, the posterior approach makes it possible to fill the defect, if necessary, with a cancellous iliac graft. Closing is obtained by reinsertion of the posterior capsule on the posterior glenoid rim by reverse Bankart repair with a horizontal mattress suture of the excess internal capsule. The infraspinatus and teres minor muscles are attached by a horizontal mattress suture, and then the posterior deltoid is reinserted into the scapular spine.

**Remark** In the case of small impression defects, closed reduction is easily obtained, outcome is often favorable, and recurrent posterior dislocation is not frequent because of spontaneous filling of the defect and posterior capsulolabral healing. Systematic repair of posterior capsular lesions does not appear to be indicated. Moreover, most stabilizing techniques are performed by anterior approach which gives them a clear advantage.

### 18.7.4 Stabilization

For impression defects between 25 and 45% of the articular surface or if reduction is unstable, surgical stabilization is essential.

The later the diagnosis, the greater the risk of post-reductional instability.

Although the choice of surgical stabilization technique mainly depends upon the size of the humeral head defect, other parameters must be taken into consideration such as the severity of contraction of the soft tissues, the permeability of the rotator cuffs, the condition of the subscapularis (torn or retracted), or the presence of posterior glenoid lesions that could affect future stability.

### 18.7.5 McLaughlin Technique

In 1952, McLaughlin reported eight cases of patients treated for recurrent posterior dislocation by subscapularis transfer. He later revised these indications to limit this procedure to locked dislocations with a humeral defect and recommended the use of a capsular plicature associated with a posterior bone block in recurrent posterior instabilities.

**Transfer of the Subscapularis Tendon** A deltopectoral incision is made, the superior and inferior portions of the subscapularis tendon are identified, and the medial insertion at the lesser tuberosity is detached. The capsule is opened, and any existing interposing fibrous scar tissue, which is frequent, is removed, to expose the anterior glenohumeral joint space and facilitate placement of retractor which is used as a lever to reduce the posterior dislocation which is blocked on the posterior glenoid surface.

The reduction should be carefully performed to prevent any further cartilage damage. Once reduction is complete, external rotation is released to explore the humeral head and evaluate the severity of the anterior defect and the trophicity of the remaining cartilage. The bottom of the defect is debrided of any interposed fibrous tissue and then abraded with a curette or a motorized drill. Several transosseous tunnels are created at the bottom of the defect, then the subscapularis which has been prepared with several nonresorbable sutures is placed in the bottom of the defect, and the sutures are knotted on the lateral portion of the humeral epiphysis.

This procedure is followed by elbow to body immobilization with the arm in 30° lateral rotation for 4 weeks, and then physical therapy is begun.

#### 18.7.5.1 Transfer of the Subscapularis Pedicled to the Lesser Tuberosity

Hughes and Neer modified the McLaughlin technique by osteotomizing the lesser tuberosity with the attached subscapularis. The first cases were published by Hawkins in 1987.

This variation to the technique has the advantage of providing better filling of the defect by the lesser tuberosity and more secure reinsertion of the subscapularis.

The approach is deltopectoral, and the long head of the biceps tendon serves as a reference for the position of the lesser tuberosity. The rotator interval and the lower edge of the tendon of the subscapularis muscle are identified. The anterior circumflex vessels are ligated. Intra-articular visualization is ensured through the rotator interval. The osteotomy of the lesser tuberosity is performed starting from the bicipital sulcus and extending to the anteromedial defect of the humeral head. The lesser tuberosity including the attached subscapularis is gradually raised to expose the glenohumeral cavity. Reduction of the dislocation can be sometimes difficult and may require extensive arthrolysis and the use of a double-angled retractor or pressing a rugine into the bone defect to help with posterior unblocking of the humeral head. These movements should be made with extreme care to prevent injuring the healthy humeral head cartilage or even fracturing the humeral epiphysis.

The lesser tuberosity is temporarily secured with K-wires. A perioperative X-ray evaluates glenohumeral congruence and the positioning of the K-wires. The tuberosity is attached to the defect with one or two cannulated cancellous screws or with nonabsorbable transosseous sutures if the quality of the tuberosity is poor or if it fragments during screwing.

If the shoulder is stable, the upper limb is immobilized in neutral or slightly external rotation for 4 weeks.

#### 18.7.5.2 Remarks

Although Neer's modified procedure may seem attractive, the osteotomy of the lesser tuberosity is sometimes difficult because of changes in the position of the anatomic structures from locked posterior dislocation. Moreover, a simple subscapularis tenotomy is easy to perform with modern and reliable methods of fixation.

For Mestdagh this procedure should be limited to impression defects <1/3 of the surface of the humeral joint. The use of the McLaughlin technique in dislocations without bone defects makes it necessary to drill a tunnel that could harm the joint on the anterior portion of the neck.

### 18.7.6 Filling the Humeral Impression Defect with a Bone Graft

In 1967 Dubousset emphasized the importance of restoring the spherical shape of the humeral head and recommended elevating the impacted cartilage and an autogenic cancellous bone graft or an iliac corticocancellous graft to fill the defect created by the impression fracture.

This therapeutic option was developed by Gerber in 1996 who recommended using a cryopreserved allograft that avoided the inconveniences of the McLaughlin procedure: disturbance of the normal shoulder anatomy, limitation of internal rotation, and difficulty in case of later shoulder arthroplasty.

#### 18.7.6.1 Allograft Technique

A deltopectoral approach is used. A subscapularis tenotomy and anterior capsulotomy are performed preserving the superior glenohumeral and coracohumeral ligaments if possible. Interposed fibrous scar tissue between the capsule and the humeral head is excised.

There should be no major bony lesions of the posterior glenoid rim or the external rotator muscles, but simple posterior capsular redundancy can be tolerated. The dislocated humeral head is reduced.

In the presence of recurrent posterior instability in internal rotation, filling the impression defect with a cryopreserved femoral head allograft is indicated. A graft is prepared that is large enough to restore sufficient sphericity to the humeral head. The defect should be debrided and prepared. The head is stabilized with two cancellous 3.5 metallic screws or even better buried absorbable screws. If the graft is stable on its own, internal fixation is not absolutely necessary (Fig. 18.9).

The anterior capsule is not repaired, and the subscapularis muscle is debrided of all adhesions

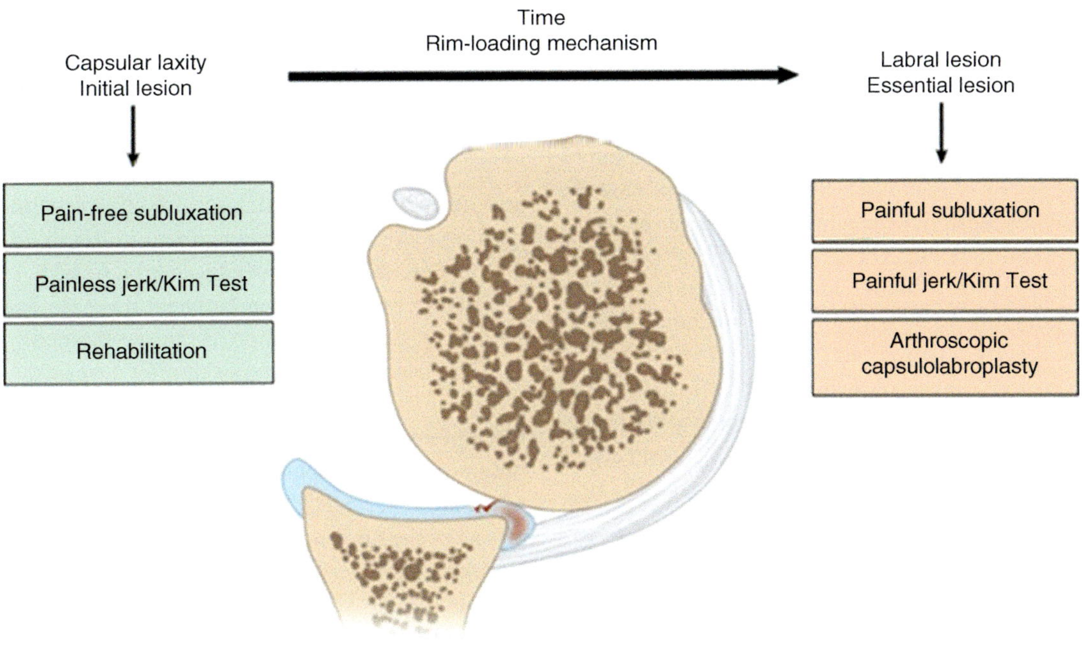


**Fig. 18.9** Radiographic control of an allograft for an anterior Hill-Sachs defect

up to the anterior surface of the scapula and sutured from one end to the other without shortening or lengthening.

The arm is immobilized in a sling with the arm across the body for 6 weeks. Passive mobilization in lateral rotation is possible during this period. Resistance exercises are not begun until the sixth week.

**Remark** Gerber does not recommend this technique if the bone appears to be osteoporotic or in the presence of degenerative lesions of the remaining cartilage of the humeral head or of the glenoid cartilage. They did not report any necrosis of the allograft after a follow-up of 68 months.

The results seem to be similar to the McLaughlin procedure without modifying the anatomy of the humeral epiphysis.

### 18.7.7 Rotational Osteotomy of the Humerus

The rotational osteotomy of the humerus has been successfully performed for the treatment of recurrent anterior instability associated with a large Hill-Sachs defect. The use of this procedure in posterior instability has only been reported by a few authors in small series.

For certain authors, excessive retroversion of the superior end of the humerus can increase the risk of posterior instability of the shoulder in medial rotation. The goal of this procedure is therefore to obtain anterior rotation of the humeral head by performing a subcapital osteotomy of the superior end of the humerus, based on the osteotomy proposed by Weber to treat anterior instability. The main interest of this procedure seems to be to prevent a humeral head defect anterior to the area of impingement with the posterior glenoid rim.

The results of this procedure have mainly been reported by Surin in 1990 in a series of 12 cases.

#### 18.7.7.1 Surgical Technique: Description by Surin

The patient is installed in the beach-chair position and the cutaneous incision is deltopectoral.

The approach to the superior metaphysis of the humerus is subperiosteal extending downward to the humeral insertion of the pectoralis major.

In the presence of locked posterior dislocation, an anterior arthrotomy is performed after tenotomy of subscapularis, and then the dislocation is reduced. If closed reduction was successful, the arthrotomy is not absolutely necessary.

The osteotomy is subcapital above the insertion of the pectoralis major, leaving a portion of the epiphysis to receive three humeral head screws that will be placed at the superior end of a T-shaped AO plate which is used for final fixation of the osteotomy (the use of an angled blade plate or a Milch-type plate is best).

Once the superior part of the plate has been screwed into the humeral head, with the forearm perpendicular to the plane of the surgical table, two K-wires are placed along the site of the osteotomy parallel to the forearm to create a 30° angle.

The osteotomy is then performed with a Gigli saw or an oscillating saw, and the humeral head is rotated externally (or internally for the diaphyseal segment) so that the two K-wires are parallel. The fracture site is compressed and the distal screws are tightened.

**Surgical Follow-Up** The upper limb is immobilized in a sling for 4 weeks, and then physical therapy of the shoulder is begun until full range of motion has been recovered. This procedure provides stable internal fixation, and the possibility of immediate passive movement of the shoulder but external rotation should not be forced.

Sports can begin again between the 12th and 16th week once bone union has been obtained.

The plate is usually removed after 1 year.

**Comments** According to the author, this osteotomy makes it possible to rotate the posterior part of the humeral head forward which prevents the effects of the humeral impression defect described by McLaughlin on the posterior glenoid rim in internal rotation while placing tension on the anterior capsule to limit posterior humeral translation.

However, this procedure has the disadvantage of limiting external rotation which can make the return to physical activities difficult and of increasing internal rotation of the limb as well as laxity of the posterior capsule which can play a role in recurrent posterior instability.

Humeral rotational osteotomy can be considered in rare cases of constitutional retroversion of the humeral head or if the impression defect is between 25 and 45% of the articular surface; however, shoulder arthroplasty is difficult after an osteotomy.

### 18.7.8 Posterior Iliac Bone Block

Although it is usually used in recurrent posterior instability, the results of posterior iliac bone block were reported by Augereau in 1982 for the treatment of locked posterior dislocations using a posterior and an anterior surgical approach.

The patient is installed in the lateral decubitus position, with the arm and scapular girdle swabbed and draped to allow for mobilization during surgery.

*An anterior deltopectoral* approach is first taken to section the coracoacromial ligament and for vertical sectioning of the subscapularis at the humeral insertion. A capsuloligamentary incision is performed along the anatomical neck of the humerus whose size is determined by the difficulty of reduction and to obtain lateral rotation. The anterior deltopectoral approach makes it possible to release anterior capsular and muscular retraction.

*The posterior approach* is a version of Gosset's technique. A transverse incision is made along the external 2/3 of the inferior scapular spine, and the posterior deltoid is detached from its scapular insertion and then reflected to the teres minor muscle. The infraspinatus is detached from outside to inside, taking care not to injure the suprascapular pedicle.

The supraspinatus is reflected upward, and the infraspinatus is carefully pushed downward to expose the posterior capsule and periosteal sleeve which are vertically incised to the projection of the humeral head. The internal capsular flap is detached at the bone to the most medial aspect (root) of the scapular spine to facilitate evaluation of the articular cartilage and confirm the presence of any posterior glenoid rim fracture.

Reduction of atraumatic dislocation requires lateral translation of the humeral head which facilitates posterior unblocking after confirming that there is no interposition of the long head of the biceps. The posterior aspect of the neck of the scapula is abraded, and a cancellous bone graft of 4.5 cm is harvested from the medial ipsilateral iliac crest and is carefully placed at the level of the root of the scapular spine under the vasculonervous pedicle. Sagittal graft stability is obtained by posteroanterior screws.

The upper limb is immobilized in a cast with the arm across the body 70° abduction, in internal or external rotation and slight adduction.

### 18.7.9 Total Shoulder Arthroplasty

Most authors agree that in the presence of posterior dislocations with bone defects of more than 45% of the articular surface, shoulder arthroplasty is indicated if the injury occurred more than 6 months before.

The presence of significant glenoid lesions may be an indication for total shoulder arthroplasty, but in other cases, hemiarthroplasty is preferable, in particular because these injuries frequently occur in patients under the age of 50.

A deltopectoral approach is used with the patient in the beach-chair position. The shoulder should be completely accessible to switch to a posterior approach in case of difficulty with reduction.

For Cheng, the posterior approach makes it possible to cut the posterior humeral head which is located behind the glenoid, thus facilitating reduction (cf schema). The posterior muscular plane (infraspinatus) is then closed, and the procedure continues in front by sectioning the remaining humeral head. The humeral cut is performed in neutral rotation or slight external rotation to limit retroversion of the shoulder replacement and the risk of posterior instability. Glenoid preparation and placement of the components follow standard procedures.

If the arthroplasty shows signs of posterior instability, the upper limb must be immobilized in neutral rotation or slight lateral rotation at 10° or 20° for several weeks to allow the posterior capsule to heal and the lateral rotator muscles to recover. Hawkins and Tanner have suggested performing a posterior plicature to close the capsular pouch and restore satisfactory capsular balance in case of instability of the arthroplasty. Although this technical option has not been validated, it is easy to perform with the posterior approach.

## 18.8 Treatment of Recurrent Posterior Instability

### 18.8.1 General Information

Difficult to diagnose, recurrent posterior instability (posterior subluxations) is much more frequent than traumatic dislocations.

The usual forms must be assessed individually because there is a psychiatric element that cannot be treated surgically. The other forms (not recurrent voluntary and involuntary) are generally assessed together because surgical treatment may be considered if conservative treatment fails.

Capsulolabral and posterior glenoid lesions (reverse Bankart lesions) are more frequent in recurrent instability with an initial episode of trauma and in involuntary atraumatic forms. Atraumatic forms more frequently involve posteroinferior capsular insufficiency.

Rare cases of constitutional morphological anomalies such as excess humeral or glenoid retroversion can favor instability and require specific treatment.

Patients with recurrent posterior instability often present with features of multidirectional laxity that must be diagnosed and treated (cf chapter on pathogenesis and clinical examination).

Physical therapy must always precede surgical treatment. Atraumatic posterior subluxations or those associated with multidirectional laxity respond better to physical therapy than recurrent instabilities secondary to trauma.

In patients with a painless Jerk Test or Kim Test, initial treatment is based on physical therapy, including restoring scapulohumeral kinematics. Conservative treatment associates pain relief; changing activities and patient education; a program to restore muscle strength and endurance to the rotator cuffs, the deltoid, and the periscapular muscles (the different bundles of the trapezius, serratus anterior, rhomboids, levator scapula, pectoralis minor); as well as restoring range of motion and neuromuscular stability. The work of the periscapular muscles and the rotator cuff muscles must be coordinated to obtain a stable glenohumeral joint.

Physical therapy should be continued for 6 months. Although residual posterior instability may persist in certain cases, it is frequently well tolerated. Although the strengthening exercises do not reduce hyperlaxity of the shoulder, they improve overall control and function of the shoulder joint (Fig. 18.10). Well-managed conservative

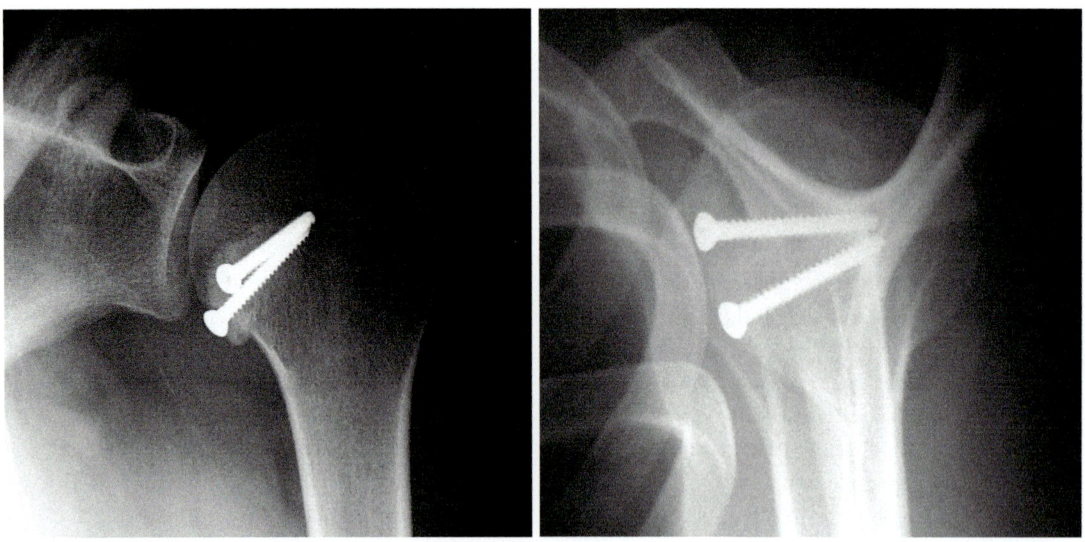

**Fig. 18.10** Natural progression and therapeutic options Kim et al.

treatment involves a long period of physical therapy, including exercises to strengthen the rotator cuff muscles, the deltoids, and the scapular stabilizers. Despite persistent hyperlaxity, the symptoms improve in these patients and they can return to their daily activities. Surgical treatment is indicated in patients with painful Jerk or Kim Tests and in those in whom well-managed conservative treatment fails.

Surgical bone repair procedures will correct, in particular, architectural deformities or posterior glenoid lesions.

Surgical soft tissue repair procedures will often be indicated because of the predominance of posterior capsulolabral lesions. Recent improvements in arthroscopic techniques and material have increased understanding of the pathogenesis of this entity, providing results that are comparable to those with open surgery.

## 18.8.2 Surgical Bone Repair Techniques

### 18.8.2.1 Posterior Bone Blocks

Initially described by Hindenach in 1947 and then Fried in 1949, the posterior iliac bone graft was made popular in France by Gosset. The principle is similar to the procedure Eden-Hybinette described for anterior instabilities and is based on iliac bone graft on the posterior portion of the neck of the scapula, preferably in an extracapsular position and laterally extending the posterior glenoid rim.

The bone graft may also be harvested from the scapular spine by the same posterior approach avoiding having to harvest from the iliac crest.

The posterior bone block should overhang to extend and enlarge the surface of the glenoid. The extension should be limited and equally distributed to the desired height of the glenoid, rather than serve as an actual block. The bone graft should be extracapsular without direct contact with the humeral head to prevent the development of degenerative glenohumeral arthropathy.

Fronek associates the iliac bone block with a posterior capsulorrhaphy if there are bone lesions of the posterior glenoid rim or if the mechanical quality of the posterior capsule is insufficient for capsular repair alone. At present indications for a posterior bone block are the two latter situations.

The position of the bone block on the vertical plane depends on the topography of the lesion (posterosuperior or posteroinferior), if the lesions are mainly found in the posteroinferior quadrant; capsule and bone repair procedures will help strengthen this weaker area.

The unique acromial bone block with a vascularized deltoid flap described by Kouvalchouk will be described separately.

#### Posterior Iliac Bone Block

Two surgical techniques are possible, either an iliac graft by open surgery or an arthroscopy procedure.

1. *Iliac bone block by open surgery*

The patient can be installed in the ventral or lateral decubitus position with the upper limb completely draped to allow for movement during surgery. The surgical field should include the ipsilateral posterior iliac crest.

The cutaneous incision is curved and 12–15 cm long, parallel to the scapular spine extending to the posterolateral edge of the acromion.

For most authors, the posterior portion of the deltoid is detached from the scapular spine, leaving enough muscle tissue to perform later repair. This approach has the disadvantage of weakening a muscle that is responsible for posterior stability of the shoulder. Splitting the deltoid in line with the fibers, as recommended by Wirth, avoids this, but does not provide as wide a surgical field. Sectioning of the deltoid can be avoided by releasing the inferior part of the posterior deltoid bundle which is reflected upward, with the upper limb in 90° abduction.

The posterior portion of the external rotator cuff muscles is exposed. The type of approach taken to gain access to the capsule depends on later positioning of the graft.

Detachment of the infraspinatus from the humerus provides better exposure of the capsule (sectioning of the teres minor is never necessary) but it may hamper later muscle function.

Careful opening of the interval separating the infraspinatus from the teres minor provides sufficient access to the inferior portion of the glenoid and is the first choice in the presence of posteroinferior instability.

In cases of posterosuperior instability, the space separating the supraspinatus from the infraspinatus should be dissected to optimize exposure of the superior glenoid and to control the suprascapular pedicle.

A vertical or horizontal capsulotomy is performed slightly outside of the joint space for intra-articular exploration.

The periosteum is sectioned at the glenoid to scrape and prepare the supra- and infraspinatus fossae. The medial capsule is released from the posterior portion of the glenoid but not completely detached.

A U-shaped bone graft, 2–4.5 cm long depending on the author, is harvested from the posterior iliac crest to be transferred to the lateral border of the scapular spine.

Mowery positions the bone graft so that it extends over the posterior border of the joint by approximately 1.5 cm in an intra-articular position. Essadki and Dumontier create a U-shaped graft to press upon the lateral border of the scapular spine with a lateral extension of 1 cm in an extracapsular position, being careful not to damage the suprascapular pedicle.

The graft is screwed to the neck of the scapula with one or two screws facing toward the tip of coracoid process and on the anterior cortex to improve stability and compression of the graft.

The surgeon confirms that there are no limitations in range of motion, conflict with the humeral head, or residual posterior instability.

The capsule is then closed and the muscular plane is carefully repaired.

Postoperatively, the upper limb is immobilized in a sling between 30 and 45°abduction in neutral rotation or in lateral rotation at 45° depending on the author. Pendulum exercises are begun after 4 weeks, and active physical therapy is begun at 6 weeks.

2. *Arthroscopic iliac bone block*

The patient is installed in the beach-chair position under general anesthesia. Axial traction is obtained with a specific device for this purpose.

The 30° arthroscope is introduced in a standard posterior portal at the soft spot for intra-articular visualization and evaluation of all injuries (labral, bicipital and rotator cuff lesions, glenohumeral chondropathies).

To improve the view, an additional anterolateral portal is created anterior to the supraspinatus in the rotator interval.

The posterior scapular neck is prepared using a radiofrequency device (taking care not to injure the suprascapular nerve). The scapular neck is abraded until cortical bone is reached. The posterior cutaneous incision is widened 2–3 cm. A horizontal split is performed between the infraspinatus and the teres minor with a radiofrequency device at the equator of the scapula. The passageway in the deltoid can be bluntly widened with the surgeon's finger.

The bone graft of 2.5–3 cm × 1 cm × 1 cm is then harvested from the ipsilateral iliac crest.

The surgeon then follows the instructions for the material to create an arthroscopic anterior coracoid bone block developed by Dr L. Lafosse (Bristow-Latarjet Instabilité de l'épaule Système; DePuy Mitek). Two 1.5 mm diameter K-wires are put in place using a drill guide, so that the tips protrude from the angled cancellous surface of the superior cortex of the iliac crest and are then remodeled with the oscillating saw to adapt it to the curve of the neck of the posterior glenoid.

The two wires are used as a guide to drill the holes in the coracoid. The K-wires and drill are removed. Both of the holes are tapped for good compression of the graft when it is tightened.

The graft is then reduced on the positioning device by cannulated 3.5 mm screws.

The prepared graft is then introduced through the posterior portal after making sure that the soft tissue passage is the correct size. The arthroscope is introduced through the anterolateral portal.

The graft is then maneuvered to the posterior glenoid neck with a positioning cannula.

The lateral surface of the iliac crest graft is aligned with the posterior glenoid rim. Once the graft is in the correct position on the glenoid neck, 2 K-wires, 2.5 mm long, are positioned using a cannula for fixation, passing by the graft and the screws. The inferior screw is then removed and a 3.2 mm cannulated drill is passed over the K-wire which has been left in the correct position on the glenoid. The drill is carefully advanced to the anterior cortex. The drill is removed and the inferior screw is reinserted taking care to leave the inferior K-wire in place. The screw should not be more than 32–36 mm long, and correct positioning must be confirmed in any screw longer than 40 mm because this means that the angle of the screw is too large in relation to the glenoid resulting in incorrect positioning of the graft and an overlap that is probably too large.

The same step is repeated for the superior screw. The K-wires are removed once the graft is in place.

If necessary, the posterior labrum and the capsule are reattached to the glenoid rim with suture anchors using a technique that is similar to the standard arthroscopic labral repair. Postoperatively patients are immobilized at 20° abduction in neutral rotation for 6 weeks. Passive mobilization of the shoulder and the hand can begin on postoperative day 1.

However, exercises should not be painful, with no internal rotation exercises. Active mobilization begins 3 weeks after surgery.

### Acromial Bone Block with a Vascularized Deltoid Pedicle: Kouvalchouk

For Kouvalchouk, this technique has the advantages of a posterior bone block and Neer's capsulorrhaphy in cases of multidirectional laxity without limiting articular range of motion or the classic complications of these grafts (necrosis, overhang, and scapulohumeral arthritis).

A postoperative evaluation has shown that harvesting the flap and mobilization of the posterior deltoid fibers do not influence the theoretical maximum strength of the posterior deltoid.

The patient is installed in the ventral decubitus position. A circular arc incision is made along the scapular spine to the acromial angle where it curves to follow the direction of the deltoid fibers. The posterior deltoid fibers are detached for 5–6 cm to the posterosuperior angle of the acromion, and then the muscle fibers are separated for 4–5 cm to compose the posterior border of the future flap. The anterior border of the flap is separated for approximately 2.5 cm in front of the posterior border. The acromial portion of the graft is created from the superior portion of the acromion to be 2 cm wide. With a chisel or a small motorized saw, the acromial block is harvested from the superior half of the bone while preserving the insertion of the muscle flap. The bone block therefore measures 2 cm × 2.5 cm and is 3–4 mm thick.

The graft has superior, cortical, and inferior cancellous sides and it is pedicled to a muscle flap; the bone graft and the flap are reflected.

The approach to the posterior capsule is obtained by a reverse L section of the infraspinatus or dissection of the muscle in line with its fibers.

The posterior capsule is opened to explore the joint. In the presence of predominantly posterior multidirectional laxity, a capsulotomy is performed using the Neer technique by drawing two capsular flaps that will then be crossed.

The posterior border of the glenoid is then abraded and prepared, and the acromial graft is attached with the cancellous side against the scapula with two cortical screw and washer constructs or with a small locking plate. The graft must be positioned at the middle inferior third of the glenoid and not extend beyond the posterior border or by only a few millimeters, except if a mechanical effect is looked for, in the presence of a posterior fracture or severe dysplasia.

The infraspinatus is secured with or without a mattress suture depending on whether myoplasty is the goal. Mobilization of the shoulder and the muscle flap must be confirmed. The deltoid is repaired and the gap left from the flap is closed by moving the posterior bundle, whose reinsertion is obtained with transosseous sutures including in the area where the acromial graft was harvested.

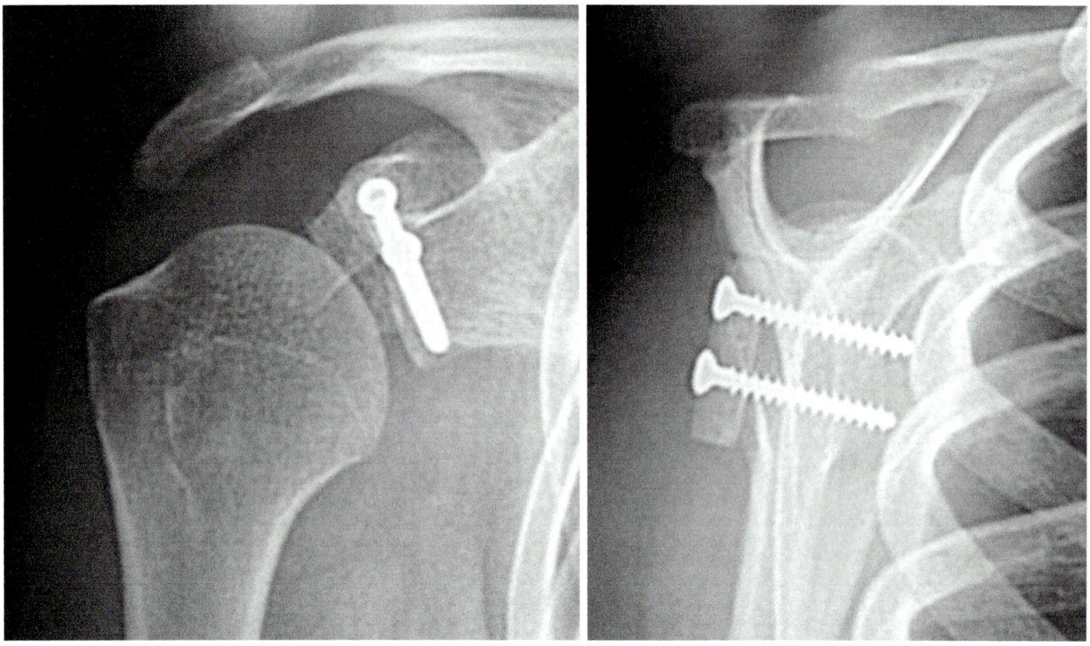

**Fig. 18.11** Control of a posterior bone graft harvested from the acromion

Postoperatively the arm is immobilized across the body with immediate physical therapy and full range of motion (Fig. 18.11).

#### 18.8.2.2 Glenoid Osteotomy

First described by Scott in 1967, and indicated for the treatment of recurrent posterior instability of the shoulder, this technique is based on augmentation of the angle of glenoid anteversion to limit posterior translation of the humeral head.

Constitutional excess retroversion or defective glenoid concavity has been shown to be the cause of posterior shoulder instability.

In a cadaveric study, Metcalf has shown that posteroinferior glenoplasty can increase the mechanical stability of the shoulder.

An MRI study in 20 patients with atraumatic recurrent posterior instability by Inui et al. confirmed the presence of posteroinferior hypoplasia of the articular surface of the glenoid.

##### Surgical Technique

The upper limb is entirely draped and left free to allow for perioperative movement.

A posterior approach is used and the Deltoid is dissected according to Rockwood or by scapular detachment of the posterior deltoid. The infraspinatus and the teres minor muscles are identified. The infraspinatus is sectioned laterally and reflected inward (if there is an associated capsulorrhaphy) or the muscle is simply split along the line of the fibers without humeral detachment.

Posterior translation of the humeral head is evaluated by placing the upper limb in a position of instability (flexion-adduction-internal rotation).

Vertical capsular incision is made 3–4 mm laterally in relation to the glenoid rim.

Endoarticular exploration. A retractor is introduced into the joint space pressing on the anterior and posterior rims of the glenoid to evaluate the direction of the glenoid.

For Rockwood the osteotomy is performed 6 mm from the glenoid rim, while Hawkins preserves a distance of 10 mm from the capsular insertion, thus preserving a lateral bone fragment that is thick enough to avoid necrosis of the fragment or a radiolucency in the glenoid.

A 3 cm-wide osteotome is gradually impacted until the glenoid fragment can be moved while preserving the anterior cortex of the scapula. The osteotome should be parallel to the glenoid axis. The end of the bone cut in the cortex of the posterior glenoid neck can be begun with an oscillating saw to precisely determine the angle of the osteotomy.

An 8 mm-thick and 30 mm-high bone graft is harvested from the ipsilateral iliac crest or the acromion. For Brewer, the mechanical quality of the acromial bone is not as good as iliac bone, and there is a risk of graft fragmentation and secondary loss of correction. The graft is forcefully inserted into the osteotomy gap. Opening of the osteotomy is facilitated by traction on the upper limb.

Several morsels of cancellous graft may be necessary to completely fill the gap.

Unless the anterior cortex is torn, the stability of the graft prevents any need for additional internal fixation. If the graft does not seem stable, additional screw or staple fixation may be used.

An associated posterior capsulorrhaphy may be performed with the glenoid osteotomy in the presence of capsular distension or posteroinferior capsular laxity.

If there is simple posterior capsular redundancy, a mattress suture of the posterior capsule is recommended by suturing the lateral capsular flap to the posterior labrum and the medial flap on top of this. This mattress suture is often facilitated by lateralization of the glenoid from the osteotomy.

In the presence of posterior inferior laxity, a T-capsuloplasty may be considered.

Closing the infraspinatus with the upper limb in neutral rotation does not affect shortening (Fig. 18.12).

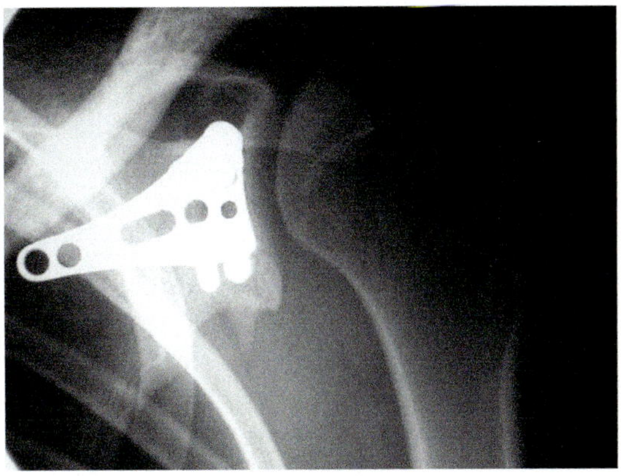

**Fig. 18.12** Control of a glenoid osteotomy

**Postoperative course** The upper limb is immobilized in neutral rotation or slight external rotation for 4–6 weeks depending on the authors.

Movements of horizontal adduction above the median line should not be allowed for 4 months to avoid soliciting the posterior capsule and to prevent recurrent stability.

No contact sports for 6 months.

**Remarks** This procedure has the unfortunate reputation of being associated with numerous complications with persistent instability, degenerative glenohumeral osteoarthritis, anterior coracoid impingement, intra-articular fractures, and insufficient correction being the most frequent.

Based on a clinical case of subcoracoid anterior impingement secondary to a posterior glenoid osteotomy, Gerber performed an experimental study in 13 cadavers. He concluded that reorienting the glenoid from 15–25° always resulted in anterior impingement between the humeral head and the coracoid process in adduction and medial rotation. This anterior graft can cause a cam effect which increases the risk of recurrent posterior instability and which can be identified during the procedure by limiting medial rotation and/or anterior elevation to 90° abduction. In these cases, the author suggests resection of the lateral half of the coracoid process (inferolateral coracoplasty) while preserving the insertions of the conjoint tendon and pectoralis minor by a small anterior deltoid dissection.

For numerous authors, the degree of correction varies, is unpredictable, and is difficult to reproduce, resulting in frequent over- or undercorrection.

Moreover, several authors have shown an absence of asymmetric glenoid version in stable and unstable shoulders so that they do not consider this possible anatomic variation to be a factor of instability.

For most authors, the indications for this osteotomy should be very restrictive and limited to posterior instability alone due to severe glenoid hypoplasia or confirmed glenoid retroversion (>30° for Wirth).

#### 18.8.2.3 Surgical Repair of the Soft Tissues

Recurrent involuntary posterior instability or instability with an initial traumatic episode may be characterized by isolated posterior capsulolabral lesions (reverse Bankart lesions) which do not require glenoid repair.

For numerous authors, the presence of an isolated Bankart lesion is not enough to cause posterior dislocation, which requires lesions of the posterior capsule and the inferior glenohumeral ligament associated with a defective rotator interval. Failure to diagnose inferior laxity is the main reason that isolated posterior capsulolabral repair techniques fail.

Thus, patients who present with recurrent posterior instability, especially voluntary, frequently have features of predominantly posteroinferior multidirectional laxity which is often classified as bidirectional instability (if the inferior component is symptomatic).

As a result, most of the capsulorrhaphy techniques used today for recurrent posterior instability take into account this inferior component and have been described in reports of multidirectional instability, based on the notions of Neer. They will be described in the chapter on multidirectional instability

##### Open Capsulomuscular Repair

The presence of isolated posterior capsuloperiosteal detachment can be an indication for capsulolabral repair by posterior approach.

Described by Rowe, who recommends the use of transosseous sutures, this repair technique is now facilitated by the use of suture anchors placed in the posterior glenoid rim which has first been abraded.

Tibone reported the results of staple capsulorrhaphy for posterior dislocation with 30% recurrence and complications including residual pain due to the presence of the staple. This technique has now been abandoned by its inventor.

These techniques do not take into account the posteroinferior capsuloligamentary laxity that has been observed by most authors, so their indications are quite limited.

##### Posterior Capsulomuscular Plication (Posterior "Putti-Platt" Repair)

The goal of this procedure is to limit posterior translation of the humeral head by performing posterior capsular plication and closing the infraspinatus with a mattress suture (vest over pants).

In the first report by Hawkins (1984), posterior instability recurred in five of the six patients who underwent surgery with this technique, leading the author to recommend physical therapy. Nevertheless, in 1996, the same author published satisfactory results in 93% of the cases with a similar technique.

In the report by Hurley, the results of posterior Putti-Platt repair were mediocre with recurrent instability in 16/22 patients.

##### Posterior Capsulomuscular Plication by Hawkins (Am J Sports Med 1996) (cf Schema)

The patient is in the lateral decubitus position, and a posterior longitudinal incision is made beginning 2 cm from the posterolateral corner of the acromion extending distally to the axillary fossa. Dissection is performed in line with the fibers of the posterior deltoid to expose the external rotator muscles. The arm is placed in neutral rotation. A vertical incision is made in the infraspinatus and the posterior articular capsule on the plane of the posterior joint space. The teres minor is preserved to protect the axillary nerve. The joint is carefully explored, and the arm is place in 20° lateral rotation for suturing of the lateral capsular flap to the posterior labrum.

In the presence of a labral lesion, the lateral capsulomuscular flap is attached to the posterior glenoid rim by suture anchors. The medial portion of the capsule and the infraspinatus are then sutured laterally on the previously mentioned plane resulting in a capsulomuscular mattress suture. After suturing, mobility in internal rotation should be possible up to 20°. The upper limb is immobilized at 20° external rotation and 20° abduction and slight extension. The arm is immobilized for 4–6 weeks depending on the type of instability (cases of atraumatic instability are immobilized for longer).

## Boyd and Sisk Procedure (1972)

These authors associate a posterior capsulorrhaphy with a transfer of the long head of the brachial biceps for traumatic and atraumatic dislocations. The biceps tendon is detached from the supraglenoid tuberosity and rerouted along the posterolateral border of the humeral neck to be reinserted into the posterior rim of the glenoid to create a dynamic forward spring of the humeral head. A posterior infraspinatus-splitting approach allows detachment of the posterior deltoid and access to the space separating the infraspinatus from the teres minor which is opened longitudinally along with the underlying capsule. The long head of the biceps is sectioned by the posterior approach and recovered in front with a small anterior counter-incision in the rotator interval. The tendon is then rerouted along the lateral humeral epiphysis and then recovered on the posterior portion of the joint. Reverse Bankart repair or a posterior capsulorrhaphy is then performed with posterior stapling where the long head of the biceps rests in an extra-articular position.

All authors seemed to have abandoned this technique.

## Arthroscopic Posterior Labral Repair and Capsulorrhaphy

Arthroscopic posterior stabilization is performed under general anesthesia with interscalenic block to optimize control of postoperative pain. After intubation the involved and contralateral shoulders are evaluated with the patient under anesthesia and in the supine position.

The patient is then installed in the lateral decubitus or the beach-chair position. The lateral decubitus position combined with axial traction of the operated limb displaces the humeral head forward and downward, facilitating exposure and repair of lesions.

Arthroscopic repair of the posterior labrum is performed using a technique with two portals. The position of the portal is essential to have full access to the posterior and inferior labrum. Thus it is created approximately 1 cm more distal and 1 cm outside of a standard posterior arthroscopic portal. There may be difficulty placing the suture anchors, and a suture hook may be needed if the portal is too superior or medial to the posterior capsule.

A needle is used to locate the modified posterior portal at 7 o'clock on the glenoid rim in a right shoulder, approximately 1–2 cm from the lateral glenoid rim.

A standard 30° arthroscope is inserted into the scapulohumeral joint through the posterior portal, and diagnostic arthroscopy is systematically performed. The anterior portal is created in the rotator interval, approximately 1 cm outside the coracoid process. The articular surface of the humeral head is evaluated as well as the other articular surfaces, the posterior labrum, the posterior capsule, the superior labrum and the insertion of the biceps tendon, the anterior capsule of the inferior labrum, the axillary pouch, the subscapularis tendon, and the rotator interval.

To improve the view and treat posterior structures, the arthroscope is inserted through the anterior portal once the lesions have been evaluated. Lesions typically associated with posterior instability are looked for cracks in the posterior labrum, detachment of the posterior labrum from the glenoid rim, lax posterior capsule, partial tear of the rotator cuff tendons, and an enlarged rotator interval. The surgeon should also look for a "Kim lesion" corresponding to a full-thickness tear of the deep glenoid portion of the labrum. An 8.25 mm-diameter cannula is used in the posterior portal to facilitate the passage and simplify the manipulation of instruments needed to repair the labrum. The posterior labrum is repaired with suture anchors that are impacted or screwed into the glenoid rim after having detached and freed the labrum of adhesions with an electrocoagulation probe, a rasp, and a hand drill.

The anchors should be placed on the cartilaginous rim of the glenoid to allow the tissue to heal in the correct position and to restore height to the posterior glenoid rim to favor re-centering of the humeral head on the scapula.

The anchors are placed along the posterior glenoid rim and the labrum is thus attached to the articular surface of the glenoid. This makes it possible to restore tension to the posterior band of the inferior glenohumeral ligament (IGHL).

The number of suture anchors used depends on the size of the labral lesion. Hours are used to describe their position and the extent of the labral tear. The first anchor is usually placed higher than the inferior part of tear (at 6 h30 for a lesion that extends to 6 o'clock), to obtain superior displacement of the IGHL complex at the same time.

The suture is put in place with a hook at 45° (Linvatec Corp., Largo, FL, USA), loaded with a relay suture (PDS 0, Ethicon, Somerville, NJ, USA) or a Lasso suture (Arthrex Inc., Naples, FL, USA). The hook is passed behind by the capsular portion of the labrum to the rim of the articular surface of the glenoid. Reinforced sutures such as FiberWire (Arthrex) are then used either separately or mounted on an anchor screwed into the glenoid. Additional suture anchors are then placed in the same way to repair the labrum up to the superior part of the lesion.

### 18.8.3 Repair of the Labrum Associated with Capsular Plication

When a loose posterior capsule is found in the preoperative assessment or diagnostic arthroscopy, this tissue is also abraded to prepare for associated capsular plication with the sutures used for repair of the posterior labrum (Fig. 18.13).

### 18.8.4 Isolated Posterior Capsular Plication

In certain cases, patients present with unidirectional posterior instability or primary posterior multidirectional instability with no posterior labral lesions, but only significant capsular laxity on the diagnostic arthroscopy. In these cases, isolated posterior capsulorrhaphy is performed with sutures similar to the procedure described above.

### 18.8.5 Rotator Interval Closure

Biomechanical studies have shown that in cases of unidirectional posterior instability, the rotator interval does not need to be closed surgically to restore stability. Nevertheless, in case of predominantly posterior multidirectional instability, it may be necessary to perform rotator interval closure. These patients are defined preoperatively by a sulcus sign >2 that does not decrease in external rotation.

Interval closure is performed with a posterior arthroscopic portal and a working portal in the rotator interval. The goal is plication of the tissue between the supraspinatus and subscapularis tendons. Thus a suture of the anterior capsule and the superior glenohumeral ligament to

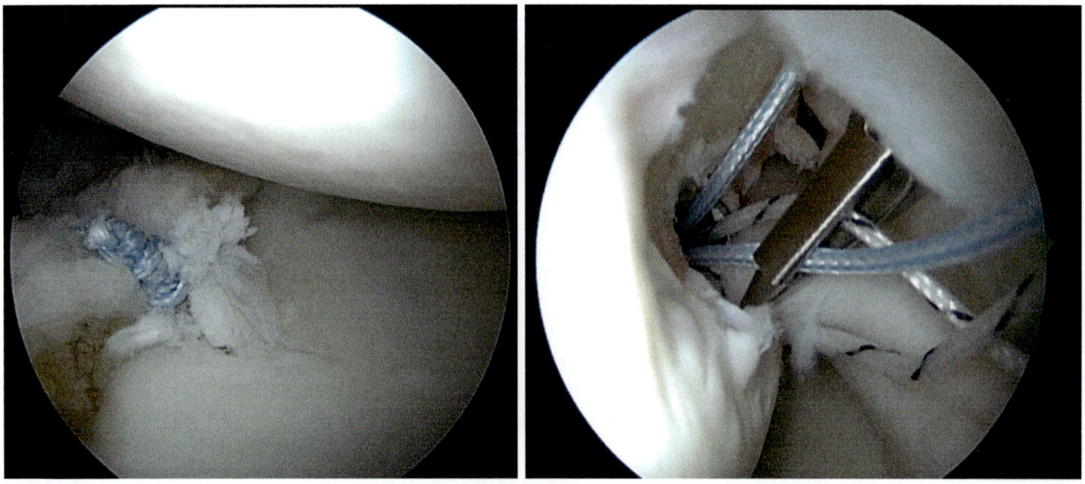

**Fig. 18.13** Arthroscopic view of posterior Bankart repair and anterior Hill-Sachs remplissage

the anterior capsule and of the medial glenohumeral ligament is performed. The closure begins medially and is obtained with a PDS Number 0 suture, which is passed through the tissue with a suture passer and recovered with an arthroscopic forceps. A knot secures closure of the interval.

### 18.8.6 Postoperative Follow-Up and Physical Therapy

Postoperatively the shoulder is placed in scapulohumeral immobilization with an abduction cushion, which immobilizes the shoulder at 30° abduction and prevents internal rotation. The day after surgery, patients begin moving the elbow, the wrist, and the fingers. Physical therapy begins at 1 week with passive anterior flexion and abduction with the scapula at 90°. Recovery of passive range of motion is continued for the next 5 weeks. At 6 weeks, immobilization is stopped and active exercises of the shoulder are begun.

**Conclusion**

Management of posterior instability of the shoulder is complex, but a thorough understanding of the pathophysiology as well as a complete clinical examination and detailed questioning of the patient makes it possible to reach a diagnosis and provide optimal management. Additional tests can improve preoperative planning. In most cases, treatment by labral repair and capsular plication provides satisfactory results.

Progress in arthroscopic techniques and improvement in arthroscopic instruments have made this approach increasingly popular and accessible. Arthroscopic posterior iliac grafts are already used in daily practice by numerous surgeons, but it should be remembered that open surgical procedures obtain good intermediate and long-term results and are still the gold standard for the management of posterior instability of the shoulder.

## References


1. Kim SH, et al. Loss of chondrolabral containment of the glenohumeral joint in atraumatic posteroinferior multidirectional instability. J Bone Joint Surg Am. 2005;8(1):92–8.
2. Kim SH, et al. The Kim test. a novel test for posteroinferior labral lesion of the shoulder—a comparison to the jerk test. Am J Sports Med. 2005;33(8):1188–92. 16000664.
3. Matsen III FA et al. Shoulder surgery: principles and procedures. Philadelphia: WB Saunders; 2004. p. 115.


## Suggested Reading


1. Barbier O, et al. Iliac bone-block autograft for posterior shoulder instability. Orthop Traumatol Surg Res. 2009;95(2):100–7. 19332402.
2. Fuchs B, et al. Posterior-inferior capsular shift for the treatment of recurrent, voluntary posterior subluxation of the shoulder. J Bone Joint Surg Am. 2001;82(1):16–24.
3. Pollock RG, et al. Recurrent posterior shoulder instability. Diagnosis and treatment. Clin Orthop. 1993;291: 85–96.
4. Robinson M, et al. Current concepts review. Recurrent posterior shoulder instability. J Bone Joint Surg Am. 2005;87(4):883–92.
5. Millett PJ, et al. Recurrent shoulder instability. J Am Acad Orthop Surg. 2006;14(8):464–76. 16885478.
6. Provencher MT, et al. Posterior and multidirectional instability of the shoulder. challenges associated with diagnosis and management. Instr Course Lec. 2008;57:133–52.
7. Harryman DT, et al. The role of the rotator interval capsule in passive motion and stability of the shoulder. J Bone Joint Surg Am. 1992;74(1):53–66.
8. Warren RF, et al. Static factors affecting posterior shoulder instability. Orthop Trans. 1984;8:89.
9. Weber SC, et al. A biomechanical evaluation of the restraints to posterior shoulder dislocation. Arthroscopy. 1989;5(2):115–21. 2736007.
10. Weishaupt D, et al. Posterior glenoid rim deficiency in recurrent (atraumatic) posterior shoulder instability. Skeletal Radiol. 2000;29(4):204–10. 10855468.
11. Lazarus MD, et al. Effect of a chondral-labral defect on glenoid concavity and glenohumeral stability. A cadaveric model. J Bone Joint Surg Am. 1996;78(1):94–102. 8550685.
12. Kim SH, et al. Kim's lesion. an incomplete and concealed avulsion of the posteroinferior labrum in posterior or multidirectional posteroinferior instability of the shoulder. Arthroscopy. 2004;20(7):712. 15346113.
13. Bradley JP, et al. Arthroscopic capsulolabral reconstruction for posterior instability of the shoulder. a prospective study of 100 shoulders. Am J Sports Med. 2006;34(7):1061–71. 16567458.

14. Neer II CS, et al. Inferior capsular shift for involuntary inferior and multidirectional instability of the shoulder. A preliminary report. J Bone Joint Surg Am. 1980;62(6):897–908. 7430177.
15. Provencher MT, et al. An analysis of the rotator interval in patients with anterior, posterior, and multidirectional shoulder instability. Arthroscopy. 2008;24(8):921–9. 18657741.
16. Kim SH, et al. Painful jerk test. a predictor of success in nonoperative treatment of posteroinferior instability of the shoulder. Am J Sports Med. 2004;32(8):1849–55. 15572311.
17. Kim SH, et al. Arthroscopic posterior labral repair and capsular shift for traumatic unidirectional recurrent posterior subluxation of the shoulder. J Bone Joint Surg Am. 2003;85(8):1479–87. 12925627.
18. Kim SH, et al. Arthroscopic capsulolabroplasty for posteroinferior multidirectional instability of the shoulder. Am J Sports Med. 2004;32(3):594–607. 15090373.
19. Rhee YG, et al. Posterior capsulolabral reconstruction in posterior shoulder instability. Deltoid saving. J Shoulder Elbow Surg. 2005;14(4):355–60. 16015233.
20. Bottoni CR, et al. Operative stabilization of posterior shoulder instability. Am J Sports Med. 2005;33(7): 996–1002. 15890637.
21. Radkowski CA, et al. Arthroscopic capsulolabral repair for posterior shoulder instability in throwing athletes compared with nonthrowing athletes. Am J Sports Med. 2008;36(4):693–9. 18364459.
22. Legan LM, et al. Tears of the glenoid labrum. MR imaging of 88 arthroscopically confirmed cases. Radiology. 1991;179(1):241–6. 2006284.
23. Gusmer PB, et al. Labral injuries. accuracy of detection with unenhanced MR imaging of the shoulder. Radiology. 1996;200(2):519–24. 8685350.
24. Chandnani VP, et al. Glenoid labral tears. prospective evaluation with MRI imaging, MR arthrography, and CT arthrography. Am J Roentgenol. 1993;161(6):1229–35.
25. Neumann CH, et al. MR imaging of the labral-capsular complex. normal variations. Am J Roentgenol. 1991;157(5):1015–21.
26. Dewing CB, et al. An analysis of capsular area in patients with anterior, posterior, and multidirectional shoulder instability. Am J Sports Med. 2008;36(3): 515–22. 18216272.
27. Shankman S, et al. Glenohumeral instability. evaluation using MR arthrography of the shoulder. Skeletal Radiol. 1999;28(7):365–82. 10478618.
28. Edelson JG. Localized glenoid hypoplasia- an anatomic variation of possible clinical significance. Clin Orthop. 1995;321:189–95.
29. Harper KW, et al. Glenoid dysplasia: incidence and association with posterior labral tears as evaluated on MRI. Am J Roentgenol. 2005;184(3):984–8.
30. Wirth MA, et al. Hypoplasia of the glenoid. A review of 16 patients. J Bone Joint Surg Am. 1993;75(8): 1175–84. 8354676.
31. Steinmann SP. Posterior shoulder instability. Arthroscopy. 2003;19(Suppl 1):102–5. 14673426.
32. Griffith JF, et al. CT compared with arthroscopy in quantifying glenoid bone loss. Am J Roentgenol. 2007;189(6):1490–3.
33. Yu J, et al. The POLPSA lesion. MR imaging findings with arthroscopic correlation in patients with posterior instability. Skeletal Radiol. 2002;31(7):396–9. 12107572.
34. Neviaser TJ. The GLAD lesion. another cause of anterior shoulder pain. Arthroscopy. 1993;9(1):22–3. 8442825.
35. Wolf BR, et al. Open posterior stabilization for recurrent posterior glenohumeral instability. J Shoulder Elbow Surg. 2005;14(2):157–64. 15789009.
36. Hottya G, et al. Tear of the posterior shoulder stabilizers after posterior dislocation. MR imaging and MR arthrographic findings with arthroscopic correlation. Am J Roentgenol. 1998;171(3):763–8.
37. Schwartz E, et al. Posterior shoulder instability. Orthop Clin North Am. 1987;18(3):409–19. 3327030.
38. Bigliani LU, et al. Shift of the posteroinferior aspect of the capsule for recurrent posterior glenohumeral instability. J Bone Joint Surg Am. 1995;77(7): 1011–120. 7608222.
39. Hawkins RJ, et al. Posterior instability of the shoulder. Instr Course Lect. 1989;38:211–5. 2703716.
40. Chaudhuri GK, et al. Rotation osteotomy of the shaft of the humerus for recurrent dislocation of the shoulder. anterior and posterior. Acta Orthop Scand. 1974;45(2):193–8. 4406974.
41. Surin V, et al. Rotational osteotomy of the humerus for posterior instability of the shoulder. J Bone Joint Surg Am. 1990;72(2):181–6. 2303504.
42. Scott Jr DJ. Treatment of recurrent posterior dislocations of the shoulder by glenoidplasty. Report of three cases. J Bone Joint Surg Am. 1967;49(3):471–6. 6022356.
43. Jones V. Recurrent posterior dislocation of the shoulder. report of a case treated by posterior bone block. J Bone Joint Surg Br. 1958;40(2):203–7. 13539103.
44. Boyd HB, et al. Recurrent posterior dislocation of the shoulder. J Bone Joint Surg Am. 1972;54(4):779–86. 5055169.
45. Gerber C, et al. Allograft reconstruction of segmental defects of the humeral head for treatment of chronic locked posterior dislocation of the shoulder. J Bone Joint Surg Am. 1996;78(3):376–82. 8613444.
46. Bisson LJ. Thermal capsulorrhaphy for isolated posterior instability of the glenohumeral joint without labral detachment. Am J Sports Med. 2005;33(12): 1898–904. 16157851.
47. Mologne TS, et al. The addition of rotator interval closure after arthroscopic repair of either anterior or posterior shoulder instability: effect on glenohumeral translation and range of motion. Am J Sports Med. 2008;36(6):1123–31.
48. Wolf EM, et al. Arthroscopic capsular plication for posterior shoulder instability. Arthroscopy. 1998;14(2): 153–63. 9531126.
49. LF MI, et al. The arthroscopic treatment of posterior shoulder instability. two-year results of a multiple suture technique. Arthroscopy. 1997;13(4):426–32. 9276047.
50. Goubier JN, et al. A 4 portal arthroscopic stabilization in posterior shoulder instability. J Shoulder Elbow Surg. 2003;12(4):337–41. 12934026.
51. Provencher MT, et al. Arthroscopic treatment of posterior shoulder instability. results in 33 patients. Am J Sports Med. 2003;33(10):1463–71.

# Arthroscopic Repair of Extended Labral Tears After a Traumatic Shoulder Dislocation

19

Felix Dyrna, Jessica DiVenere, and Augustus D. Mazzocca

## Contents


19.1 **Epidemiology and Patient History** ...... 169

19.2 **Diagnostic Imaging** .................. 169

19.3 **Physical Examination** ................ 170

19.4 **Alarm Signals for an Extended Labral Tear** ........................ 171

19.5 **Surgical Technique** .................. 171

19.6 **Rehab Protocol** ...................... 173

19.7 **Complications** ...................... 174

19.8 **Results and Outcomes in the Literature for Extended Labral Tears** ............ 174

**References** .............................. 175



F. Dyrna, MD (✉) • J. DiVenere, BS
Orthopaedic Sports Medicine Division, University of Connecticut Health, 263 Farmington Avenue, Farmington, CT 06001, USA
e-mail: dyrna@tum.de

A.D. Mazzocca, MS, MD
Orthopaedics Sports Medicine Division, University of Connecticut Health, University of Connecticut Athletics, Farmington, CT, USA


## 19.1 Epidemiology and Patient History

Extended traumatic labral tears are rare, but if present they need to be addressed as such.

Lo et al. [2] reported within a case series of 297 surgically repaired Bankart lesions that 2.4% of their patients had extended, triple labral lesions. Similar results were published by Owens et al. [6] with 229 consecutive included labral repairs, of which 6.5% were described as triple labral lesions. In our study population [3] of 149 consecutive performed arthroscopic stabilizations, we found 23 (15%) extended 270° labral tears. The patient cohort consists of mainly young males between 16 and 35. The injury is based on a traumatic event during contact sports or fall from significant heights. Patients will present with bi- or multidirectional instability and pain during consultation.

## 19.2 Diagnostic Imaging

Plain radiographs including AP, supraspinatus outlet, and axillary views should be obtained to exclude bony lesions like glenoid rim fractures or extended Hill-Sachs lesions. Radiographs should be followed by a diagnostic MRI to elucidate the degree of labral injury but even more important to show possible additional pathologies like HAGL lesions, rotator cuff tears, or cartilage


© ISAKOS 2017


A.B. Imhoff, F.H. Savoie III (eds.), *Shoulder Instability Across the Life Span*,
DOI 10.1007/978-3-662-54077-0_19

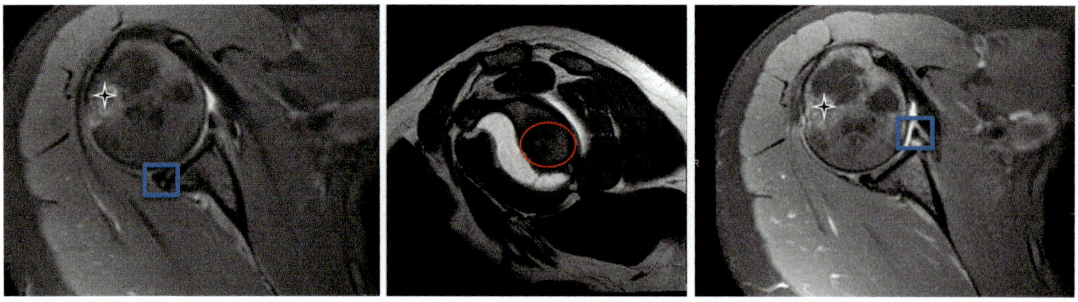

**Fig. 19.1** Diagnostic MRI showing anterior and posterior labral lesions in blue box on axial sections; sagittal projection is confirming no significant glenoid bone loss estimated by Sugaya [7] measuring method 1. Star indicates Hill-Sachs bone edema

lesions (Fig. 19.1). Axial and sagittal projections are helpful to identifying anterior and posterior labral tear extensions. In this circumstance, a CT scan can also be helpful to address and evaluate bony defects and should be considered if any of the previous taking images show evidence of glenoid rim or humeral head defects [7]. Furthermore, patients with significant recurrent instability after an original traumatic dislocation are prone to have bony defects and may receive a CT scan.

## 19.3 Physical Examination

Most important is to evaluate the degree and direction of the instability to reflect and interpret the imaging findings. This will direct the surgical strategy and help balance the shoulder stability. All patients should be examined regarding their range of motion, strength, and sensibility before evaluating their instability. A variety of tests can be used to address the instability components and directions like anterior-inferior or posterior load shift, apprehension, relocation, posterior jerk, and Kim test.

The load and shift test evaluates the translation of the humerus in relation to the glenoid and is graded in four stages from 0 to 3. The patient is placed supine on the edge of a bench and the arm is positioned in 90° of abduction. An axial load to the humerus is applied with one hand, while the other hand is used to translate the anterior and posterior humerus.

For the jerk test, patients are sitting or standing with the surgeon behind them. Patient's scapula is fixed with one hand; the affected arm is positioned at 90° abduction and internally rotated. Pushing the elbow posteriorly provides an axial load to center the humerus, and a horizontal motion of the arm across the body is performed. A positive test is indicated by a sudden click as the humeral head slides off the back of the glenoid. When the arm is returned to the original position, a second click may be observed, as the humeral head is returning to the glenoid.

For the Kim test, patients are in a sitting position and the arm in 90° of abduction. The surgeon stands behind the patient holding on to the elbow with one hand, and the other hand is holding on to lateral aspect of the proximal humerus. Simultaneously, an axial loading force to the elbow and upward elevation is applied over the elbow, while the other hand pushes the proximal humerus posteroinferiorly. Posterior shoulder pain is considered as a positive test result, and an additional click can occur but is not mandatory for a positive result.

All directions should be evaluated with appropriate tests as extended labral tears result in bidirectional instability. A general impression for mobility and laxity should also be evaluated in order to include findings into preoperative planning for possible capsule shifts. The sulcus sign is helpful for this evaluation. Therefore, the arm is pulled caudally in neutral rotation and the lateral aspect underneath the acromion is inspected for any dimpling which can be measured and graded. The test is repeated in external rotation to evaluate the rotator interval and in internal rotation to address the posterior capsule more specifically. Lastly, examination under anesthesia should be performed to confirm clinical findings. We prefer to divide this into two separate steps, first after the still-awake patient received the nerve block where the position of patient and arm can be changed freely and a second look with the patient asleep to fully understand the direction and extension of the instability.

## 19.4 Alarm Signals for an Extended Labral Tear

Patient should have a history of traumatic dislocation that resulted in symptomatic anterior-inferior or bidirectional instability. Appropriate physical examination findings included 2+ or greater anterior-inferior or posterior-inferior load shift, symptomatic apprehension test with positive relocation, symptomatic posterior jerk test, and a positive Kim test, and this is confirmed by MRI imaging showing extended anterior, inferior, and posterior labral tears while ruling out significant bone loss. Surgeons should expect a more extended injury with the combination of abovementioned clinical and imaging findings. This may influence surgery setup to favor lateral decubitus position to perform a posterior stabilization, and surgery time may be planed for an extended case.

## 19.5 Surgical Technique [3, 9]

The procedure starts with the performance of an examination under anesthesia. Therefore, the patient is positioned supine, and all previously performed clinical tests are repeated, and the contralateral shoulder is examined for comparison. Afterward, the patient is positioned in the lateral decubitus and secured with a bean/sand bag or vacuum mattress. The involved arm is prepared and draped utilizing an overhead traction device with 5 lbs of longitudinal traction and 7 lbs of abduction/distraction (Fig. 19.2). The surface anatomy is marked with a sterile marker, and initial anterosuperior viewing portal is established. The posterior portal can then be created under arthroscopic visualization with a spinal needle and switching stick to determine the optimal entrance trajectory and location of the posterior anchor. This way the posterior portal can be placed more laterally to achieve the optimal angle for anchor placement. We recommend the use of cannulas in both portals for suture management purposes to avoid soft tissue bridges and prevent fluid extravasation. An additional anteroinferior portal can be created directly above the subscapularis midway between the humeral head and the

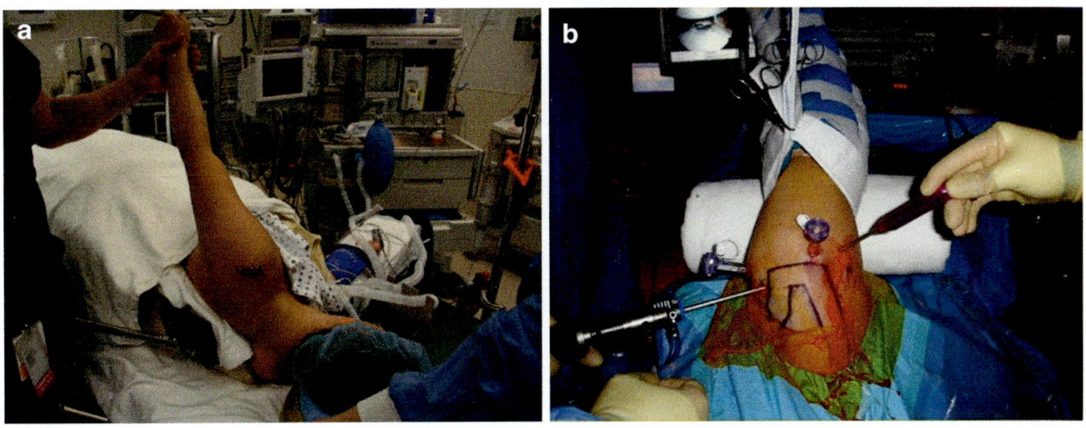

**Fig. 19.2** (**a**) Patient positioned in lateral decubitus utilizing a vacuum mattress. (**b**) The affected shoulder in distraction with anterosuperior, posterior, and anteroinferior portal placement. The scope is primarily positioned in the front to start with the posterior repair

glenoid for better triangulation. As for every Bankart lesion, the labrum first has to be mobilized precisely using a sharp elevator along the lesion's entirety. The labral footprint is then to be prepared using a hand rasp and motorized burr, decorticating the glenoid neck to improve the healing capacity. We typically repair the labrum in a posterior to anterior fashion wherein the number of suture anchors is determined by the extent of the tear. In accordance with what is performed for simple anteroinferior instability cases, the anchors can be placed every 10–12 mm along the glenoid rim. For a standard Bankart repair in a right shoulder, this would represent three or four anchors placed at the 5-o'clock, 4-o'clock, 3-o'clock, and 2-o'clock positions anteriorly and two or three anchors placed at the 7-o'clock, 8-o'clock, and sometimes 9-o'clock positions posteriorly. The posteroinferior anchor can be placed through a percutaneous insertion to provide a perpendicular angle to the glenoid. A suture passing instrument helps grasping tissue inferiorly and passing the suture underneath the capsulolabral complex to shift tissue from inferior to superior for each individual anchor. We prefer to put a shuttle suture prior to the anchor in place because we believe accurate placement of suture is necessary for adequate capsular retensioning which we believe is the most important part of the procedure, especially inferiorly (Fig. 19.3). This ensures that the shuttle suture is placed caudal to the planed anchor position so that subsequent shuttling of the permanent suture housed within the anchor knot tying will cause an inferior to superior shift of the capsulolabral complex. The same suture-first technique is applied to a second anchor and so forth. In traumatic injuries such as these, the extended labral detachment is also composed of a capsular laxity component. In such cases, we perform a capsu-

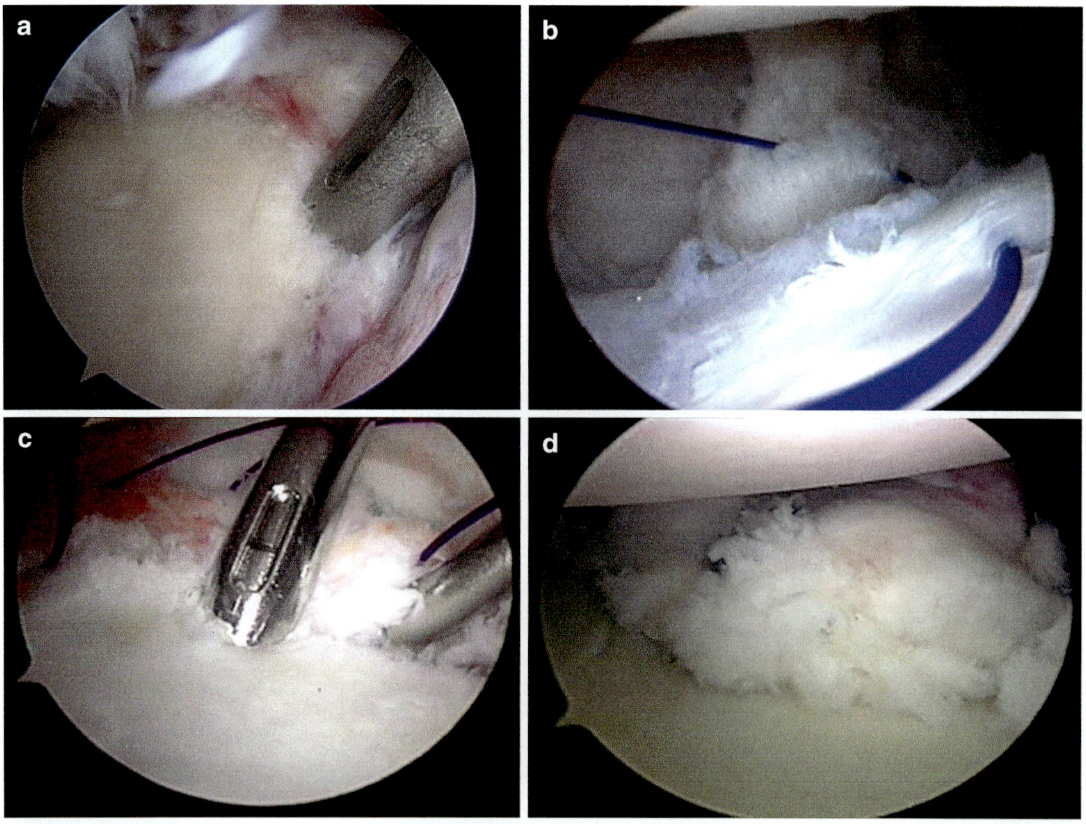


**Fig. 19.3** (**a**) Arthroscopic view of first posterior placed anchor (**b**) Pass PDS suture through the posterior capsule labral complex (**c**) Use this stitch for traction and retensioning of the inferior glenohumeral ligament (**d**) This way correct anchor placement can be planed

lorrhaphy approximately 10 mm away from the labrum. There is a balance between retensioning of the posterior band of the inferior glenohumeral ligament complex, without extensive plication to avoid overtightening and subsequent loss of internal rotation. Postoperatively, while the patient is still on the operating room table, we examine internal rotation to make sure there is no restriction. Once the posterior labrum is repaired, the scope is switched to the posterior portal, and the anterior and inferior labrum can be addressed. Anchors are placed percutaneously through the subscapularis starting inferior and moving superior similar to the posterior repair (Fig. 19.4). With consideration of tissue quality, laxity, and previous clinical findings, a capsule shift or plication can be integrated into the either anterior or posterior repair. The same applies for a rotator interval closure. The closure is performed by passing a suture through the middle glenohumeral ligament and the superior glenohumeral ligament and tying them at the end of the procedure (Fig. 19.5).

## 19.6 Rehab Protocol

Patients are immobilized in a shoulder sling with an abduction pillow for 6 weeks postoperatively. Formal physical therapy can be initiated between 7 and 10 days postoperatively. Passive external rotation to 30° and forward elevation to 180° are permitted in the first 4 weeks. Weeks 4 to 12 focus on active assisted and active motion in all

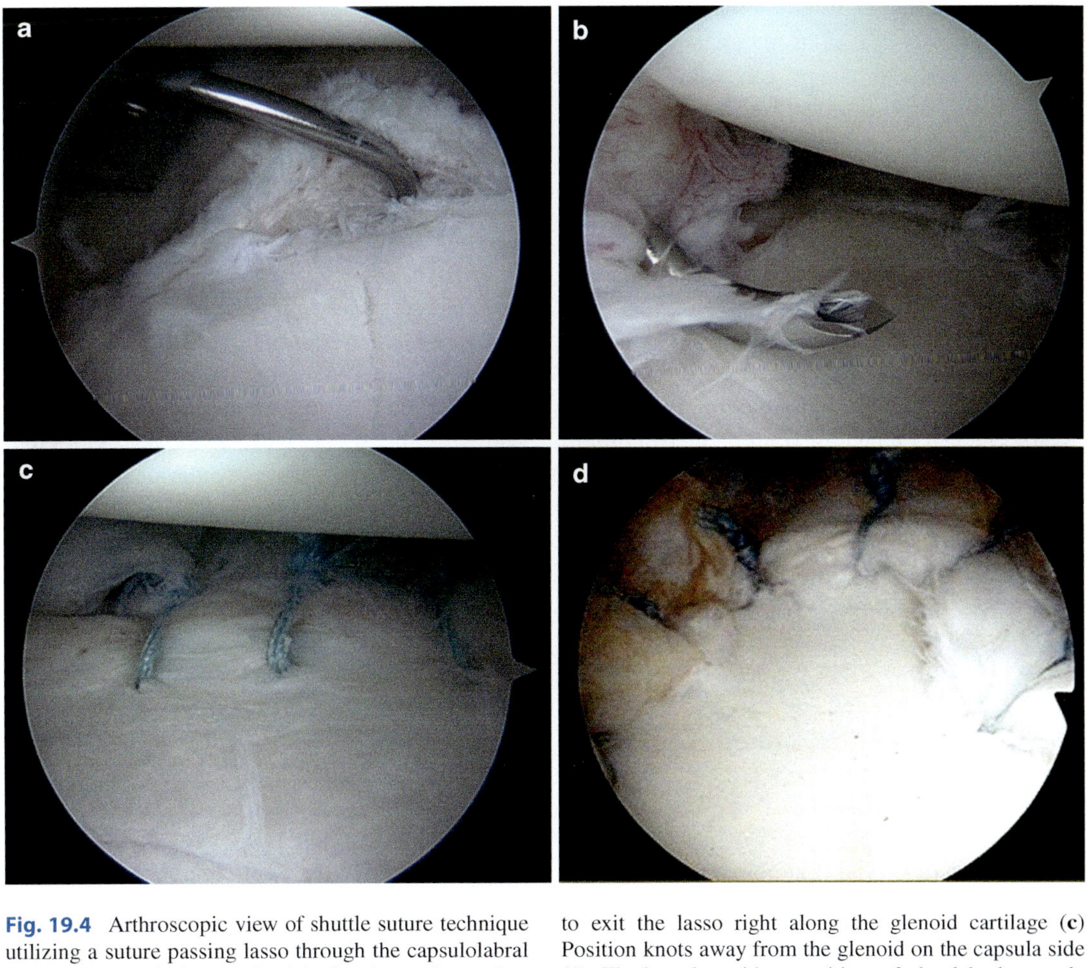


**Fig. 19.4** Arthroscopic view of shuttle suture technique utilizing a suture passing lasso through the capsulolabral complex to repair the anterior labral lesion and complete the procedure. (**a**) Usage of a lasso device (**b**) Make sure to exit the lasso right along the glenoid cartilage (**c**) Position knots away from the glenoid on the capsula side (**d**) Final reults with reposition of the labral capsule complex

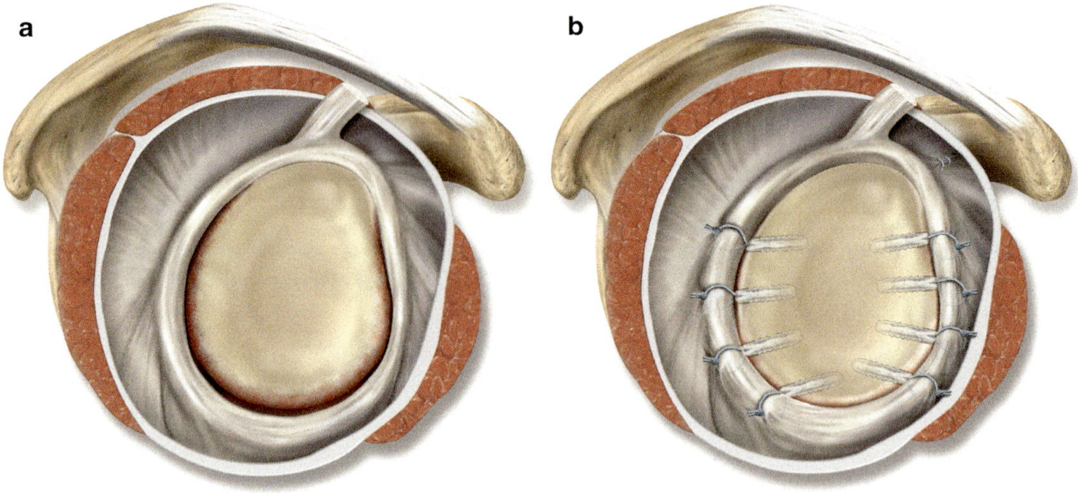


**Fig. 19.5** The extended labrum tear is shown including the anterior, inferior, and posterior quadrant. The final repaired results in a complete refixation of all quadrants with anchor positioned anterior and posterior as well as an inferior to superior capsule labral shift. (**a**) First repair the posterior tear completely (**b**) Finilize the repair with the anterior stbilization

planes as well as scapular stabilization. At the conclusion of 12 weeks, progressive rotator cuff strengthening and sport-specific training is initiated, with return to full activities typically at 6–9 months.

## 19.7 Complications

There are no intraoperative complications nor any adverse events described.

But considering the extent of injury and necessary surgical procedure, a high rate of complications and failures is published within the postoperative period. The complication rate ranges from 15–35%. Main complications are recurrent shoulder dislocations up to 15% and subluxation, followed by postoperative stiffness and pain [2, 3, 8].

## 19.8 Results and Outcomes in the Literature for Extended Labral Tears

The results after a multiple quadrant labral tear are treated arthroscopically to restore stability and improve shoulder function significantly. Nevertheless, a higher recurrence rate is reported if compared to single quadrant lesions. Systematic reviews [4, 5] show a failure rate between 4–20% for arthroscopic anterior-inferior shoulder stabilization. In comparison, a bidirectional instability case series was published by Gartsman et al. [1], showing a 7% failure rate. Further studies on multi-quadrant labral lesions report failure rates ranging from 15 to 35% [2, 3, 8]. The extensive nature of these lesions can also lead to loss of motion, due to over constraining surgery since it is a balance act between stability and stiffness considering the additional capsule laxity caused by the traumatic dislocation. Functional outcome scores as the WOSI, ASES, ROWE, or SANE score did not differ between anterior-inferior stabilizations and extended labral repairs, all resulting in satisfactory outcomes and improved function. Given the extensive nature of these lesions, patients tend to be more mindful of their shoulder after extended labral repairs [3]. Despite the surgical procedure, the return to sport rate has been high as Tokish et al. [8] report that all athletes returned to the preinjury level of sports activity, similar to our case series [3]. Patients with an extended labral tears represent a unique subpopulation of shoulder instability. The clinical outcome after arthroscopic repair observed in this patient group is comparable with that reported for arthroscopically treated labral lesions associated with traumatic anterior-inferior or bidirectional instability. The extensive nature of these injuries may explain a higher failure rate. In conclusion, arthroscopic repair of these extensive labral injuries can be effectively addressed.

## References


1. Gartsman GM, Roddey TS, Hammerman SM. Arthroscopic treatment of bidirectional glenohumeral instability: two- to five-year follow-up. J Shoulder Elbow Surg. 2001;10(1):28–36. doi:10.1067/mse.2001.109324.
2. Lo IKY, Burkhart SS. Triple labral lesions: pathology and surgical repair technique-report of seven cases. Arthroscopy. 2005;21(2):186–93. doi:10.1016/j.arthro.2004.09.022.
3. Mazzocca AD, Cote MP, Solovyova O, Rizvi SHH, Mostofi A, Arciero RA. Traumatic shoulder instability involving anterior, inferior, and posterior labral injury: a prospective clinical evaluation of arthroscopic repair of 270° labral tears. Am J Sports Med. 2011;39(8):1687–96. doi:10.1177/0363546511405449.
4. Mohtadi NGH, Bitar IJ, Sasyniuk TM, Hollinshead RM, Harper WP. Arthroscopic versus open repair for traumatic anterior shoulder instability: a meta-analysis. Arthroscopy. 2005;21(6):652–8. doi:10.1016/j.arthro.2005.02.021.
5. Petrera M, Patella V, Patella S, Theodoropoulos J. A meta-analysis of open versus arthroscopic Bankart repair using suture anchors. Knee Surg Sports Traumatol Arthrosc. 2010;18(12):1742–7. doi:10.1007/s00167-010-1093-5.
6. Pollock RG, Owens JM, Flatow EL, Bigliani LU. Operative results of the inferior capsular shift procedure for multidirectional instability of the shoulder. J Bone Joint Surg. 2000;82-A(7):919–28.
7. Sugaya H. Techniques to evaluate glenoid bone loss. Curr Rev Muscoskelet Med. 2014;7(1):1–5. doi:10.1007/s12178-013-9198-3.
8. Tokish JM, McBratney CM, Solomon DJ, LeClere L, Dewing CB, Provencher MT. Arthroscopic repair of circumferential lesions of the glenoid labrum. J Bone Joint Surg Am. 2009;91(12):2795–802. doi:10.2106/JBJS.H.01241.
9. Wang RY, Mazzocca AD, Arciero RA. Arthroscopic Management of 270° Labral Tears. Oper Tech Orthop. 2008;18(1):46–52. doi:10.1053/j.oto.2008.07.005.

# Part III

# Instability in the Middle Ages (Age 25–50)

# Spectrum of Instability in the Middle-Age Range

# 20

A.B. Imhoff, K. Beitzel, and A. Voss

## Content

References ........ 180

In the middle-age group with a population in the ages between 25 and 50, it is important to distinguish between an active population with a high demand on shoulder activity and the ones with less pretense. The incidence rate reported for traumatic anterior shoulder dislocation in the United States within NEISS (National Electronic Injury Surveillance System) was 47.76, 25.69 and 17.59 per 100,000 persons/year at risk within the age groups 20–29, 30–39, and 40–49, with a higher risk for young age and male sex [17] and an overall prevalence of 2% [6] with a less common posterior instability (2–10% of all shoulder instabilities) [1, 2, 10]. The risk for recurrent anterior shoulder dislocation is mostly depending on age, sex, time of initial dislocation, and damage to the capsule-labral complex or the bony anatomy and decreased with time from the initial dislocation [13]. Compared to young population (<20 years), the recurrence rate of shoulder dislocation is much lower in the age between 23 and 29 with 56% and even lower in patients over 30 years with a rate of 27–30% [7, 14]. Through aging and changes in static and dynamic shoulder stabilizers, there is a certain stiffening, due to collagen changes in the capsular complex and changes in daily life and sports activities. This may be an explanation for decreasing recurrence rate in the aging population. Due to this loosening of elastic characteristics, the impact of a traumatic shoulder event

A.B. Imhoff (✉) • K. Beitzel • A. Voss
Department of Orthopaedic Sports Medicine, Technical University of Munich, Munich, Germany
e-mail: Imhoff@tum.de

© ISAKOS 2017
A.B. Imhoff, F.H. Savoie III (eds.), *Shoulder Instability Across the Life Span*,
DOI 10.1007/978-3-662-54077-0_20

may have more effect on the static stabilizers with glenoid and humeral bony deficiency and fractures. Patients with recurrent instability and dislocation with a total time-out of the joint (cumulative time from dislocation to reduction) of more than 5 h will have a significant glenoid bone loss [3, 5]. Therefore, it is important to differentiate between the high-active person in the middle and late 20s with a higher recurrence rate and the less-active patients at the end of their 40s. It has been proposed that the active group may benefit from early surgical intervention due the increasing risk to suffer from bony deficiency resulting in a chronic instability with a degenerative arthropathy as the final result [8]. The incidence of humeral and glenoidal cartilage lesions in unstable shoulders is reported to be 24% (acute instability), 25% (chronic instability) [4], and 57% [16], respectively. There is no association between the direction of instability and the degree of cartilage damage and no specific defect location, neither on the humeral side nor on the glenoidal side. The results in the study from Cameron et al. showed a more severe osteoarthritis (OA) the longer the shoulder was unstable with a higher prevalence for OA [4], and it is undoubted that there is an increased risk for glenohumeral OA development after shoulder stabilization [11, 12, 15, 18].

The less-active and older patient population may benefit from a first-line conservative treatment, unless bony deficiency and fractures on glenoid and humeral side do not substantially increase the risk of recurrent dislocation. It has been shown that the older population suffers more from nerve lesions and fractures of the proximal part of the humerus due to the tendency to dislocate the shoulder by falling on the outstretched arm apart from a blow against the shoulder [9]. As a consequence of this finding, soft tissue repair is becoming less important compared to fracture treatment.

In conclusion the following chapters will focus on treatment of shoulder instability in the middle-age patient, aimed to point out the specifics of this population in regard to their activity level.

## References


1. Antoniou J, Duckworth DT, Harryman 2nd DT. Capsulolabral augmentation for the management of posteroinferior instability of the shoulder. J Bone Joint Surg Am. 2000;82(9):1220–30.
2. Bock P, Kluger R, Hintermann B. Anatomical reconstruction for Reverse Hill-Sachs lesions after posterior locked shoulder dislocation fracture: a case series of six patients. Arch Orthop Trauma Surg. 2007;127(7):543–8. doi:10.1007/s00402-007-0359-y.
3. Burkhart SS, Lo IKY, Brady PC, Denard PJ. Philosophy of instability repair. In: The cowboys companion. Philadelphia: Wolters Kluwer - Lippincott Williams & Wilkins; 2012.
4. Cameron ML, Kocher MS, Briggs KK, Horan MP, Hawkins RJ. The prevalence of glenohumeral osteoarthrosis in unstable shoulders. Am J Sports Med. 2003;31(1):53–5.
5. Denard PJ, Dai X, Burkhart SS. Increasing preoperative dislocations and total time of dislocation affect surgical management of anterior shoulder instability. Int J Shoulder Surg. 2015;9(1):1–5. doi:10.4103/0973-6042.150215.
6. Hovelius L, Augustini BG, Fredin H, Johansson O, Norlin R, Thorling J. Primary anterior dislocation of the shoulder in young patients. A ten-year prospective study. J Bone Joint Surg Am. 1996;78(11):1677–84.
7. Hovelius L, Olofsson A, Sandstrom B, Augustini BG, Krantz L, Fredin H, Tillander B, Skoglund U, Salomonsson B, Nowak J, Sennerby U. Nonoperative treatment of primary anterior shoulder dislocation in patients forty years of age and younger. a prospective twenty-five-year follow-up. J Bone Joint Surg Am. 2008;90(5):945–52. doi:10.2106/JBJS.G.00070.
8. Hovelius L, Saeboe M. Neer Award 2008: Arthropathy after primary anterior shoulder dislocation–223 shoulders prospectively followed up for twenty-five years. J Shoulder Elbow Surg. 2009;18(3):339–47. doi:10.1016/j.jse.2008.11.004.
9. Kroner K, Lind T, Jensen J. The epidemiology of shoulder dislocations. Arch Orthop Trauma Surg. 1989;108(5):288–90.
10. Mc LH. Posterior dislocation of the shoulder. J Bone Joint Surg Am. 1952;24 A(3):584–90.
11. Morrey BF, Janes JM. Recurrent anterior dislocation of the shoulder. Long-term follow-up of the Putti-Platt and Bankart procedures. J Bone Joint Surg Am. 1976;58(2):252–6.
12. O'Driscoll SW, Evans DC. Long-term results of staple capsulorrhaphy for anterior instability of the shoulder. J Bone Joint Surg Am. 1993;75(2):249–58.
13. Olds M, Ellis R, Donaldson K, Parmar P, Kersten P. Risk factors which predispose first-time traumatic anterior shoulder dislocations to recurrent instability in adults: a systematic review and meta-analysis.

Br J Sports Med. 2015;49(14):913–22. doi:10.1136/bjsports-2014-094342.
14. Robinson CM, Howes J, Murdoch H, Will E, Graham C. Functional outcome and risk of recurrent instability after primary traumatic anterior shoulder dislocation in young patients. J Bone Joint Surg Am. 2006;88(11):2326–36. doi:10.2106/JBJS.E.01327.
15. Rosenberg BN, Richmond JC, Levine WN. Long-term followup of Bankart reconstruction. Incidence of late degenerative glenohumeral arthrosis. Am J Sports Med. 1995;23(5):538–44.
16. Werner A, Lichtenberg S, Nikolic A, Habermeyer P. Intraarticular pathology of atraumatic shoulder dislocations. An arthroscopic study. Unfallchirurg. 2003;106(2):110–3. doi:10.1007/s00113-002-0480-x.
17. Zacchilli MA, Owens BD. Epidemiology of shoulder dislocations presenting to emergency departments in the United States. J Bone Joint Surg Am. 2010;92(3):542–9. doi:10.2106/JBJS.I.00450.
18. Zuckerman JD, Matsen 3rd FA. Complications about the glenohumeral joint related to the use of screws and staples. J Bone Joint Surg Am. 1984;66(2):175–80.

# The Association of Bankart and Rotator Cuff Tear in Patients Aged 25–50

21

Francesco Franceschi, Edoardo Franceschetti, and Enrique Alberto Salas

## Contents

| | | |
|---|---|---|
| 21.1 | **Introduction** | 183 |
| 21.2 | **Literature Overview Summary: What Is Known** | 184 |
| 21.3 | **Anatomy** | 184 |
| 21.4 | **Indication for Surgery** | 184 |
| **Conclusion** | | 185 |
| **References** | | 185 |

F. Franceschi (✉) • E. Franceschetti
Department of Orthopaedic and Trauma Surgery, Campus Bio-Medico University of Rome, Via Alvaro del Portillo, 200, 00128, Trigoria, Rome, Italy
e-mail: f.franceschi@unicampus.it

E. A. Salas
Universidad Central de Venezuela, Caracas, Venezuela

## 21.1 Introduction

In the patient age 25–50 it is important to distiguish between the patients less than 40 and those over 40 years of age. First time dislocation in the patient over 40 years of age is often associated with significant rotator cuff and neurologic injury, and also may have a much higher risk of developing degenerative changes.

Traumatic supraspinatus tears in middle-age patients younger than 40 years are rare events, with few reports in the literature [1–4]. Posttraumatic shoulder pain in this patient population is routinely attributed to instability or fracture, and the diagnosis of a rotator cuff tear can often be overlooked due to the patient's age.

When compared with the more mature shoulder, the young, healthy supraspinatus tendon is a robust tendon that is able to absorb a significant amount of energy before tendon failure. The weakest structural link in the shoulder in this patient population is often the bone as opposed to the tendon. As a result, shoulder trauma in younger patients likely results in more fractures than supraspinatus tears [5].

In older individuals, the dynamic stabilizers are more likely to fail (rotator cuff), whereas in young individuals it is more often the static restraints that fail (labrum). Additionally, with increasing age,

© ISAKOS 2017
A.B. Imhoff, F.H. Savoie III (eds.), *Shoulder Instability Across the Life Span*, DOI 10.1007/978-3-662-54077-0_21

the incidence of preexisting, degenerative tears of the rotator cuff is increasing.

Based on pathological findings seen during arthroscopy in young, first-time dislocators, it is now evident that both age and severity of labral detachment are important factors in determining the chance of recurrence [6–8]. Results from these studies suggest that early arthroscopic labral stabilization reduces the chance of recurrence in these select individuals [6, 9].

Unlike the younger population, older individuals typically have a different spectrum of intra-articular pathology associated with first-time traumatic dislocations [10–13]. This may explain the difference in recurrence rates between these two populations.

Unlike the younger population, the older individual is more at risk for rotator cuff injury during a first-time dislocation [7, 10–13]. McLaughlin [14] referred to this as a posterior mechanism of injury as opposed to an anterior mechanism seen in younger individuals. His point was that in the older individual, it is more likely for the dynamic stabilizers (e.g., rotator cuff) to fail, whereas in the younger individual, it is the static restraints (e.g., labrum and capsule) that typically fail.

Morbidity secondary to rotator cuff lesions can be as debilitating in these patients as recurrence is in the young.

## 21.2 Literature Overview Summary: What Is Known

There are no studies in literature regarding the association of Bankart and rotator cuff tear in patients aged less than 40 years. Neviaser et al. [10] reported a 100% rate of rotator cuff tears in patients older than 40 years with a primary traumatic anterior dislocation. However, this was a preselected group of patients, making the true incidence impossible to determine. In their study, most rotator cuff tears were initially misdiagnosed as axillary nerve injuries. They also reported a 30% recurrence rate and emphasized the importance of the rotator cuff to glenohumeral stability.

This is consistent with Itoi et al. [15] who used a cadaver model to describe the importance of the rotator cuff muscles, and the long head of the biceps, as dynamic stabilizers of the shoulder.

Ribbans et al. [13] reported a 63% rotator cuff tear rate in primary traumatic dislocation in a small number of patients older than 50 years. Hawkins and Mohtadi [12] reported a 90% rotator cuff tear rate in a similar patient population.

## 21.3 Anatomy

McLaughlin and MacLellan [14] suggested that anterior dislocation of the shoulder occurs either by disruption of the glenohumeral ligament (anterior mechanism) or by rupture of the rotator cuff (posterior mechanism). They believed that failure of the posterior support was more likely in patients who are older than 40 years, because the tendinous structure usually degenerates and weakens with age. Rupture of the musculotendinous cuff, particularly of the supraspinatus, infraspinatus, and teres minor, can permit anterior dislocation of the humeral head on an intact anterior soft tissue hinge and thus may be termed the posterior mechanism of anterior dislocation [16].

Hsu et al. [17] demonstrated in a cadaveric study that the displacement of the humeral head increases with an increase in tear size with or without translational forces applied and that a rotator interval tear is more crucial than a critical area tear from the viewpoint of instability.

## 21.4 Indication for Surgery

The association between Bankart and tear of the rotator cuff is rare in patients under the age of 40. In this category of patients, the presence of a Bankart represents the main cause of recurrence which is much more frequent as the younger the patient; therefore, the surgical repair treatment of the Bankart lesion will be indicated in any case. If there is a rupture of the rotator cuff, repair is to be made.

Even now, the management of shoulder dislocations in elderly patients is a subject of controversy. Recommendations vary from predominately conservative treatment [18] to more aggressive surgical protocols [18]. Pevny et al. [18] showed that patients treated surgically had 84% excellent/good results, compared with 50% excellent/good results when treated nonoperatively. Bassett and Coffield [19] also reported better results after surgical cuff repair in terms of functional outcome and pain relief following acute dislocations. Operation is suggested by many authors, but there is discussion as to which structure should be repaired, only Bankart repair, only rotator cuff repair, or both. The Itoi's results indicate that repair of a Bankart lesion is probably not necessary in older patients [15]. In the elderly, cuff tears are commonly associated with anterior dislocation and repair of the cuff alone may be sufficient to achieve stability. Voos et al. [20] showed good clinical outcomes, restoration of motion, and high degree of patient's satisfaction doing arthroscopic treatment of both labrum lesion and rotator cuff.

Although data from this study do not permit to conclude whether repair of the sole cuff tear can achieve shoulder stability nor whether shoulder stabilization alone can resolve the instability, therefore, treatment of both lesions should be performed arthroscopically, because the arthroscopic technique allows to treat capsular-labral and cuff lesions in the same procedure. In these patients it is important to manage both lesions. However, with advancing age the labrum can be stablized without a capsular with less risk of recurrence as in the younger patients. We therefore recommend a direct repair of the labrum while leaving some inferior capsular laxity to decreased the risk of post operative stiffness.

The techinque involves visuaization via a superior portal through the rotator cuff tear and stable fixation of the labral lesions. The arthroscope is then moved into the subacromial area. A bursoscopy is performed and a stable rotator cuff repair performed by the authors favored technique.

A decompression, biceps tenodesis, and distal clavicle excision can be added as needed but in many of these patients with combined lesions these additional procedurers.

In addition, rehabilitation in these patients should follow rotator cuff guidelines as that would be the major factor in long term function.

**Conclusion**

The association between Bankart and tear of the rotator cuff is a rare event. In the age group between 25 and 50 years, it is appropriate to distinguish two subcategories, patients younger than 40 years and patients with age above 40 years. In patients under the age of 40 years, the Bankart lesions are associated more frequently to fractures of the humeral greater tuberosity rather than rupture of the rotator cuff. In these patients, the presence of a Bankart lesion predisposes to recurrence, and therefore there is no doubt about the surgical treatment. When present the association between the two lesions is recommended repair of both lesions, but there is a need for studies to substantiate this hypothesis. In patients aged superior, the coexistence of both lesions to 40 years is more common and denotes the failure of the posterior stabilization mechanism described by McLaughlin. The work of Itoi shows that in this kind of patients, the repair of the lip is not necessary since the recurrence rate is not as high as in younger. In this area, further studies are needed.

## References


1. Gerstman BA, Malanga GA, Ferrer S. Rotator cuff tear in a 12-year-old baseball pitcher: a case report. PM R. 2009;1(7):687–90.
2. Battaglia TC, Barr MA, Diduch DR. Rotator cuff tear in a 13-year-old baseball player: a case report. Am J Sports Med. 2003;31(5):779–82.
3. Tarkin IS et al. Rotator cuff tears in adolescent athletes. Am J Sports Med. 2005;33(4):596–601.
4. Itoi E, Tabata S. Rotator cuff tears in the adolescent. Orthopedics. 1993;16(1):78–81.
5. Weiss JM et al. Rotator cuff injuries in adolescent athletes. J Pediatr Orthop B. 2013;22(2):133–7.
6. Arciero RA et al. Arthroscopic Bankart repair versus nonoperative treatment for acute, initial anterior shoulder dislocations. Am J Sports Med. 1994;22(5):589–94.
7. Baker CL, Uribe JW, Whitman C. Arthroscopic evaluation of acute initial anterior shoulder dislocations. Am J Sports Med. 1990;18(1):25–8.
8. Norlin R. Intraarticular pathology in acute, first-time anterior shoulder dislocation: an arthroscopic study. Arthroscopy. 1993;9(5):546–9.

9. Wheeler JH et al. Arthroscopic versus nonoperative treatment of acute shoulder dislocations in young athletes. Arthroscopy. 1989;5(3):213–7.
10. Neviaser RJ, Neviaser TJ, Neviaser JS. Anterior dislocation of the shoulder and rotator cuff rupture. Clin Orthop Relat Res. 1993;291:103–6.
11. Sonnabend DH. Treatment of primary anterior shoulder dislocation in patients older than 40 years of age. Conservative versus operative. Clin Orthop Relat Res. 1994;304:74–7.
12. Hawkins RJ, Mohtadi NG. Controversy in anterior shoulder instability. Clin Orthop Relat Res. 1991; 272:152–61.
13. Ribbans WJ, Mitchell R, Taylor GJ. Computerised arthrotomography of primary anterior dislocation of the shoulder. J Bone Joint Surg Br. 1990;72(2): 181–5.
14. McLaughlin HL, MacLellan DI. Recurrent anterior dislocation of the shoulder. II. A comparative study. J Trauma. 1967;7(2):191–201.
15. Itoi E et al. Dynamic anterior stabilisers of the shoulder with the arm in abduction. J Bone Joint Surg Br. 1994;76(5):834–6.
16. Craig EV. The posterior mechanism of acute anterior shoulder dislocations. Clin Orthop Relat Res. 1984;190:212–6.
17. Hsu HC et al. Influence of rotator cuff tearing on glenohumeral stability. J Shoulder Elbow Surg. 1997;6(5):413–22.
18. Pevny T, Hunter RE, Freeman JR. Primary traumatic anterior shoulder dislocation in patients 40 years of age and older. Arthroscopy. 1998;14(3):289–94.
19. Bassett RW, Cofield RH. Acute tears of the rotator cuff. The timing of surgical repair. Clin Orthop Relat Res. 1983;175:18–24.
20. Voos JE et al. Outcomes of combined arthroscopic rotator cuff and labral repair. Am J Sports Med. 2007;35(7):1174–9.

# SLAP

# 22

Carina Cohen, Bernardo Terra, Benno Ejnisman, Dan Guttmann, and Andreas Voss

## Contents


| | | |
|---|---|---|
| 22.1 | **Introduction** | 187 |
| 22.2 | **Biomechanics** | 189 |
| 22.3 | **Mechanism of Trauma** | 190 |
| 22.4 | **Classification** | 190 |
| 22.5 | **History and Physical Exam** | 194 |
| 22.6 | **Radiological Evaluation** | 194 |
| 22.7 | **Treatment** | 194 |
| 22.7.1 | Conservative Treatment | 194 |
| 22.7.2 | Operative Treatment | 194 |
| 22.8 | **Authors Preferred Operative Technique** | 197 |
| 22.9 | **Postoperative Treatment** | 197 |
| 22.10 | **Outcomes and Failures of SLAP Repairs** | 198 |
| **References** | | 199 |


C. Cohen, MD (✉) • B. Terra, MD
B. Ejnisman, MD
Department of Orthopaedic Sports Medicine (CETE), Federal University of São Paulo (UNIFESP), São Paulo, Brazil
e-mail: cacohen18@gmail.com

D. Guttmann, MD
Taos Orthopaedic Institute Research Foundation, Taos, NM, USA

A. Voss, MD
Department of Orthopaedic Sports Medicine, Technical University of Munich, Munich, Germany

## 22.1 Introduction

Initially described in 1985 by Andrews et al. [1], injuries to the superior glenoid labrum and biceps origin are a well-recognized cause of shoulder pain and dysfunction. In the nearly three decades since their description, our understanding of the anatomy, pathogenesis, diagnosis, and treatment of superior labrum anterior-posterior (SLAP) lesions has evolved together with widespread advances in shoulder arthroscopic surgery. According to the following studies, 11–57% of the patients with recurrent dislocation had combined Bankart and SLAP lesions [2]. A concomitant SLAP lesion occurs in up to 22% of anterior instabilities [3], the presence of which greatly increases shoulder instability [4, 5]. Snyder et al. provided the first classification of SLAP tears based on intraoperative findings [6]. However, more extensive labral tears do occur, some of which may be a progression of preexisting SLAP lesions or its combination with a Bankart lesion categorized by Maffet et al. [7] as the type V SLAP lesion that is characterized by superior extension of an anteroinferior labral tear involving a Bankart lesion and is thought to be caused by traumatic instability [8].

Cadaveric and arthroscopic studies have better defined the histology, anatomic variation, and vascularity of the superior labrum and long head of the biceps origin. Histologically, the glenoid labrum is characterized as being composed of

© ISAKOS 2017
A.B. Imhoff, F.H. Savoie III (eds.), *Shoulder Instability Across the Life Span*,
DOI 10.1007/978-3-662-54077-0_22

fibrous tissue and fibrocartilage (Fig. 22.1) [9]. Its vascularity has a radial and circumferential pattern and comes from branches of the suprascapular artery, circumflex scapular, and posterior circumflex humeral arteries (Fig. 22.2). The innermost portion of the labrum is avascular, and the superior and anterosuperior regions have less vascular supply than the posterior and inferior regions. In all regions, there is no significant contribution from the underlying glenoid bone into the labrum [9, 10]. The upper labrum has a triangular shape, but may have a meniscoid aspect. Forty to sixty percent of the insertion of the cable along the biceps originates from supraglenoid tubercle, with the remainder entering directly from the upper labrum, especially in the most posterior portion [11].

Anatomical variations are common in the anterior labral region and should be distinguished from pathological conditions. Variations include a sublabral foramen [12] or absence of the anterior labrum, both of which are commonly associated with a robust middle glenohumeral ligament (Buford complex) present in 1.5% of people [13, 14] (Fig. 22.3).

The glenoid labrum is the fibrocartilage of the shoulder joint. It comprises three sides and one edge: the superficial side is free and responsive to the humeral head; the articular side adheres to

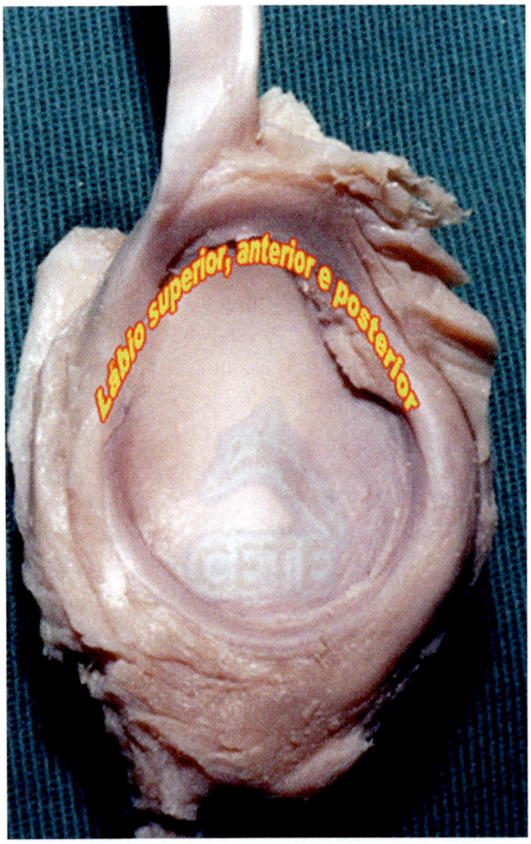


**Fig. 22.1** Anatomy of the glenoid cavity showing the superior labral complex, anterior, posterior, and inferior

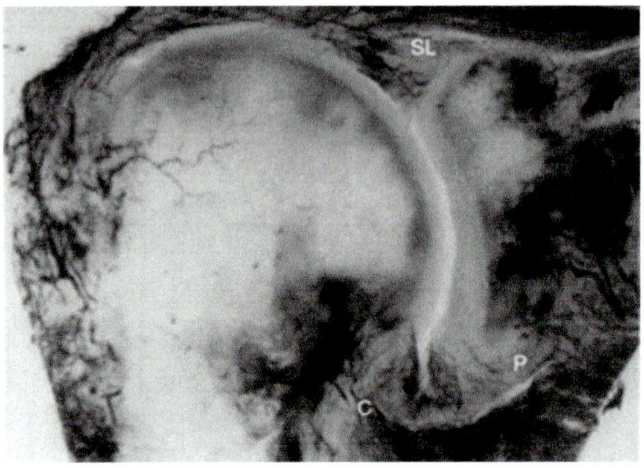


**Fig. 22.2** Anatomy showing the vasculature of the superior labrum complex (From: Cooper et al. [9])

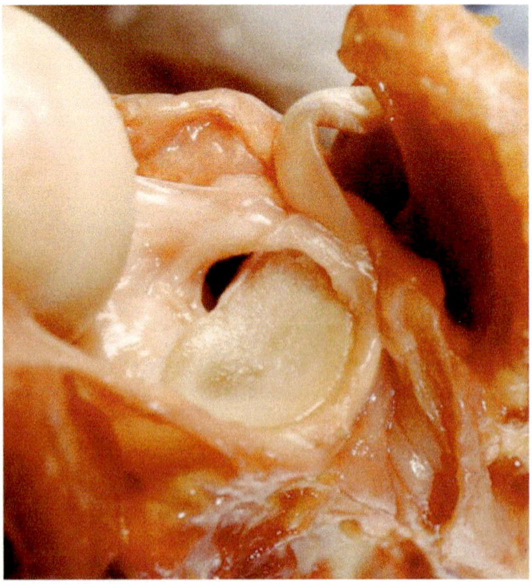

**Fig. 22.3** Anatomical variations of the labral complex. Above: foramen sublabral. Below: Buford complex (medial glenohumeral ligament in rope entering the base of the long biceps cable and hypoplastic anterior labrum)

the edge of the glenoid cavity; and the peripheral side is in continuity with the joint capsule (providing vascularization) and the shoulder ligament insertion. The axial edge is free. The form varies according to the region: the articular side does not adhere to the edge of the glenoid cavity in the superior region, where it is free (meniscus-like aspect); it is wide and voluminous and adheres to the edge of the glenoid cavity in the inferior and posterior region (region of the inferior glenohumeral ligament insertion), on which the strongest forces act. The insertion of the long head of the biceps tendon is to both the supraglenoid tubercle and the superior part of the labrum. The proportion and orientation of biceps fibers connected to the labrum vary greatly between individuals [9].

## 22.2 Biomechanics

The labrum has several functions and three in particular: it increases the contact area between the humeral head and scapula, by 2 mm anteroposteriorly and 4.5 mm supero-inferiorly; it contributes to the "viscoelastic piston" effect, maintaining −32 mmHg intra-articular negative pressure; this is especially effective against traction stress and, to a lesser extent, against shear stress; it provides the insertion for stabilizing structures (capsule and glenohumeral ligaments), as a fibrous "crossroad" [15]. Labrum and ligaments are in synergy in a genuine complex, each structure's contribution varying with the position of the limb: in abduction and external rotation (ABER), the inferior glenohumeral ligament (IGHL) absorbs 51% of the stress, the superior glenohumeral ligament (SGHL) 22%, and the MGHL 9% [16].

Biomechanical studies have sought to elucidate the function of an intact superior labrum/biceps complex and confirm the pathogenesis of injuries [17]. The function of the biceps is controversial and many authors have looked at this. The long head of the biceps tendon (LHBT) is felt to act as a humeral head depressor, aiding in glenohumeral compression and anterior and posterior glenohumeral stabilization and can limit external rotation [18, 19]. Giphart et al., however, found that there was no significant effect of the LHBT on glenohumeral kinematics [20].

A variety of mechanisms of injury are proposed in the pathogenesis of SLAP lesions, especially traction tension loads on the arm, compressive forces, and repeated microtrauma in throwing athletes. During the overhead throwing motion in the baseball pitch, SLAP lesions are often seen in the late and deceleration phase [21]. The increased lateral rotation in this late stage creates an increase in torsional stress in the insertion of the biceps, resulting in the dynamic peel-back mechanism and injury to the posterosuperior labrum [22]. In the last decade, understanding of the biomechanics and pathophysiology of the athletic shoulder has significantly improved. Especially in overhead athletes and throwers, several pathologic mechanisms have been identified which could not be explained by the traditional concepts of instability and impingement. Glenohumeral instability and posterior capsule contracture are believed to play a crucial role in the etiology of the painful athletic shoulder. Instability and contractures related to sports are frequently underappreciated. These may initiate a vicious cycle of secondary internal impingement, muscular dysfunction, and damage to intra-articular structures. The results can be devastating and may even end the athlete's career [23].

The term "instability" constitutes a spectrum of disorders, which includes hyperlaxity, subluxation, and dislocation. Principally, glenohumeral instability can be classified according to its etiology, degree, frequency, and direction. The classic categorization of affected individuals into two groups with traumatic and atraumatic instability represented by the mnemonics TUBS (traumatic, unidirectional, Bankart lesion, surgical treatment) and AMBRII (atraumatic, multidirectional, bilateral, rehabilitation, inferior capsular shift, rotator interval closure) has been supplemented by a further grouping that is mainly comprised of overhead athletes with so-called micro-instability (microtraumatic instability) and that has been labeled with the acronym AIOS (acquired instability in overstressed shoulder). However, it should be emphasized that congenital or acquired hyperlaxity, micro-instability, and traumatic instability can overlap particularly in athletes engaged in overhead sports [24, 25].

## 22.3 Mechanism of Trauma

Snyder et al. [6] described the most common mechanisms of SLAP lesions as compression injuries of the upper limb and traction injuries of the superior labrum biceps tendon complex with the shoulder in hyperextension. A three-part series of articles by Burkhart and colleagues looked at the association of kinetic chain disorders and scapular dyskinesia on SLAP injuries. The peel-back mechanism is associated with SLAP tears, with associated posteroinferior contraction and migration of rotation from the center toward the posterosuperior portion of the glenohumeral joint. With associated anteroinferior relaxation, there is a change in the biceps vector and elevated shearing in peel-back forces during the throwing cycle [21, 22, 26, 27].

Traumatic glenohumeral instability is also implicated as an associated etiology. It is typically initiated by a specific traumatic event, followed by other episodes of dislocation or subluxation usually in an anteroinferior direction when a sudden force overwhelms the anterior capsular structures. This occurs while the athlete's arm is in an abducted, externally rotated, and extended position. The resulting combination of injuries represents the source of chronic instability, particularly those involving the inferior glenohumeral ligament (IGHL). Most studies agree that the IGHL is the most important passive stabilizer of the shoulder joint [28, 29]. The IGHL is formed by an anterior and a posterior band, which represents a thickening of the capsule connecting the inferior labrum to the glenoid and the humeral neck. The anteroinferior labrum and the anterior band of the IGHL together form the anteroinferior labro-ligamentous complex. The labrum is thought to serve as an insertion site for the IGHL and to provide stability to the glenohumeral joint by deepening the glenoid fossa [30]. Although generally common in contact collision sports, this type of instability is rarely observed in throwers or overhead athletes. When present, however, this type of instability can cause secondary damage to the rotator cuff and the superior and posterior labrum [31].

According to Soslowsky et al., inferior subluxation of the shoulder resulted in type II SLAP lesions [32]. Lo and Burkhart concluded that anterior lesions led to injuries of the superior and posterior labrum, because a history of trauma was observed in shoulders when they were positioned in abduction and external rotation [33]. They believe that recurrent anteroinferior instability is mainly responsible for the SLAP lesions.

These authors also suggest that more extensive lesions are a result of an increased number of dislocations, secondary to progression of a simple injury. However, this is not always the case, since extensive lesions have also been noted with low numbers of dislocations in the presence of high-energy trauma [34]. Durban et al. suggest that the severity of the lesions is a result of the initial high-energy trauma leading to the anterior shoulder instability with SLAP lesions [35]. Therefore, primary lesions of complex labral tears, such as type V SLAP lesions, should be examined thoroughly.

## 22.4 Classification

In 1985, Andrews postulated that a SLAP lesion, an anteroposterior tear of the superior labrum, was caused by overloading and traction of the long head of the biceps tendon during the follow-through phase of throwing [1]. Snyder categorized SLAP lesions into four types and suggested that type II SLAP lesions were the most common injuries and were primarily responsible for pain and restricted mobility of the shoulder joint in overhead athletes [6]. Maffet then added more types to this classification, because 38% of the SLAP lesion patients did not fall into the classification by Snyder. The authors use the Morgan and Maffet modifications [7] (Figs. 22.4, 22.5, 22.6, 22.7, and 22.8):

- Type I: Lip fibrillation with a local degeneration. Commonly seen in middle-aged, usually asymptomatic
- Type II: More common. Detachment of the upper lip/biceps glenoid complex with an abnormal mobility. Important to differentiate the meniscoid appearance and the medial insertion of the glenoid lip (usually symptomatic). Subdivided into types A (anterior), B (predominantly posterior), and C (combined)
- Type III: Bucket handle injury with an intact biceps. May cause mechanical symptoms depending on the size of the lesion
- Type IV: Bucket handle injury extending into the biceps tendon
- Type V: Association with Bankart lesion
- Type VI: SLAP with an unstable labrum flap
- Type VII: Association with the middle glenohumeral ligament injury
- Type VIII: Association with a posterior labrum injury
- Type IX: Circumferential labral injury (360°)
- Type X: Association with a superior glenohumeral ligament injury

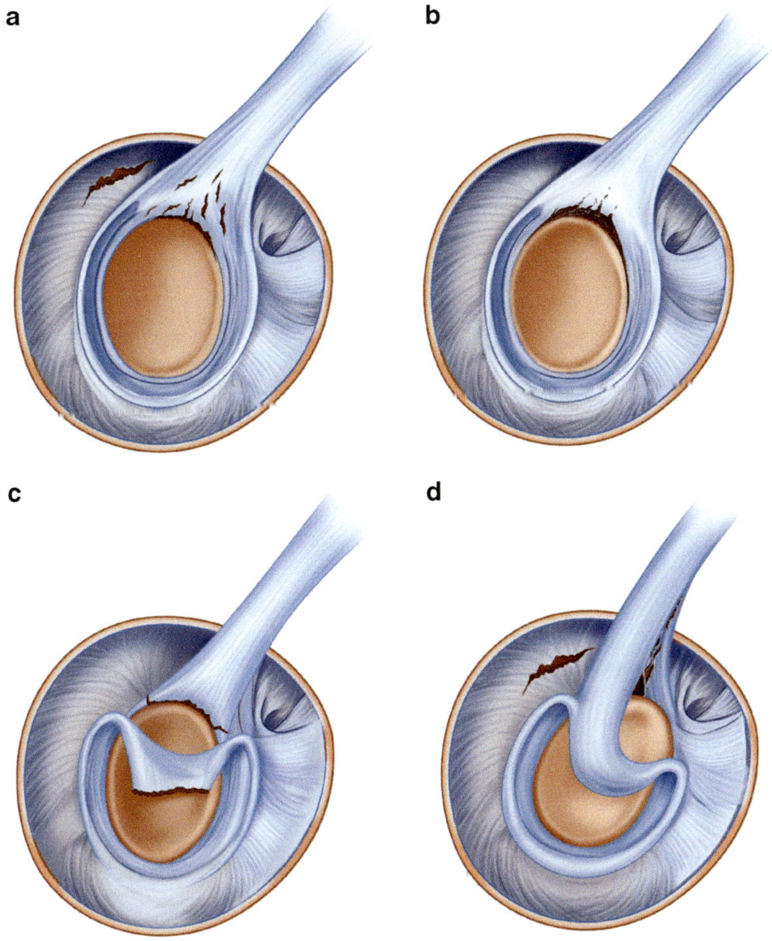


**Fig. 22.4** Snyder classification of the four types of injury. (**a**) type I; (**b**) type II; (**c**) type III; (**d**) type IV

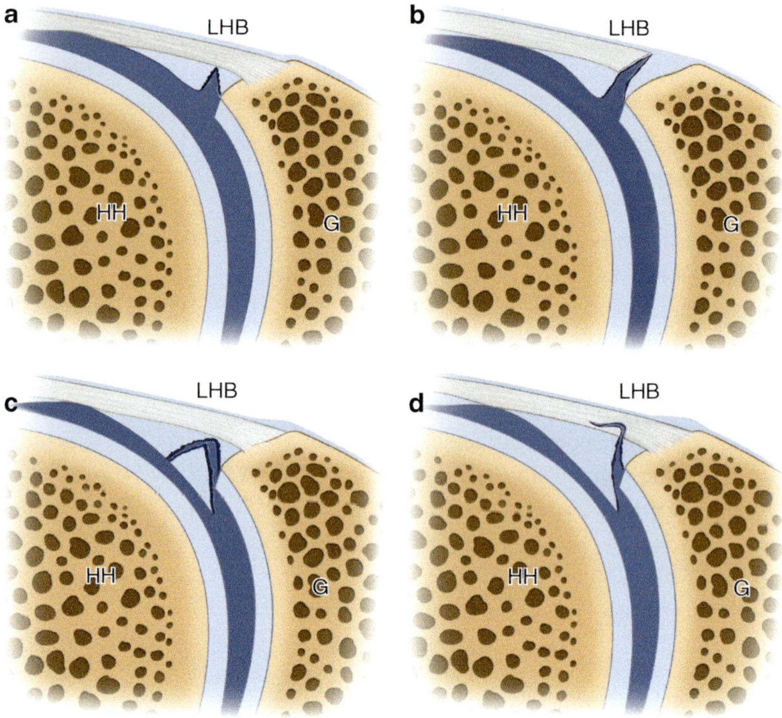


**Fig. 22.5** SLAP lesions: classification according to Snyder. (**a**) Type I: Lip fibrillation. (**b**) Type II: Detachment of the upper lip/biceps glenoid complex. (**c**) Type III: Bucket handle injury with an intact biceps. (**d**) Type IV: Bucket handle injury extending into the biceps tendon (*LBC* labral-bicipital complex, *HH* humeral head, *G* glenoid)

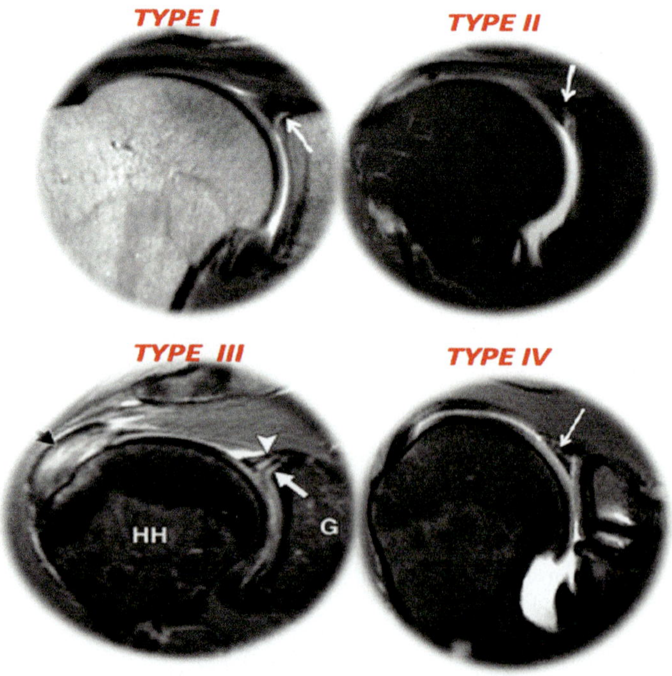


**Fig. 22.6** Four types of SLAP. Coronal oblique MRI with arrows pointing superior labrum lesions types I to IV. Type I: Lip fibrillation. Type II: Detachment of the upper lip/biceps glenoid complex. Type III: Bucket handle injury with an intact biceps. Type IV: Bucket handle injury extending into the biceps tendon. *HH* humeral head, *G* glenoid (From: Woertler and Waldt [62])

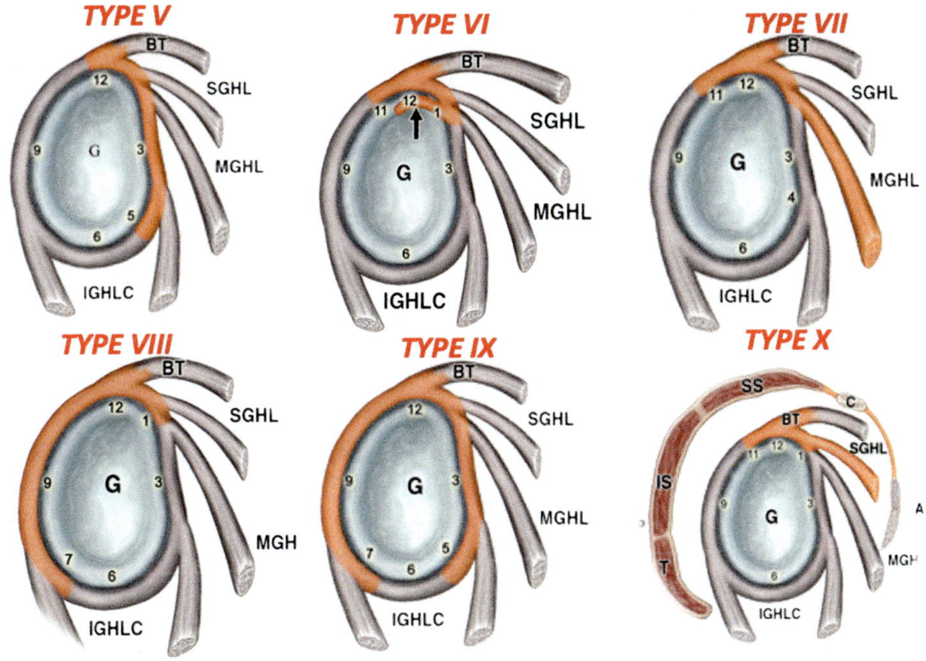


**Fig. 22.7** Type V to type X SLAP lesions (*BT* biceps tendon, *G* glenoid, *SGHL* superior glenohumeral ligament, *MGHL* medium glenohumeral ligament, *IGHL* inferior glenohumeral ligament, *SS* supraspinal, *IS* infraspinal, *T* teres minor)

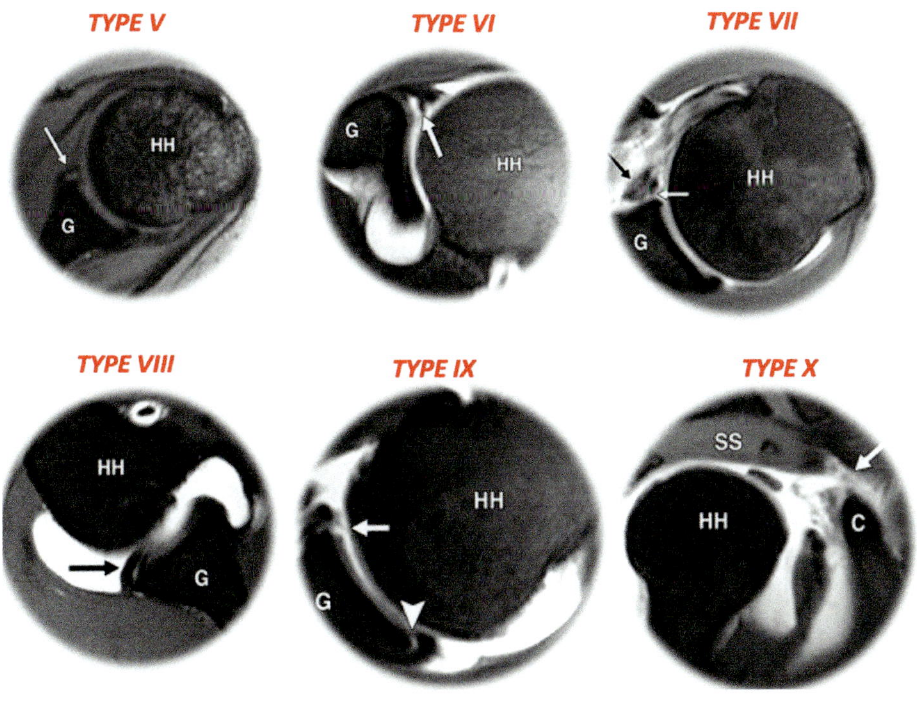


**Fig. 22.8** Types V to X of SLAP (Maffet-Morgan modification) seen in MR arthrogram, pointed by the *arrows*. Type V: Association with Bankart lesion. Type VI: SLAP with an unstable labrum flap. Type VII: Association with the middle glenohumeral ligament injury. Type VIII: Association with the posterior labrum injury. Type IX: Circumferential labral injury (360°). Type X: Association with superior glenohumeral ligament injury. *HH* humeral head, *G* glenoid, *SS* supraspinal muscle, *C* coracoid process (From: Woertler and Waldt [62])

## 22.5 History and Physical Exam

A complete clinical history with detailed mechanism of trauma description is essential. Symptoms associated with Bankart lesions typically do not include chronic pain but rather functional limitations that arise from symptoms of instability. In contrast, SLAP lesions frequently present with pain. We believe the combination of both lesions involves a great degree of energy with the arm in abduction and external rotation, where simultaneously the biceps labral complex is subjected to shear and torsional forces.

There are many tests that have been described in the literature. These include O'Brien's test, Speed's test, Yergason's test, pain provocation test, biceps load test, biceps load test type II, crank test, and many more. Recent literature [36] has looked at a combination of tests to get the optimal sensitivity and specificity. And these often involve the combination of O'Brien's, Hawkin's, Speed's, Neer's, and Jobe's test. High specificity tests include pain provocation and Yergason's test. The authors feel that a combination of several tests is optimal for an accurate diagnosis.

The use of SLAP tests and assessments for traumatic anterior instability in combination with radiologic imaging can improve accuracy, but arthroscopy is the gold standard for both diagnosis and treatment of SLAP tears [37].

## 22.6 Radiological Evaluation

The high diagnostic accuracy of magnetic resonance (MR) arthrography in the detection of labro-ligamentous lesions has been demonstrated in several studies with a sensitivity of 88–96% and a specificity of 91–98% [38]. For the detection of lesions of the superior, middle, and inferior glenohumeral ligaments, Chandnani and coworkers reported sensitivities and specificities of 88–100% [39]. The sensitivities and specificities of unenhanced MR imaging for the diagnosis of labro-ligamentous injuries vary widely in the literature. A direct comparison with MR arthrography has not yet been performed in a larger series. The role of standard MR imaging in the diagnostic work-up of shoulder instability is questionable, particularly in regard to chronic cases and the identification of associated pathology. The advantages of MR arthrography result from capsular distension with separation of anatomic structures and improved delineation of tears following introduction of contrast media. MR arthrography thereby allows a more confident identification of pathology from the common anatomic variations of labral morphology, as well as the congenital variants of the glenohumeral ligaments and the labro-ligamentous unit, such as the Buford complex. MR arthrography (MRA) is the current gold standard imaging method to detect SLAP tears [39, 40].

We can clearly see a SLAP type II lesion in association with a Bankart lesion using MR arthrography (Fig. 22.9).

## 22.7 Treatment

### 22.7.1 Conservative Treatment

Nonoperative treatment continues to have a role for patients who have mild symptoms and/or with contraindications to a surgical procedure. Nonoperative treatment usually focuses on associated shoulder injuries and the results of clinical examination. The aim of therapy is capsular mobilization, rotator cuff strengthening, scapular and humeral head stabilization, and the use of nonsteroidal anti-inflammatory drug (NSAID) medications [37, 41]. There is no study, which the authors are aware of, that investigates the effectiveness of conservative treatment with SLAP lesions.

### 22.7.2 Operative Treatment

Although the exact contribution of the biceps and superior labrum to anterior shoulder stability is unclear, several authors have noted that SLAP lesions can contribute to glenohumeral joint instability. Rodosky et al., in a biomechanical study, found that superior labral detachment placed increased strain on the inferior glenohu-

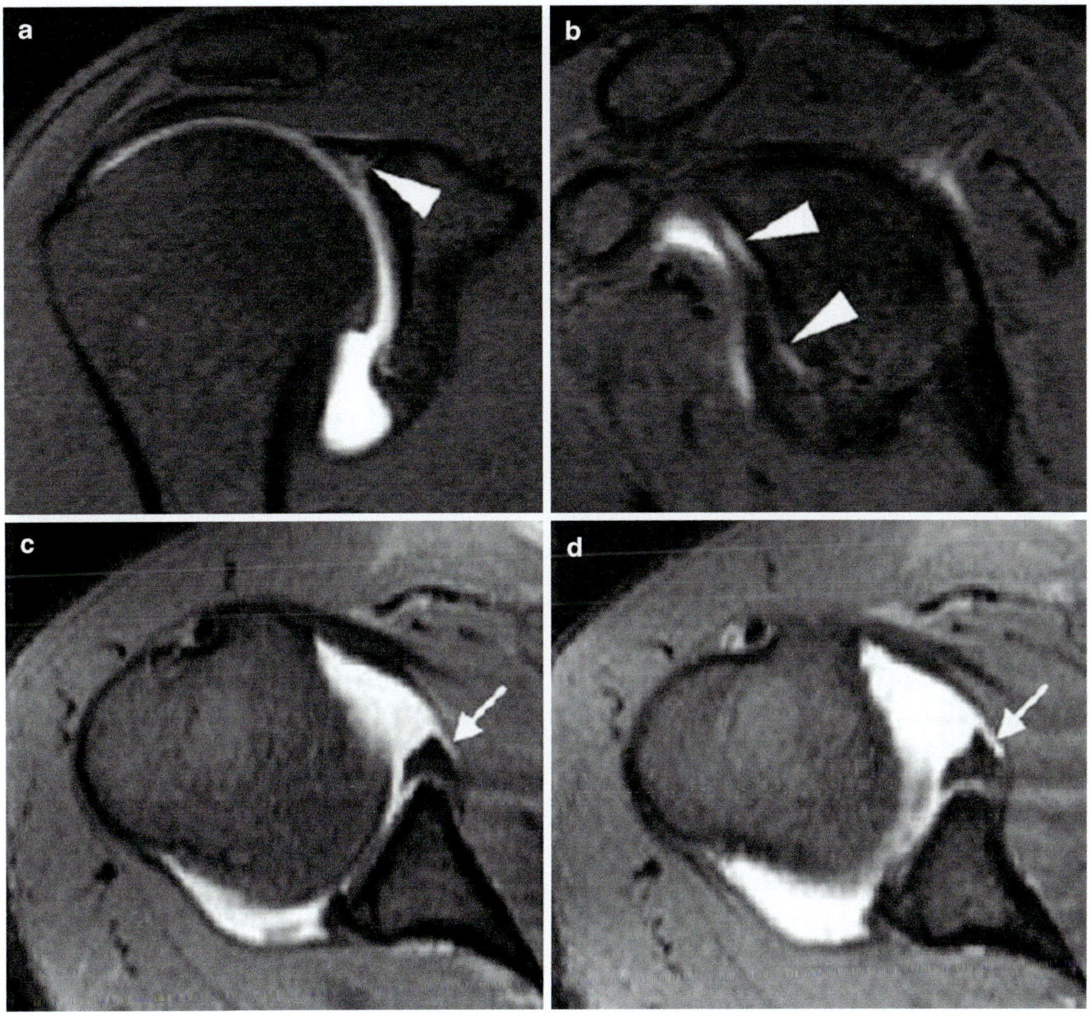


**Fig. 22.9** SLAP type II lesion in association with a Bankart lesion in traumatic anterior glenohumeral instability. (**a**) Coronal oblique fat-suppressed T1-weighted MR arthrogram shows superior extension of contrast media into the superior labrum and biceps anchor (*arrowhead*). (**b**) Corresponding sagittal oblique MR arthrogram reveals tearing of the entire anterior labrum (*arrowheads*) extending from inferior to superior. (**c**, **d**) Corresponding transverse MR arthrograms demonstrate detachment of the anterior labrum that continues as a classic Bankart lesion anteroinferiorly (*arrows*) (From: Woertler and Waldt [62])

meral ligament and decreased the shoulder's resistance to torsional forces [42]. They considered superior labral detachment to be detrimental to anterior shoulder stability. Pagnani et al. in 1995 showed significantly increased anteroposterior and supero-inferior glenohumeral translation when the insertion of the biceps was destabilized [43]. In their analysis of 139 cases of SLAP tears, Kim et al. noted that type III and type IV lesions were significantly associated with a Bankart lesion and a high-demand occupation [25]. Similarly, Snyder et al. noted that 43% of their patients with type IV SLAP tears had a concurrent Bankart lesion [11]. When confronted with a combined Bankart and type IV SLAP lesion, we make an effort to repair all pathoanatomy present including the superior labrum and biceps tendon split to preserve its stabilizing function.

Some authors believe that reattachment of concomitant SLAP lesions depends on the age and functional demand of the patient, noting that biceps tenodesis or tenotomy had varied results. Most studies show that with combined repairs, there is a significant difference in ranges of motion, functional scores, and recurrence rates when compared to an isolated Bankart repair [44, 45]. However, other authors have noted several limitations especially in external rotation among those who underwent the combined procedure [46].

The treatment of LHBT pathology lies along a spectrum ranging from simple debridement to tenotomy to one of many procedures developed for tenodesis. The decision to perform a tenodesis versus primary SLAP repair has evolved over recent years as the rate of SLAP repair has declined in response to discouraging outcomes in some patient populations. The location of tenodesis remains a topic of controversy, as does the debate between arthroscopic and open techniques.

In cases where the biceps tendon is involved and/or the SLAP tear is very degenerative and has a low potential for healing, a biceps tenotomy or tenodesis has been more recently recommended, rather than a SLAP repair [47]. Additionally it has been shown that operative treatments of SLAP tears that involve debridement were often unsuccessful [48, 49].

In 1993 Burkhart and Fox described the arthroscopic repair of a type IV SLAP lesion as a component of anterior instability [50]. They repaired the Bankart lesion first with a Caspari arthroscopic transglenoid reconstruction followed by suture repair of the SLAP tear. With the authors' technique, a reduction of the bucket handle tear of the superior labrum first is performed. This reduction provides a template for the Bankart reconstruction. After completion of the Bankart reconstruction, the SLAP tear is then addressed. The authors believe this to be an effective technique in the arthroscopic management of a patient with anterior shoulder instability and an associated SLAP IV lesion.

No agreement has been reached on whether Bankart lesion repair should precede SLAP lesion repair or vice versa. Warner et al. recommended to perform a Bankart lesion repair prior to SLAP lesion repair, but did not provide a specific reason [51]. Lo and Burkhart passed a suture through the SLAP lesion, closed the Bankart lesion, and then finished the SLAP lesion repair in the cases of triple labral lesions (anterior, posterior, and superior labral tears) [33]. Based on the authors' experience, performing a Bankart lesion repair first, in cases of complex labral lesions, could lengthen the operative time. This would cause swelling of the soft tissues, especially those located superior to the SLAP lesion, and therefore potentially disrupt clear visualization during SLAP lesion repair. In addition, inferior and medial displacement of the superior and anteroinferior labrum caused by chronic dislocations necessitated to include an inferior area of the labrum in the repair in order to obtain enough mobility of the labrum. However, when stabilization of the unstable SLAP lesions is performed first, the bowstring effect of the labrum contributed to the maintenance of tension on the labrum and anatomical reduction of the anteroinferior labrum. Accordingly, Bankart lesion repair could be performed more efficiently. Repairs of relatively extensive labral tears such as combined Bankart and SLAP lesions can result in restrictions on the range of motion. According to Warner et al., no difference was found with regard to external rotation when the shoulder was placed in the neutral position or at 90° abduction [51]. However, slower range of motion recovery was noted in the combined Bankart and SLAP lesion patients compared to the isolated Bankart lesion patients. The authors attributed this to the difference in the extent of the lesions and intra-articular adhesion (could also be tightening up rotator interval/anterior tissue). Limited joint mobility is a relatively common complication in patients with isolated SLAP lesion repair. Oh et al. reduced the risk of postoperative stiffness by avoiding closure of the anterosuperior labrum during SLAP lesion repair to reduce tension in the rotator interval [52]. Therefore, the delay in recovery of the range of motion was caused by closure of the anterosuperior labrum in patients at the authors' institution.

Although controversial, arthroscopic portals created for SLAP repair can affect postoperative function of the shoulder. According to

Cohen et al., trans-rotator cuff portals resulted in a 25% of reduction in function compared to the rotator interval portal [2]. Therefore, the authors believe that the stiffness observed in 10 of 15 patients with posterior labral tears might have been caused by the use of a trans-rotator cuff portal (port of Wilmington) resulting in postoperative pain or impingement. Future studies are needed to determine the optimal clinical outcome after combined Bankart and SLAP lesion repairs.

## 22.8 Authors Preferred Operative Technique

Surgery is performed with the patient in the beach-chair position under general anesthesia. A posterior portal is first established to identify intra-articular lesions. An anteroinferior portal is then placed. Next, an anterosuperior portal is made at the anterolateral corner of the acromion. A probe is passed through an anterosuperior-positioned cannula to determine the extent of the Bankart lesion and the presence of a SLAP lesion. Before the repair of the SLAP lesion, confirmation is necessary that anatomical reduction of the medially displaced anteroinferior labrum can be obtained with tension when trial reduction of the superior labrum is performed. Then, the anteroinferior labral tissue is released from the articular surface, and the glenoid is abraded. The first suture anchor is placed around the 5-o'clock position. A second anchor is placed through the anteroinferior portal, approximately 7 mm proximal to the first anchor. A minimum of three anchors is used for the repair. After completion of the Bankart repair, the SLAP tear is addressed. The glenoid underneath the superior labrum detachment is prepared. The anchor is inserted at a 45° angle just medial to the glenoid articular surface. Upon insertion, the eyelet is rotated, so one set of sutures is anterior and the other set is posterior. After suture passing through or around the labrum, a secure arthroscopic knot is tied. Care is taken to place the knot on top of the superior labrum away from the articular surface. Alternatively, a knotless technique may be used (preferred by DG). After repair of the superior labrum to the glenoid, the split in the biceps tendon is addressed if a SLAP IV is present (with either repair or tenodesis).

In failed SLAP repairs or in older patients who have a degenerative labrum, our recommendation is to perform open or arthroscopic biceps tenodesis rather than the isolated SLAP repair/reinsertion. Some authors have shown that tenodesis had better results in terms of satisfaction and return to previous level activities in young active and competitive athletes [53, 54].

## 22.9 Postoperative Treatment

Postoperatively, a shoulder immobilizer is used for approximately 4 weeks. For the first 3 weeks, there are no active biceps exercises. Range of motion is allowed with table slides and gentle range of motion to approximately 90° of flexion and gentle internal/external rotation as tolerated. Over the next 3–6 weeks, range of motion is advanced to full.

From the eighth postoperative week, full-range active exercise and strength training is started. From the tenth postoperative week, patients begin strength training of their biceps. A gradual return to throwing sports over the next 2–3 months is allowed when muscle strength and range of motion return to normal. Special attention is focused on the mechanics of throwing and the kinetic chain.

In biceps tenodesis, passive range of motion may start earlier approximately 1–2 weeks postoperatively and active range of motion in week 4. Strengthening phase starts approximately in 6–8 weeks postoperatively, and advanced strengthening phase starts around week 10 until return to full recreational and strenuous work activities [55]. In biceps tenotomy, active range of motion is allowed in weeks 2–4 postoperatively. Strengthening phase starts approximately in 4–6 weeks postoperatively, and advanced strengthening phase starts after 6 weeks until full recovery [56].

## 22.10 Outcomes and Failures of SLAP Repairs

Provencher et al. [57] found that 36.8% of SLAP repairs had problems postoperatively and were unable to return to work or sports successfully. He also found that patients greater than 36 years of age had a high risk for failure. Using ASES scores (<75), return to full military duties, and no need for revision procedures to mark successful cases, the investigators found that 66 patients (36.8%) had failures. Of these, 50 patients with failures opted for corrective surgery including 42 patients who underwent biceps tenodesis, four patients had biceps tenotomy, and four patients required debridement.

Age was a major factor in whether the repair was successful. The mean age in the failures was 39 years of age; successes were 29 years of age. Additionally there was no association with etiology, smoking history, or preoperative outcome scores.

Waterman et al. [58] investigated a total of 192 patients with SLAP repairs who were identified with a mean follow-up of 50.0 months. Isolated SLAP repair occurred in 31.3% ($n = 60$) versus 68.8% ($n = 132$) with concomitant procedures. At final follow-up, 37% ($n = 71$) of patients reported some subjective activity-related shoulder pain. Postoperative return to duty occurred in 79.6% ($n = 153$). Thirty-seven percent still had some pain, and 31 patients (16.1%) were classified as surgical failure and required revision. Of these, the majority of patients undergoing biceps tenodesis (76%) returned to active duty, as compared with revision SLAP repair (17%).

In a French study, Boileau et al. compared type II SLAP repairs with biceps tenodesis as an alternative to SLAP repair. He found that the patients who had a SLAP repair were disappointed and still had pain in 60% of cases and only 20% were back to the previous sports level, whereas in patients who had a tenodesis of the biceps, 93% were satisfied or very satisfied and 87% returned to previous sports level [54].

Chalmers et al. [59] recently described motion analyses with simultaneous surface electromyographic measurements in 18 baseball pitchers. Of these 18 players, seven were uninjured (controls), six were pitching after SLAP repair, and five were pitching after subpectoral biceps tenodesis. There were no significant differences between controls and postoperative patients with respect to pitching kinematics. Interestingly, compared with the controls and the patients who underwent open biceps tenodesis, the patients who underwent SLAP repair had altered patterns of thoracic rotation during pitching. The clinical significance of this finding and the impact of this finding on pitching efficacy are not currently known.

A retrospective analysis was performed of patients who had surgery for an isolated type II SLAP lesion between 2008 and 2011 [60]. There were 25 patients: 15 underwent biceps tenodesis, with a mean follow-up of 31 months and 10 underwent SLAP repair, with a mean follow-up of 35 months. The mean age was 47 years in the tenodesis group and 31 years in the repair group. At the latest follow-up, both groups showed significant improvements in subjective shoulder value and pain score. No difference was observed in American Shoulder and Elbow Surgeons score, patient satisfaction, or return to preinjury sporting level. Analysis of the indications for treatment showed that in the large majority, tenodesis was performed in older patients (>35 years) and patients who showed degenerative or frayed labrums, whereas SLAP repairs were performed in younger and more active patients with healthy-appearing labral tissue. There was only one failure in the tenodesis group, and in the SLAP repair group, there were two cases of postoperative stiffness; all were treated nonoperatively. In this study, both biceps tenodesis and SLAP repair can provide good to excellent results if performed in appropriately selected patients with isolated type II SLAP lesions.

Mollon and colleagues recently reviewed the literature [61]. They were not aware of any high-quality studies comparing revision SLAP repair and biceps tenodesis in the management of failed SLAP repair. They suggested that, therefore, there is an expanding role of tenodesis in the failed SLAP repair and potentially a treatment for the primary SLAP patient. They identified a 10.1% incidence of subsequent surgery after isolated SLAP repair, often related to an additional diagnosis, suggesting that clinicians should consider other potential causes of shoulder pain when considering surgery for patients with SLAP lesions. In addition, the number of isolated SLAP repairs performed has decreased over time, and management of failed SLAP repair has shifted toward biceps tenodesis or tenotomy over revision SLAP repair in more recent years.

The authors are not aware of any high-quality studies comparing revision SLAP repair and biceps tenodesis in the management of failed SLAP repair. This makes a case for an expanding role of tenodesis in the failed SLAP repair and potentially a treatment for the primary SLAP patient.

## References


1. Andrews JR, Carson Jr WG, McLeod WD. Glenoid labrum tears related to the long head of the biceps. Am J Sports Med. 1985;13(5):337–41.
2. Cohen DB, Coleman S, Drakos MC, Allen AA, O'Brien SJ, Altchek DW, et al. Outcomes of isolated type II SLAP lesions treated with arthroscopic fixation using a bioabsorbable tack. Arthroscopy. 2006;22(2):136–42.
3. Yiannakopoulos CK, Mataragas E, Antonogiannakis E. A comparison of the spectrum of intra-articular lesions in acute and chronic anterior shoulder instability. Arthroscopy. 2007;23(9):985–90.
4. Mihata T, McGarry MH, Tibone JE, Fitzpatrick MJ, Kinoshita M, Lee TQ. Biomechanical assessment of Type II superior labral anterior-posterior (SLAP) lesions associated with anterior shoulder capsular laxity as seen in throwers: a cadaveric study. Am J Sports Med. 2008;36(8):1604–10.
5. Hantes ME, Venouziou AI, Liantsis AK, Dailiana ZH, Malizos KN. Arthroscopic repair for chronic anterior shoulder instability: a comparative study between patients with Bankart lesions and patients with combined Bankart and superior labral anterior posterior lesions. Am J Sports Med. 2009;37(6):1093–8.
6. Snyder SJ, Karzel RP, Del Pizzo W, Ferkel RD, Friedman MJ. SLAP lesions of the shoulder. Arthroscopy. 1990;6(4):274–9.
7. Maffet MW, Gartsman GM, Moseley B. Superior labrum-biceps tendon complex lesions of the shoulder. Am J Sports Med. 1995;23(1):93–8.
8. Virk MS, Arciero RA. Superior labrum anterior to posterior tears and glenohumeral instability. Instr Course Lect. 2013;62:501–14.
9. Cooper DE, Arnoczky SP, O'Brien SJ, Warren RF, Di Carlo E, Allen AA. Anatomy, histology, and vascularity of the glenoid labrum. An anatomical study. J Bone Joint Surg Am. 1992;74(1):46–52.
10. Abrassart S, Stern R, Hoffmeyer P. Arterial supply of the glenoid: an anatomic study. J Shoulder Elbow Surg. 2006;15:232–8.
11. Snyder SJ, Banas MP, Karzel RP. An analysis of 140 injuries to the superior glenoid labrum. J Shoulder Elbow Surg. 1995;4(4):243–8.
12. Rao AG, Kim TK, Chronopoulos E, McFarland EG. Anatomical variants in the anterosuperior aspect of the glenoid labrum: a statistical analysis of seventy-three cases. J Bone Joint Surg Am. 2003;85:653–9.
13. Williams MM, Snyder SJ, Buford Jr D. The Buford complex–the "cord-like" middle glenohumeral ligament and absent anterosuperior labrum complex: a normal anatomic capsulolabral variant. Arthroscopy. 1994;10(3):241–7.
14. Nam EK, Snyder SJ. The diagnosis and treatment of superior labrum, anterior and posterior (SLAP) lesions. Am J Sports Med. 2003;31(5):798–810.
15. Clavert P. Glenoid labrum pathology. Orthop Traumatol Surg Res. 2015;101(1 Suppl):S19–24.
16. Itoi E, Kuechle DK, Newman SR, Morrey BF, An KN. Stabilising function of the biceps in stable and unstable shoulders. J Bone Joint Surg Br. 1993;75(4):546–50.
17. Elser F, Braun S, Dewing CB, Giphart JE, Millett PJ. Anatomy, function, injuries, and treatment of the long head of the biceps brachii tendon. Arthroscopy. 2011;27(4):581–92.
18. Albers, Biomechanical Investigation of the long head of the biceps tendon of the dog, LMU Munich 2002.
19. Ruchay, An anatomical-histological investigation considering the collagen fibers distribution and the clinical relevance in comparison to the glenohumeral joint, dissertation, Erlangen 2008.
20. Giphart JE, Elser F, Dewing CB, Torry MR, Millett PJ. The long head of the biceps tendon has minimal effect on in vivo glenohumeral kinematics: a biplane fluoroscopy study. Am J Sports Med. 2012;40: 202–12.
21. Burkhart SS, Morgan CD, Kibler WB. The disabled throwing shoulder: spectrum of pathology Part I: pathoanatomy and biomechanics. Arthroscopy. 2003;19(4): 404–20.
22. Burkhart SS, Morgan CD. The peel-back mechanism: its role in producing and extending posterior type II SLAP lesions and its effect on SLAP repair rehabilitation. Arthroscopy. 1998;14(6):637–40.
23. Norwood LA, Del Pizzo W, Jobe FW, Kerlan RK. Anterior shoulder pain in baseball pitchers. Am J Sports Med. 1978;6(3):103–5.
24. Beltran J, Rosenberg ZS, Chandnani VP, Cuomo F, Beltran S, Rokito A. Glenohumeral instability: evaluation with MR arthrography. Radiographics. 1997;17(3):657–73.
25. Kim SJ, Jahng JS, Lee JW. Arthroscopic transglenoid Bankart suture repair with modifications of Caspari's technique. Yonsei Med J. 1997;38(5):294–300.

26. Burkhart SS, Morgan CD, Kibler WB. The disabled throwing shoulder: spectrum of pathology. Part II: evaluation and treatment of SLAP lesions in throwers. Arthroscopy. 2003;19(5):531–9.
27. Burkhart SS, Morgan CD, Kibler WB. The disabled throwing shoulder: spectrum of pathology Part III: The SICK scapula, scapular dyskinesis, the kinetic chain, and rehabilitation. Arthroscopy. 2003;19(6):641–61.
28. O'Brien SJ, Neves MC, Arnoczky SP, Rozbruck SR, Dicarlo EF, Warren RF, Schwartz R, Wickiewicz TL. The anatomy and histology of the inferior glenohumeral ligament complex of the shoulder. Am J Sports Med. 1990;18:449–56.
29. Warner JJ, Deng XH, Warren RF, Torzilli PA. Static capsuloligamentous restraints to superior-inferior translation of the glenohumeral joint. Am J Sports Med. 1992;20:675–85.
30. O'Connell PW, Nuber GW, Mileski RA, Lautenschalger E. The contribution of glenohumeral ligaments to anterior stability of the shoulder joint. Am J Sports Med. 1990;18:579–84.
31. Meister K. Injuries to the shoulder in the throwing athlete. Part one: biomechanics, pathophysiology, classification of injury. Am J Sports Med. 2000;28:265–75.
32. Soslowsky LJ, Malicky DM, Blasier RB. Active and passive factors in inferior glenohumeral stabilization: a biomechanical model. J Shoulder Elbow Surg. 1997;6(4):371–9.
33. Lo IK, Burkhart SS. Triple labral lesions: pathology and surgical repair technique-report of seven cases. Arthroscopy. 2005;21(2):186–93.
34. Kim DS, Yi CH, Kwon KY, Oh JR. Relationship between the extent of labral lesions and the frequency of glenohumeral dislocation in shoulder instability. Knee Surg Sports Traumatol Arthrosc. 2013;21(2):430–7.
35. Durban CMC, Kim JK, Kim SH, Oh JH. Anterior Shoulder Instability with or without a SLAP Lesion. Clin Orthop Surg. 2016;8(2):168–74.
36. Parentis MA, Glousman RE, Mohr KS, Yocum LA. An evaluation of the provocative tests for superior labral anterior posterior lesions. Am J Sports Med. 2006;34(2):265–8.
37. Snyder SJ, Karzel RP, Pizzo WD, Ferkel RD, Friedman MJ. Arthroscopy classics. SLAP lesions of the shoulder. Arthroscopy. 2010;26(8):1117.
38. Tirman PF, Smith ED, Stoller DW, Fritz RC. Shoulder imaging in athletes. Semin Musculoskelet Radiol. 2004;8(1):29–40.
39. Chandnani VP, Gagliardi JA, Murnane TG, et al. Glenohumeral ligaments and shoulder capsular mechanism: evaluation with MR arthrography. Radiology. 1995;196:27–32.
40. Jee WH, McCauley TR, Katz LD, Matheny JM, Ruwe PA, Daigneault JP. Superior labral anterior posterior (SLAP) lesions of the glenoid labrum: reliability and accuracy of MR arthrography for diagnosis. Radiology. 2001;218(1):127–32.
41. Paxinos A, Walton J, Rutten S, Muller M, Murrell GA. Arthroscopic stabilization of superior labral (SLAP) tears with biodegradable tack: outcomes to 2 years. Arthroscopy. 2006;22(6):627–34.
42. Rodosky MW, Harner CD, Fu FH. The role of the long head of the biceps muscle and superior glenoid labrum in anterior stability of the shoulder. Am J Sports Med. 1994;22(1):121–30.
43. Pagnani MJ, Deng XH, Warren RF, Torzilli PA, Altchek DW. Effect of lesions of the superior portion of the glenoid labrum on glenohumeral translation. J Bone Joint Surg Am. 1995;77(7):1003–10.
44. Cho HL, Lee CK, Hwang TH, Suh KT, Park JW. Arthroscopic repair of combined Bankart and SLAP lesions: operative techniques and clinical results. Clin Orthop Surg. 2010;2(1):39–46.
45. Kim DS, Yi CH, Yoon YS. Arthroscopic repair for combined Bankart and superior labral anterior posterior lesions: a comparative study between primary and recurrent anterior dislocation in the shoulder. Int Orthop. 2011;35(8):1187–95.
46. Takase K. Risk of motion loss with combined Bankart and SLAP repairs. Orthopedics. 2009;32(8). pii: orthosupersite.com/view.asp?rID=41913. doi: 10.3928/01477447-20090624-05.
47. Braun S, Minzlaff P, Imhoff AB. Subpectoral tenodesis of the long head of the biceps tendon for pathologies of the long head of the biceps ten-don and the biceps pulley. Oper Orthop Traumatol. 2012;24:479–85.
48. Cordasco FA, Steinmann S, Flatow EL, Bigliani LU. Arthroscopic treatment of glenoid labral tears. Am J Sports Med. 1993;21(3):425–31.
49. Altchek OW, Warren FR, Wickiewicz TL, Ortiz G. Arthroscopic labral debridement – a three-year follow-up study. Am J Sports Med. 1992;20:702–6.
50. Burkhart SS, Fox DL. Case report: arthroscopic repair of a type IV SLAP lesion–the red-on-white lesion as a component of anterior instability. Arthroscopy. 1993;9(5):488–92. discussion 93–7.
51. Warner JJ, Kann S, Marks P. Arthroscopic repair of combined Bankart and superior labral detachment anterior and posterior lesions: technique and preliminary results. Arthroscopy. 1994;10(4):383–91.
52. Oh JH, Kim SH, Lee HK, Jo KH, Bae KJ. Transrotator cuff portal is safe for arthroscopic superior labral anterior and posterior lesion repair: clinical and radiological analysis of 58 SLAP lesions. Am J Sports Med. 2008;36(10):1913–21.
53. Kim SH, Ha KI, Kim SH, Choi HJ. Results of arthroscopic treatment of superior labral lesions. J Bone Joint Surg Am. 2002;84(6):981–5.
54. Boileau P, Parratte S, Chuinard C, Roussanne Y, Shia D, Bicknell R. Arthroscopic treatment of isolated type II SLAP lesions: biceps tenodesis as an alternative to reinsertion. Am J Sports Med. 2009;37(5):929–36.
55. Biceps Tenodesis Protocol – Brigham and Women's Hospital. Reg B. Rehabilitation Department. Wilcox III RB.
56. Biceps Tenotomy Protocol – Brigham and Women's Hospital. Reg B. Rehabilitation Department. Wilcox III RB.

57. Provencher MT, McCormick F, Dewing CB, Solomon DJ. A prospective analysis of 179 type 2 superior labrum anterior and posterior repairs: outcomes and factors associated with success and failure. Am J Sports Med. 2013;41(4):880–6.
58. Waterman BR, Arroyo W, Heida K, Burks R, Pallis M. SLAP repairs with combined procedures have lower failure rate than isolated repairs in a military population: surgical outcomes with minimum 2-Year follow-up. Orthop J Sports Med. 2015;3:2325967115599154.
59. Chalmers PN, Trombley R, Cip J, Monson B, Forsythe B, Nicholson GP, Bush-Joseph CA, Cole BJ, Wimmer MA, Romeo AA, Verma NN. Postoperative restoration of upper extremity motion and neuromuscular control during the overhand pitch: evaluation of tenodesis and repair for superior labral anterior-posterior tears. Am J Sports Med. 2014;42:2825–36.
60. Ek ETH, Shi LL, Tompson JD, Freehill MT, Warner JP. Surgical treatment of isolated type II superior labrum anterior-posterior (SLAP) lesions: repair versus biceps tenodesis. J Shoulder Elbow Surg. 2014;23:1059–65.
61. Mollon B, Mahure SA, Ensor KL, Zuckerman JD, Kwon YW, Rokito AS. Subsequent shoulder surgery after isolated arthroscopic SLAP repair. Arthroscopy. 2016;32(10):1954–1962.e1.
62. Woertler K, Waldt S. MR imaging in sports- related glenohumeral instability. Eur Radiol. 2006;16(12):2622–36.

# 23 Biceps Injuries: What to Do and Where?

Stephen C. Weber

## Contents


23.1 **Brief Introduction** .......... 203

23.2 **Literature Overview Summary** .......... 203

23.3 **Anatomy, Examination, and Imaging** .... 206

23.4 **Indication and Technique** .......... 206

23.5 **Specific Points in Rehabilitation** .......... 206

23.6 **Complications and Tips to Avoid Them** .......... 207

23.7 **Conclusion Summary** .......... 207

**References** .......... 208


S.C. Weber, MD
Assistant Professor, Department of Orthopedics,
Johns Hopkins University,
Baltimore, Maryland, USA
e-mail: webersc@earthlink.net

## 23.1 Brief Introduction

The biceps has been recognized as a pain generator for some time [3, 10, 17, 29–31, 39, 43]. This diagnosis came into disfavor with the work of Becker and Cofield [1] who showed generally poor results with isolated biceps tenodesis in an era without MRI or arthroscopy. Subsequent reports have generally been more favorable, and the biceps has been increasingly recognized as a pain generator in the shoulder. Increasingly debate has focused on differing techniques and locations for biceps tenodesis.

## 23.2 Literature Overview Summary

The arthroscopic subpectoral biceps tenodesis was first developed by Dr. Richard Caspari as a unique surgical exposure for his arthroscopic Gallie procedure and first published in 1993 [44]. Numerous other centers have adopted this technique as their own since [19, 23–25, 28, 34, 35, 46]. While generally successful, this represented an open technique, and other authors represented arthroscopic techniques that could be performed without a short incision. This included tenotomy [2, 6, 11, 13, 40], proximal soft tissue tenodesis [7, 9, 18, 38], proximal fixation to the bone [5, 12, 23, 36], and arthroscopic distal biceps fixation to the bone [15] or soft tissue [42]. Post [32] first raised the concern that leaving a diseased

© ISAKOS 2017
A.B. Imhoff, F.H. Savoie III (eds.), *Shoulder Instability Across the Life Span*,
DOI 10.1007/978-3-662-54077-0_23

biceps tendon in the bicipital groove would lead to persistent pain. This concept was resurrected by Sanders et al. [35]. They represented that a proximal tenodesis that did not release the sheath carried a 20.6% revision rate, as opposed to a 6.8% revision rate with release. This was at odds with all the reported results with proximal tenodesis. Both Brady et al. [5] and our data [18] showed excellent long-term results with proximal tenodesis. Comparative studies remain few. Werner et al. performed a level four retrospective review [45] showing more stiffness in the proximally tenodesed group but similar outcomes. Gombera et al. [15] compared an arthroscopic distal tenodesis technique to open subpectoral tenodesis. ASES, patient satisfaction scores, and outcomes were the same in both groups. No increase in stiffness was noted. One serious neurovascular injury was noted in the open group.

While outcomes have generally been good with open subpectoral tenodesis, serious complications such as fracture [37], neurologic injury [33], and failure of fixation [20] can occur. Given the paucity of data directly comparing the two techniques, it seemed to evaluate this more thoroughly. To this end, we instituted a study evaluating the long-term follow-up of proximal versus distal biceps tenodesis. Two series previously reported were retrospectively compared in regard to outcome of proximal [18] and distal biceps tenodesis [44]. This data was further studied to establish operative times for the biceps tenodesis, total operative times, parenteral narcotics in the post-anesthesia recovery (PAR), oral narcotics in PAR, and total PAR time. A narcotic calculator was used to convert differing parenteral and oral narcotics to morphine and hydrocodone equivalents. The proximal tenodesis data was further subdivided into those with concomitant rotator cuff repairs and those with simple arthroscopic procedures such as debridement and acromioplasty.

Those patients with proximal tenodesis and no rotator cuff repair were tenodesed as described by Castagna [7] with modifications previously presented [18]. A spinal needle was used to pass sutures through the biceps of #2 Ticron and then tied in the subacromial space. With a rotator cuff tear, the biceps was tenodesed to the anterior suture anchor as originally described by Gartsman [12]. Another pathology was corrected as indicated.

Open subpectoral tenodesis was performed as described previously [44, 46]. A unicortical screw and spiked washer was used to fix the biceps at the distal bicipital groove.

Demographic data is shown in Table 23.1. No significant differences were noted retrospectively comparing the two groups. Demographics were generally consistent with other studies on this subject in regard to age and male preponderance.

Operative times and perioperative morbidity data is shown in Table 23.2. It can be seen that proximal tenodesis involved significantly less operative time, both for the tenodesis procedure

**Table 23.1** Preoperative demographics, proximal versus distal tenodesis

| | Distal tenodesis | Proximal tenodesis |
|---|---|---|
| Age | 49.37 | 63.0 |
| R/L | 30/14 | 58/34 |
| Male/female | 39/5 | |
| Preop UCLA | 18.93 | 17.61 |
| Preop SST | 3.21 | 5.82 |

**Table 23.2** Operative times and perioperative morbidity in proximal and distal biceps tenodesis

| | Distal w/o RCR | Proximal +RCR | Proximal w/o RCR |
|---|---|---|---|
| Total operative time | 85.0 (17.79) | 55.88 (16.51)* | 50.0 (15.49) ** |
| Biceps operative time | 35.0 (7.07) | 11.23 (3.84) # | 10.63 (4.18) ## |
| Parental PAR ms equivalents | 12.50 (9.57) | 17.55 (15.64) *** | 12.15 (14.14)*** |
| Oral PAR narco equivalents | 4.58 (3.16) | 5.23 (2.58) *** | 4.44 (2.32) *** |
| PAR times | 73.75 (16.53) | 70.58 (18.19) *** | 65.90 (17.43)*** |

*$P < 0.03$, **$p < 0.017$, #$p < 0.017$, ##$p < 0.0001$, ***$p$ = N.S

alone and also for the entire operative procedure. Perioperative morbidity was not statistically different despite the additional surgical approach and violating the proximal humeral bone with distal tenodesis in regard to PAR narcotic consumption and total PAR times. This was true for both the combined proximal tenodesis and when comparing the isolated tenodesis to the isolated distal tenodesis.

Final outcomes are shown in Table 23.3. There were no complications in the arthroscopic group. Only two patients complained of minimal deformity. In the subpectoral group, there were no failures of fixation with screw and washer technique. No neurologic injuries occurred. There was one superficial infection, which was successfully managed with oral antibiotics. Operative times both for the actual tenodesis and the overall procedure were significantly less for arthroscopic tenodesis. Perioperative morbidity was the same for both procedures at all times evaluated. No increase in stiffness was noted at any time with proximal tenodesis.

Cost was significantly different between the two treatments. Assuming a facility charge of $650/15 min, this would be a mean cost increase of over $600 per case. Proximal tenodesis implant costs are negligible, as it would be either a suture and spinal needle or a suture of an anchor already used for the rotator cuff repair. While the subpectoral technique described here is the original technique described using a screw and ligament washer [43] with minimal implant charges, the more widely used interference screw technique would result in significant additional charges. Cost of a biocomposite (30% biphasic calcium phosphate and 70% PLDLA) screw was 299.25

**Table 23.3** Outcome measures, proximal versus distal tenodesis

| | Distal tenodesis | Proximal tenodesis |
|---|---|---|
| UCLA | 32.37 (3.25) | 30.12 (4.31) |
| SST | 10.25 (1.29) | 10.17 (1.89) |
| Forward flexion | 164.02 (10.32) | 165.90 (9.45) |
| External rotation | 72.74 (7.42) | 68.32 (8.14) |

marked up to 1147.37 and a biotenodesis screw (PLLA) 271.75 marked up to 947.62. While cost is always difficult to assess, this calculation would mean an increased cost of 1647.37, billed to the patient in a hospital setting and absorbed by the surgery center in an outpatient setting.

The controversy of proximal versus distal biceps tenodesis has been an issue since originally reviewed by Sanders et al. [35]. They first raised concerns about reoperation rates for proximal biceps tenodesis. Careful review of this paper however showed that revision surgery rarely resulted in a satisfactory outcome. Gregory et al. [16] represent the only publication on revision biceps tenodesis. While improvement was noted, 5/21 had unsatisfactory results, and lack of data prevented analysis of the technique of the proximal tenodesis failures. Werner et al. [45] represent the only other level four study comparing proximal and distal tenodesis, which also showed increased stiffness between the two techniques using an arthroscopic interference screw. Follow-up was as little as 4.5 months. While stiffness was increased short term, there was no long-term difference in outcomes. While their and this paper represent level three data only, the combination of a relative absence of any comparative data suggesting superior outcomes with distal biceps tenodesis and the numerous level four case series with excellent results (5,712,18) with proximal tenodesis suggests that the cost of distal tenodesis, especially with interference screw fixation, may be unnecessary. Gombera et al. [15] recently presented their results with arthroscopic versus open tenodesis. Both techniques were distal, however, and one serious neurologic injury occurred in the open subpectoral group. They concluded that open tenodesis might have an increased risk of complications. Although numerous concerns have been raised about "hidden lesions" of the biceps [14, 15, 21, 27, 45] creating symptoms post proximal tenodesis, their clinical relevance remains unclear absent studies that show increased complications with proximal tenodesis that are corrected with subsequent distal tenodesis.

Complications with open subpectoral tenodesis were rare in our series [44, 46], consistent with other series of experienced surgeons performing this technique [4, 23–25, 28, 34]. Problems do occur with open subpectoral tenodesis, however. Neurologic injury is not unheard of, as what occurred in the series of Gombera [15] and also reported in four cases by Rhee [33]. Dickens [8] showed that numerous structures were "at risk" with this approach. Iatrogenic fractures continue to be reported. While not reported in our series [46] or Ngo's [28], they continue to occur [37], and the Rush team reports a biomechanical study showing a 30% decrease in strength with placement of an 8 mm drill hole [26]. This would be further compounded by the expected bone resorption that would occur around a PLLA implant with time. Koch et al. [20] reported a disturbing rate of failure of interference screw fixation, the reason of which was unclear. They did point out that in vitro mechanical strength superiority could be offset by biologic factors that cause the tenodesis to fail. None of these complications are reported with arthroscopic tenodesis.

It is important to understand that failed shoulder surgery exists with and without proximal tenodesis. The patient with a poor result can be a frustration to the surgeon looking for a solution. The data suggesting that these patients will benefit from revision to distal tenodesis is minimal despite the attractive basic science and clinical speculation about retention of the biceps within the groove [14, 21, 22, 27, 32, 35], and revision surgery to subpectoral tenodesis on this basis should be offered with caution at this time. While widely quoted, Sanders et al.'s study showed that few of the patients revised to distal tenodesis were actually improved [35].

## 23.3 Anatomy, Examination, and Imaging

Anatomy and examination are well covered in the previous chapter (Previgliano JP et al. 3.4.2). Clinical evaluation of the painful biceps can be challenging, as many of the clinical tests such as Yerguson's and Speed's test show relatively low specificity and sensitivity. Imaging can be similarly difficult. While the dislocated and ruptured biceps can be easily diagnosed with MRI, partial biceps ruptures and associated SLAP lesions can be difficult to reliably image [39]. For the most part, partial biceps ruptures remain a diagnosis obtained at the time of arthroscopy.

## 23.4 Indication and Technique

Indications for treatment of complete ruptures remain largely surgeon preference. While complete ruptures can be well tolerated in older, lower-demand patients, both iatrogenic ruptures and surgically tenotomized biceps tendons can cause both significant deformity and pain [6]. While biceps tenodesis was in disfavor after the seminal work of Becker and Cofield for many years [1], the biceps has been increasingly recognized as an important pain generator in the shoulder. A widely quoted "50% partial rupture" was used for some time in regard to treating biceps pathology. Given the progression of disease and oftentimes poor results with conservative management of biceps lesion, indications for treatment of proximal biceps pathology have become increasingly generous [4].

## 23.5 Specific Points in Rehabilitation

Rehabilitation of biceps surgery is often dictated by the need to manage other surgeries performed concomitantly, such as rotator cuff or Bankart repair. Isolated biceps tenodesis rarely results in postoperative stiffness, and for this reason aggressive early motion is normally not indicated. Both proximal [18] and distal [44, 46] in our series were managed in a sling with pendulum exercises for 3 weeks, followed by gentle active ROM for an additional 3 weeks. Weight lifting or sports were not permitted for 3 months.

## 23.6 Complications and Tips to Avoid Them

Complications with proximal biceps tenodesis are uncommon, usually related to failure of the tenodesis with recurrent deformity. Distal biceps tenodesis also has few complications in our experience [44, 46]. Despite this, rare worrisome neurologic complications with this technique continue to be reported [33]. While the approach is relatively straightforward for subpectoral tenodesis, the surgeon must be certain to stay lateral to the conjoined tendon to avoid neurologic injury. Placing sharp retractors around the humerus medial to the tenodesis site can also raise concerns, and generally a blunt retractor such as an Army is adequate for medial exposure. Fracture at the distal tenodesis site continues to be reported [37]; this is a concern where large, bioabsorbable implants are used, which can leave a significant cystic defect in the bone. While large bioabsorbable implants have been reported successful in numerous other studies [4, 19, 24–26, 28], the subpectoral tenodesis as initially described [44] used a screw and spiked washer, with no reported fractures at long-term follow-up. Cutting of the tendon with subsequent failure of the tenodesis with interference screws has also been reported [20], so care must be used in handling and fixation if this technique is chosen.

## 23.7 Conclusion Summary

In summary, both proximal and distal tenodeses show good result at long-term follow-up. Morbidity between the two procedures is not significantly different based on our study, and complications were low with both techniques. The time of surgery and potential implant costs clearly favor proximal tenodesis and may be a deciding factor in the choice of procedures. Rare serious complications with subpectoral tenodesis continue to be reported; these issues may also favor arthroscopic tenodesis.

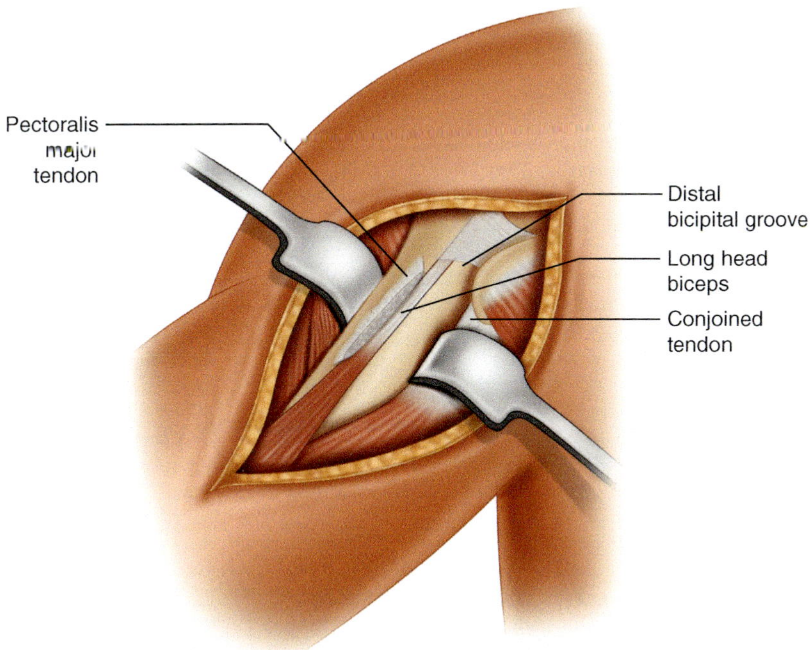


surgical approach for mini-open subpectoral biceps tenodesis

## References


1. Becker DA, Cofield RH. Tenodesis of the long head of the biceps brachii for chronic bicipital tendonitis. Long term results. J Bone Joint Surg Am. 1989;71:376–81.
2. Bicknell RT, Chuinard D, Boileau P. Arthroscopic biceps tenotomy and tenodesis of massive irreparable rotator cuff tears. Presented, 26th annual meeting AANA, San Francisco, CA, 2007.
3. Boileau P, Parratte S, Chuinard C, et al. Arthroscopic treatment of isolated type II SLAP lesions: biceps tenodesis as an alternative to reinsertion. Am J Sports Med. 2009;37(5):929–36.
4. Boileau P, Krishnan SG, Coste JS, et al. Arthroscopic biceps tenodesis: a new technique using bioabsorbable interference screw fixation. Arthroscopy. 2002;18(9):1002–12.
5. Brady PC, Narbona P, Adams CR, et al. Arthroscopic proximal biceps tenodesis at the articular margin: evaluation of outcomes, complications, and revision rate. Arthroscopy. 2015;31(3):470–6.
6. Cameron ML. The incidence of "popeye" deformity and muscle weakness following tenotomy for recalcitrant biceps tendonitis. Proc Am Acad Orthop Surg. 2003;5:442.
7. Castagna A, Sacchi G, D'Ortona A, Bungaro P. Rottura del capo lungo del bicipite, lesioni SLAP e conflitto suuperio-interno: trattamento chirurgico. G It Ort Trauma. 2002;28(Supp I):644–52.
8. Dickens JF, Kilcoyne K, Tintle S, Guliani J, Rue JP. Subpectoral bicep tenodesis: an anatomic study and evaluation of at risk structures. Am J Sports Med. 2012;40(10):2337–41.
9. Elkousy HA, Fluhme DJ, O'Connor DP, et al. Arthroscopic biceps tenodesis using the percutaneous, intra-articular trans-tendon technique: preliminary results. Orthopedics. 2005;28(11):1316–9.
10. Froimson AJ, Oh I. Keyhole tenodesis of biceps origin at the shoulder. Clin Orthop. 1975;112:245–9.
11. Frost A, Zafar MS, Maffulli N. Tenotomy versus tenodesis in the management of pathologic lesions of the tendon of the long head of the biceps brachii. Am J Sports Med. 2009;37(4):828–33.
12. Gartsman GM, Hammerman SM. Arthroscopic biceps tenodesis: operative technique. Arthroscopy. 2000;16(5):550–2.
13. Gill TJ, McIrvin E, Mair SD, Hawkins RJ. Results of biceps tenotomy for treatment of pathology of the long head of the biceps brachii. J Shoulder Elbow Surg. 2001;10(3):247–9.
14. Gilmer BB, Demers AM, Guerrero D, Reid JB, Lubowitz JH, Guttman D. Arthroscopic versus open comparison of long head of biceps tendon visualization and pathology in patients requiring tenodesis. Arthroscopy. 2015;31(1):29–34.
15. Gombera MM, Kahlenberg CA, Nair R, Saltzman MD, Terry MA. All-Arthroscopic suprapectoral versus Open subpectoral Tenodesis of the Long Head of the Biceps Brachii. Presented, 2015 Specialty Day, AOSSM.
16. Gregory JM, Harwood DP, Gochanour E, Sherman SL, Romeo AA. Clinical outcomes of revision biceps tenodesis. Int J Shoulder Surg. 2012;6:45–50.
17. Hichcock HH, Bechtol CO. Painful shoulder: observations on role of tendon of long head of biceps brachii in its causation. J Bone Joint Surg Am. 1948;30:263–73.
18. Kauffman JI, Weber SC, Higgins D. Arthroscopic biceps tenodesis: experience with the Castagna technique. Proc Am Acad Orthop Surg. 2004;5:525.
19. Klepps S, Hazrati Y, Flatlow E. Arthroscopic biceps tenodesis. Arthroscopy. 2002;18:1040–5.
20. Koch BS, Burks RT. Failure of biceps tenodesis with interference screw fixation. Arthroscopy. 2012;28(5):735–40.
21. Lutton DM, Gruson KI, Harrison AK, et al. Where to tenodese the biceps: proximal or distal? Clin Orthop Relat Res. 2011;469(4):1050–5.
22. McDonald LS, Dewing CB, Shupe PG, Provencher MT. Disorders of the proximal and distal aspects of the biceps muscle. J Bone Joint Surg Am. 2013;95:1235–45.
23. Mazzocca AD, Bicos J, Santangelo S, et al. The biomechanical evaluation of four fixation techniques for proximal biceps tenodesis. Arthroscopy. 2005;21(11):1296–306.
24. Mazzocca AD, Cote MP, Arciero CL, et al. Clinical outcomes after subpectoral biceps tenodesis with an interference screw. Am J Sports Med. 2008;36(10):1922–9.
25. Mazzocca AD, Rios CG, Romeo AA, et al. Subpectoral biceps tenodesis with interference screw fixation. The subpectoral portion as the optimal tenodesis site. Arthroscopy. 2005;21(7):896.
26. Mellano CR, Shin JJ, Mascerhanas R, Shewman E, Wang VM, Romeo AA, Verma NN, Forsthe B. Subpectoral Biceps Tenodesis with Peek Interference Screw. A biomechanical Analysis of Humerus Fracture Risk. Presented 2015 AOSSM Specialty Day, Las Vegas, NV. 30% decrease in strength.
27. Moon SC, Cho NS, Rhee YG. Analysis of "Hidden Lesions" of the extra-articular biceps after subpectoral biceps tenodesis. Am J Sports Med. 2014;43(1):63–8.
28. Nho SJ, Reiff SN, Verma NN, et al. Complications associated with subpectoral biceps tenodesis: low rates of incidence following surgery. J Shoulder Elbow Surg. 2010;19(5):764–8.
29. Osbahr DC, Diamond AB, Speer KP. The cosmetic appearance of the biceps muscle after long-head biceps tenotomy versus tenodesis. Arthroscopy. 2002;18:483–7.
30. Peterson CJ. Spontaneous medial dislocation of the long biceps brachii. Clin Orthop. 1989;21:224–7.
31. Pfahler M, Branner S, Refior HJ. The role of the bicipital groove in tendinopathy of the long biceps tendon. J Shoulder Elbow Surg. 1999;8:419–24.
32. Post M, Brenca P. Primary tendonitis of the long head of the biceps. Clin Orthop. 1989;246:117–25.
33. Rhee PC, Spinner RJ, Bishop AT, Shin AY. Iatrogenic brachial plexus injuries associated with open subpectoral

biceps tenodesis: a report of 4 cases. Am J Sports Med. 2013;41(9):2048–53.
34. Romeo AA, Mazzoca AD, Tauro JC. Arthroscopic biceps tenodesis. Arthroscopy. 2004;20(2):206–13.
35. Sanders B, Lavery KP, Pennington S, et al. Clinical success of biceps tenodesis with and without release of the transverse humeral ligament. J Shoulder Elbow Surg. 2012;21(1):66–71.
36. Scheibel M, Schroder RJ, Chen J, Bartsch M. Arthroscopic soft tissue tenodesis versus bony fixation anchor tenodesis of the long head of the biceps tendon. Am J Sports Med. 2011;39(5):1046–52.
37. Sears BW, Spencer EE, Getz CL. Humeral fracture following subpectoral biceps tenodesis in two active healthy patients. J Shoulder Elbow Surg. 2011; 20:e7–11.
38. Sekiya JK, Elkousy HA, Rodosky MW. Arthroscopic biceps tenodesis using the percutaneous intra-articular transtendon technique. Arthroscopy. 2003;19(10):1137–41.
39. Sethi N, Wright R, Yamaguchi K. Disorders of the long head of the biceps tendon. J Shoulder Elbow Surg. 1999;8:644–54.
40. Slenker NR, Lawson K, Ciccotti MG, et al. Biceps tenotomy versus tenodesis: clinical outcomes. Arthroscopy. 2012;28(4):576–82.
41. Su WR, Budoff JE, Chiang CH, Lee CJ, Lin CL. Biomechanical study comparing biceps wedge tenodesis with other proximal long head of the biceps tenodesis techniques. Arthroscopy. 2013;29(9):1498–505.
42. Verma NN, Drakos M, O'Brien SJ. Arthroscopic transfer of the long head biceps to the conjoint tendon. Arthroscopy. 2005;21(6):764.
43. Warren RF. Lesions of the long head of the biceps tendon. Instr Course Lect. 1985;30:204–9.
44. Weber SC. Arthroscopic "Mini-Open" technique in the treatment of ruptures of the long head of the biceps. Arthroscopy. 1993;9(3):365.
45. Werner BC, Cody CL, Holzgrefe RE, Tuman JM, Hart JM, Carson EW, Diduch DR, Miller MD, Brockmeyer DF. Arthroscopic suprapectoral and open suprapectoral biceps tenodesis. Minimal 2-year clinical outcomes. Am J Sports Med. 2014;42(11):2584–90.
46. Wiley WB, Meyers JF, Weber SC, et al. Arthroscopic assisted mini-open biceps tenodesis: surgical technique. Arthroscopy. 2004;20(4):444–6.

# The Unstable and Painful Long Head of the Biceps

# 24

Juan P. Previgliano and Guillermo Arce

## Contents

**24.1 Background** .......... 211
**24.2 Preoperative Assessment** .......... 212
**24.3 Anatomic and Arthroscopic Findings** .......... 212
**24.4 Discussion** .......... 215
**Bibliography** .......... 215

## 24.1 Background

Many papers address the biomechanics, injury patterns, and repair techniques of the superior labrum anterior and posterior (SLAP) avulsion from the glenoid, but the biceps instability due to conditions other than the SLAP has not been deeply studied.

The non-SLAP biceps pathology is a frequent finding for shoulder dedicated orthopedic surgeons. Biceps pathology is not uncommon, but to achieve the right diagnosis and to proceed with a successful treatment is still a challenge.

The long head of the biceps tendon (LHBT) is known as a factor which leads to residual pain after shoulder surgery.

Nevertheless, we have successful surgical techniques, before performing them, we need a clear decision-making criteria to tailor the surgical treatment to each particular patient and injury. The non-SLAP biceps instability must be fully addressed pre and intra-operatively in order to proceed with the adequate surgical treatment of the biceps pathology.

Many anatomic structures contribute to stabilize the biceps. The coraco-humeral ligament (CHL), superior gleno-humeral ligament (SGHL), subscapularis (SUBS), supraspinatus (SSP), bicipital groove, and the transverse ligament (TL) are the main restraints. The coraco-humeral ligament (CHL) is one of the main biceps tendon restraints. It arises from the coracoid base

J. Previgliano, MD (✉) • G. Arce, MD
Department of Orthopaedic Surgery, Instituto Argentino de Diagnóstico y Tratamiento, Marcelo T. de Alvear 2439, Buenos Aires 1425, Argentina
e-mail: previgjp@intramed.net

© ISAKOS 2017
A.B. Imhoff, F.H. Savoie III (eds.), *Shoulder Instability Across the Life Span*, DOI 10.1007/978-3-662-54077-0_24

and ends at the bicipital groove with a medial branch (MCHL) and a lateral branch (LCHL) at both sides of the biceps trough.

We are able to look at the structures from the joint through the scope, and from the front with open dissections, but is hard to establish biceps pulley conditions and anatomy.

The objective of this chapter is to define the surgical anatomy of the long head of the biceps tendon, to describe the tips to achieve the right diagnosis of instability or degenerative changes, and to try to outline arthroscopic basis for a comprehensive surgical treatment of LHBT disorders.

## 24.2 Preoperative Assessment

The Abbot and Saunders Test for preoperative diagnosis of the non-SLAP biceps instability is very useful. To perform the test we move the arm from abduction and external rotation to adduction and internal rotation. Pain and locking during this maneuver demonstrate biceps tendon instability.

By rotating the arm from external to internal rotation, we try to get a bow string effect of the tendon out of its pulley. Bennett developed a modified test. The patient's arm is brought from ABD-ER to ADD-IR in a full passive ROM.

Impingement tests like Neer's or Hawkins' do not have a strong correlation with biceps pathology or instability. It is not cleary known if primary impingement is an important component for biceps tendon instability. If the impingement syndrome contributes to biceps tendinopathy, the friction is secondary to rotator cuff failure. Overuse, trauma, and degenerative disease are the main causes of tendon failure. The Speed's and O'Brien's Tests are also positive in many cases of biceps tendon instability.

Imaging studies demonstrating biceps tendon instability are inconsistent due to the dynamic nature of the tendon problem. With high resolution MRI slices, MCHL or subscapularis partial tears can be found and are often correlated with biceps disease. Increased fluid at the anterior bursa and bicipital sheath demonstrates tendon instability or degenerative changes.

## 24.3 Anatomic and Arthroscopic Findings

The main structure to evaluate biceps instability is the SGHL-CHL complex (Fig. 24.1) The CHL arises from the coracoid base, and its insertion at the lesser and greater tuberosities defines two branches (Fig. 24.2), the medial CHL at the lesser tuberosity and the lateral CHL at the greater tuberosity. The MCHL is the number one biceps stabilizer to prevent subluxation or dislocation (Fig. 24.3). The close relationship between the MCHL and the subscapularis determines the frequent involvement of both structures together in many cases.

The arthroscopic evaluation of the involved anatomic structures is very important. Coraco-humeral ligament, subscapularis and supraspinatus attachments close to the biceps groove need to be assessed during the diagnostic arthroscopy. The patient's arm need to be placed in 80 degrees of forward flexion and mild external rotation in order to obtain the best view of these structures from the posterior portal.

The roof of the pulley is reinforced by subscapularis and supraspinatus tendon expansions. Therefore, we may consider the subscapularis fiber insertions not only at the lesser tuberosity but at the greater as well. The supraspinatus fibers

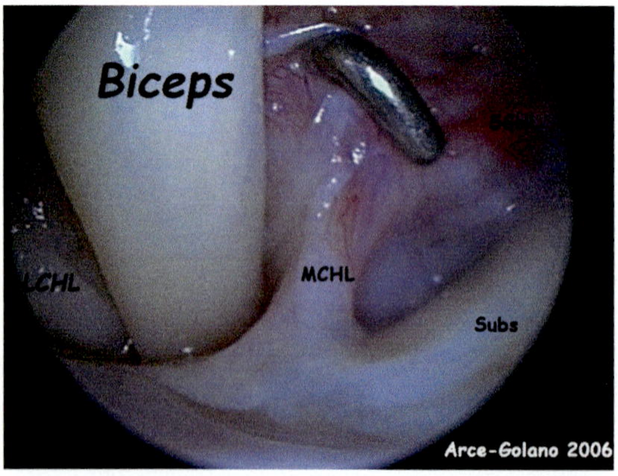


**Fig. 24.1** Left shoulder. Arthroscopic view from the posterior portal. Biceps Pulley. *Subs* subscapularis, *MCHL* medial branch of the coracohumeral ligament. *LCHL* lateral branch of the coracohumeral ligament, *SGHL* superior glenohumeral ligament

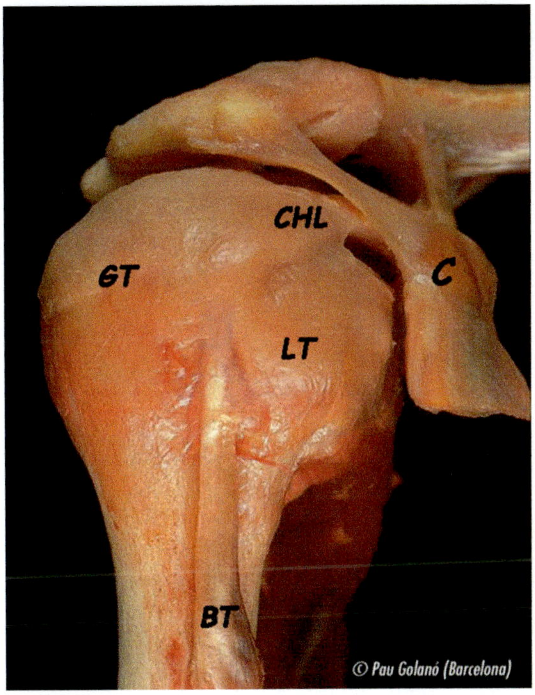


**Fig. 24.2** Right shoulder. Specimen dissection. *C* coracoid, *CHL* coracohumeral ligament, arising from the coracoid base, *LT* lesser tuberosity, *GT* greater tuberosity, *BT* biceps tendon. (Pau Golano picture with permission)

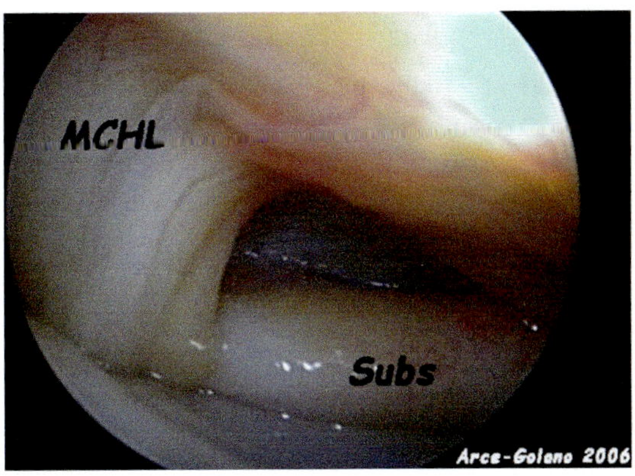


**Fig. 24.3** Left shoulder. Arthroscopic view from the posterior portal. *MCHL* medial coracohumeral ligament, *Subs* subscapularis. The MCHL constitutes part to the Comma Tissue in cases of SUBS ruptures

contribute in less proportion to the pulley's lateral wall and roof. The clinical implications of these anatomic findings are that when we repair a supraspinatus cuff tear, we should try to fix it at the edge

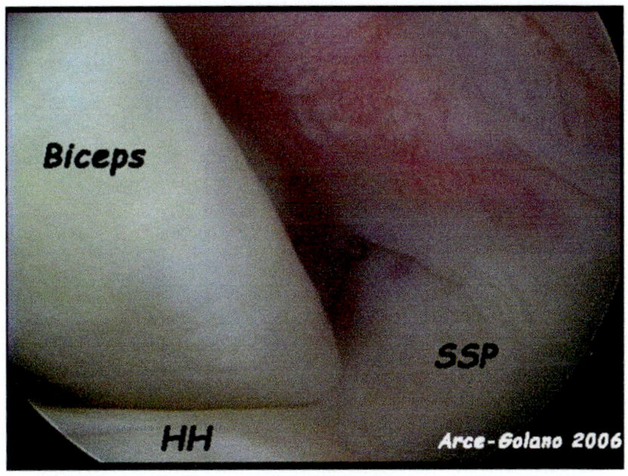


**Fig. 24.4** Right shoulder. Arthroscopic view from the posterior portal. Pulley's lateral wall. SSP Supraspinatus, HH Humeral Head

of the bicipital groove. Non anatomic SSP repairs may lead to lateral biceps tendon instability and postoperative symptoms. (Fig. 24.4).

Base on these anatomic features, the medial sling (MCHL and Subscapularis) and the lateral sling (LCHL and Supraspinatus) need to be repaired at their natural footprint at the edge of the bicipital groove in order to recover biceps tendon stability.

These structures should be evaluated not only with a static view but also with dynamic maneuvers during the arthroscopic procedure.

For lateral stability, the greater tuberosity's bony shape and the LCHL are the main structures to assess.

The transverse ligament and a well-vascularized tendon sheath are the main restraints of the lower pulley (Fig. 24.5). The subscapularis and the lesser tuberosity are other contributors.

It is very important to get used to seeing the biceps pulley anatomy in every case of shoulder arthroscopy. In this way, small changes of the normal anatomy can be identified (Fig. 24.6).

Motley described the Ramp Test to evaluate biceps tendon stability and part of the extra-articular portion of the biceps tendon. With a nerve hook, pulling from the tendon downward, we assess the tendon quality and stability (Fig. 24.7).

Two groups of biceps instability were described by Habermayer and Walch. The classification is

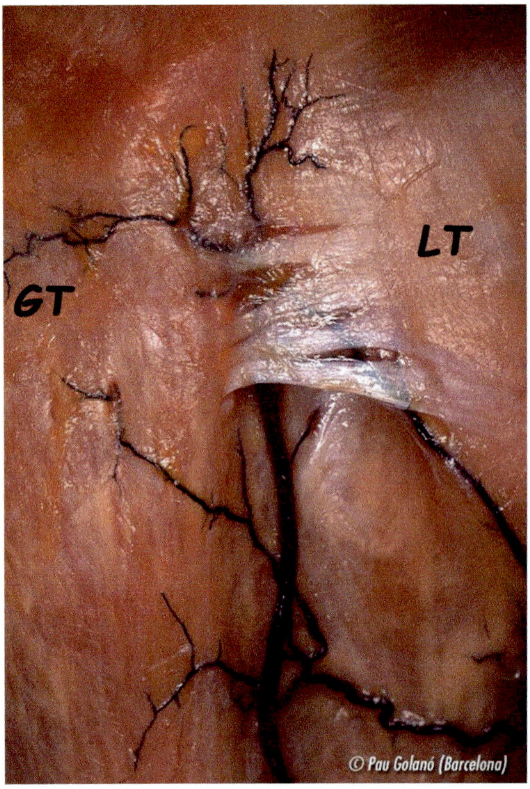


**Fig. 24.5** Right Shoulder. Specimen dissection. Lower pulley restraints. GT Greater tuberosity. LT Lesser tuberosity. Transverse ligament. Biceps pulley vascularity comes from the ascending branch of the anterior circumflex artery. (Pau Golano's picture with permission)

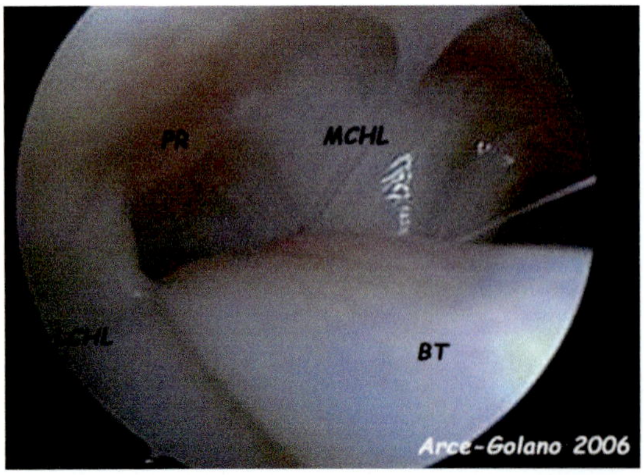


**Fig. 24.6** Left Shoulder. Arthroscopic view from the posterior portal. Arthroscopic biceps pulley anatomy. *BT* biceps tendon, *MCHL* medial coraco-humeral ligament, *LCHL* lateral coraco-humeral ligament, *PR* pulley's roof

based on the injury location. Subluxations due to ligament ruptures could be at the proximal pulley, central part of it, or at the distal groove. Tendon

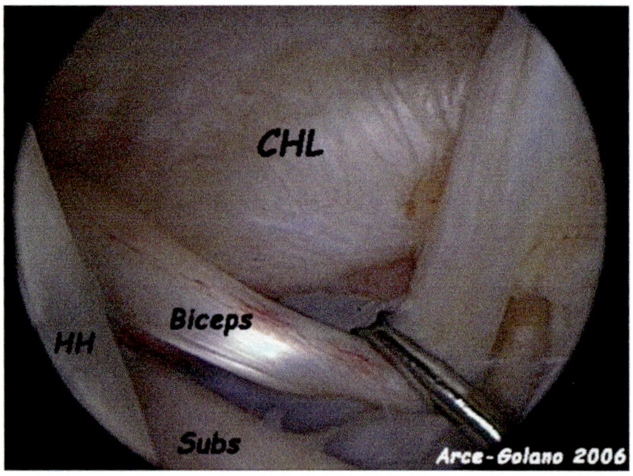


**Fig. 24.7** Left shoulder. Arthroscopic view from the posterior portal. The Ramp Test. The nerve hook pulls the biceps downward, tendon status and stability can be evaluated. CHL Coraco-humeral ligament. HH Humeral Head

**Table 24.1** Bennett's Classification. Structures involved in biceps tendon instability.

| Type | Structures involved |
|---|---|
| I | Subs |
| II | MCHL |
| III | Subs + MCHL |
| IV | SSP + LCHL |
| V | Subs + MCHL + SSP + LCHL |

dislocations could be extra- or intraarticular depending on the structures involved and torn.

Bennett's classification is based on anatomy, tendons, and ligaments injured (Table 24.1).

Bennett et al. described the surgical anatomy and defined the different biceps instability patterns. Out of 165 procedures with 27% subscapularis tears, the SGHL-MCHL complex was torn in 47% of them. The SGHL-MCHL complex or the LCHL rupture as a single lesion was less frequently found.

Based on the surgical anatomy and the arthroscopic findings, in order to have some guidelines for decision making, we developed a table of major and minor criteria for non-SLAP biceps conditions (Table 24.2). If one major or two minor criteria are found in any particular case, the biceps tendon need to be surgically treated by tenotomy or tenodesis depending on patient expectations and demands.

Burkhart et al. described the Coma Sign which corresponds to the retracted MCHL. It serves as a

**Table 24.2** Decision Making Criteria for Biceps Tendon Instability

| Major criteria | Minor criteria |
|---|---|
| 1. SGHL-MCHL complex rupture | 1. Clinical signs |
| 2. SUBS rupture | 2. LCHL rupture |
| 3. Severe tendinopathy | 3. SSP rupture |
| | 4. Mild tendinopathy |
| | 5. Lesser T. fracture |

landmark to identify the superolateral corner of the subscapularis. The subscapularis repair is the key to successful biceps pulley reconstructions. Bennett reported encouraging results of biceps tendon pulley repairs with out tenotomy or tenodesis. This procedure is only indicated for young and high demand throwing athletes in whom the biceps tendon may have an important role. Balanced repairs of the biceps restraints without persistent tendon instability or pulley stenosis are difficult to achieve. Tenotomy or tenodesis are the procedures of choice in most of the cases.

## 24.4 Discussion

The description of the surgical anatomy and arthroscopic findings is the first step to install an adequate surgical treatment of the biceps conditions.

Biceps instability must be defined with a pre-operative accurate diagnosis based on a complete physical exam, imaging studies and the arthroscopic findings of the structures involved.

Depending on the patient conditions, performance or expectations, biceps pulley reconstructions, tendon debridement, tenotomy, or tenodesis are indicated to customize the surgical treatment to each particular case.

We present the surgical anatomy of the biceps tendon stabilizers and propose a table of Decision Making Criteria in order to approach biceps tendon instability. These proposals should be validated by well analyzed surgical outcomes.

## Bibliography


1. Bennet W. Subescapularis, medial, and lateral head coracohumeral ligament insertion anatomy: arthroscopic appearance and incident of "Hidden" rotator interval lesions. Arthroscopy. 2001:173–80.
2. Bennet W. Visualization of the anatomy of the rotator interval and bicipital sheath. Arthroscopy. 2001;17(1):107–11.
3. Bennet W. Arthoscopic bicipital sheath repair: two-year followup with pulley lesions. Arthoscopy. 2004;20:964–73.
4. Bennet W. Arthoscopic repair of isolated subescapularis tears: a prospective cohort with 2- to 4- year follow-up. Arthroscopy. 2003;19:131–43.
5. Bennet W. Arthroscopic repair of anterosuperior (supraespinatus/subescapularis) rotator cuff Tears: a prospective cohort with 2- to 4 year follow-up. Classification of biceps subluxation/instability. Arthroscopy. 2003;19:21–33.
6. Favorito P, Harding W, Heidt Jr RS. Complete arthroscopic examination of the long head of the biceps tendon. Arthroscopy. 2001;17:430–2.
7. Fitzpatrick M, Warren RF. The Anatomy, pathology, and definitive treatment of rotator interval lesions: current conceps. Arthroscopy. 2003;19:70–9.
8. Glockner SM. Shoulder pain: a diagnostic dilemma. Am Fam Physician. 1995;51:1677–87.1690-2
9. Itoi E, An KN. Stabilising function of the biceps in stable and unstable shoulder. J Bone Joint Surg Br. 1993;75:546–50.
10. Seung-Ho K, Seon-Woo K. Electromyographic activity of biceps brachii muscle in shoulder with anterior instability. Arthroscopy. 2001;17:864–8.
11. Motley G, Speer K. An arthoscopic technique for confirming intra-articular subluxation of the long head of the biceps tendon: the ramp test. Arthroscopy. 2002;18:E4.
12. Rodosky NW, Harner CD, Fu FH. The role of the long head of the biceps muscle and superior glenoid labrum in anterior stability of the shoulder. Am J Sports Med. 22:121–30.
13. Spang J, Karas S. The hagl lesion: an arthroscopic technique for repair of humeral avulsion of the glenohumeral ligaments. Athroscopy. 2005;21:498–502.
14. Sarrat P, Carrasset S. Coracotrochineal conflict or anteromedial conflict of the shoulder. Contribution of arthoscanners. J Radio. 1994;75:609–17.
15. Wolf R, Weichel D. Long head biceps tenotomy versus tenodesis: a cadaveric biomechanical analysis. Arthroscopy. 2005;21:182–5.

# Subscapularis Tears and Instability 25

Geoffrey D. Abrams

## Contents


| | | |
|---|---|---|
| 25.1 | **Background** | 217 |
| 25.2 | **Subscapularis Tears and Shoulder Stability** | 218 |
| 25.3 | **Pathophysiology of Subscapularis Tears** | 218 |
| 25.4 | **Clinical Presentation** | 218 |
| 25.5 | **Imaging** | 219 |
| 25.6 | **Management of Subscapularis Tears** | 220 |
| 25.7 | **Postoperative Rehabilitation** | 223 |
| 25.8 | **Results** | 223 |
| **Conclusion** | | 223 |
| **References** | | 224 |


G.D. Abrams
Department of Orthopedic Surgery, Stanford University, Veterans Administration, Palo Alto, CA, USA
e-mail: gabrams@stanford.edu

## 25.1 Background

The subscapularis is an important contributor to normal shoulder function. It receives innervation from the upper and lower subscapular nerves (C5, C6, C7) and originates on the subscapular fossa of the scapula and inserts on the lesser tuberosity of the humerus. It is the sole anterior rotator cuff muscle-tendon unit and acts to internally rotate and adduct the humerus as well as provide anterior stability to the glenohumeral joint [1]. Along with the other rotator cuff muscles, the subscapularis provides an important dynamic force couple to keep the humeral head centered upon the glenoid, allowing for shoulder stability and proper kinematics [2]. In addition, the superolateral aspect of the subscapularis tendon is confluent with the superior glenohumeral and coracohumeral ligaments, forming a pulley that stabilizes the long head of the biceps tendon.

Historically, the presence of subscapularis tears was thought to be low. In 1934, Codman reported a 3.5% rate of subscapularis tears in a series of 200 patients with rotator cuff tears [3]. Warner et al. reported a subscapularis tear rate of 4.6% in another series of 407 patients who had supraspinatus and infraspinatus tears and underwent open rotator cuff repair [4]. More recently, however, with the increased use of arthroscopic approaches for rotator cuff repair, subscapularis tears have been increasingly recognized. Arai

© ISAKOS 2017
A.B. Imhoff, F.H. Savoie III (eds.), *Shoulder Instability Across the Life Span*,
DOI 10.1007/978-3-662-54077-0_25

et al. noted a prevalence of 27% in a series of patients with supraspinatus tears [5], while Barth et al. found a prevalence of 29% [6]. A more recent series, which also proposed a detailed tear classification system, noted an incidence of over 50% [7]. Isolated subscapularis tears remain less common, occurring in approximately 5% of patients undergoing rotator cuff repair [8] and are usually associated with traumatic injury to the shoulder [9, 10]. Subscapularis tears are often associated with biceps tendon pathology given their close anatomic relationship [11, 12].

## 25.2 Subscapularis Tears and Shoulder Stability

With its location in the anterior aspect of the glenohumeral joint, the subscapularis plays an important role in anterior shoulder stability [13–15]. It has been shown that, particularly in external rotation of the humerus, the subscapularis provides the most significant anterior stabilization force in both a cadaveric and computational model of shoulder kinematics [16]. Numerous clinical reports have supported these biomechanical findings. Wirth et al. reported that out of 221 patients who underwent open stabilization for recurrent anterior instability, 14 had an irreparable injury to the subscapularis [17]. The authors concluded that subscapularis deficiency was a significant contributor to recurrent instability. Neviaser et al. reported on 31 patients with an average age of 57 years who had inability to abduct the arm following a first-time glenohumeral dislocation. Eight patients were found to have full-thickness tearing of the subscapularis, and all of these patients developed recurrent anterior instability [14].

## 25.3 Pathophysiology of Subscapularis Tears

Except in settings of acute trauma, a majority of subscapularis tears are degenerative in nature. Like other tendons, degeneration can be separated into intrinsic and extrinsic factors. Intrinsic tendon degeneration is macroscopically characterized by healthy, white, firm fibroelastic tendon giving way to gray, soft, and fragile tissue [18]. Histopathologically, this correlates to mucoid degeneration and fibrocartilage metaplasia of healthy elongated tenocytes, with normal parallel-organized collagen fibers replaced by disoriented and frayed fibers [19, 20]. From a molecular standpoint, this process coincides with upregulated apoptosis pathways associated with oxidative stress [21]. This degenerative process is characteristically devoid of inflammatory cells within the tendon itself [21] but instead is associated with chronic synovial inflammation leading to the increased presence of catabolic factors within the joint [22].

Extrinsic causes of degeneration of the subscapularis tendon relate to subcoracoid and anterior-superior impingement [23–26]. Subcoracoid impingement occurs when the subscapularis tendon passes through a narrowed coracohumeral space, usually less than 10 mm. This narrowed space causes mechanical abrasion on the tendon leading to degeneration, similar to the classic extrinsic mechanism proposed by Neer for degeneration of the supraspinatus tendon [27]. A number of recent reports have found an association between a narrowed coracohumeral distance and degenerative tears of the subscapularis [23, 26], with one study proposing a critical coracohumeral distance of only 6 mm [23]. Anterior-superior impingement occurs when subscapularis tendon fibers become abraded by the anterior-superior glenoid or become impinged between this portion of the glenoid and the humeral head [28, 29]. In contrast to bursal-sided pathology within the tendon from subcoracoid impingement, this is more likely to lead to articular-sided tearing of the subscapularis.

## 25.4 Clinical Presentation

Patients having subscapularis tears will typically complain of anterior shoulder pain and weakness, particularly with internal rotation of the arm. As isolated subscapularis tears are rare, one must remember that concomitant posterosuperior rotator cuff and/or biceps pathology may also be present. Physical examination may demonstrate tenderness over the lesser tuberosity and anterior shoulder, pain or decreased strength with resisted internal rotation, and increased passive external rotation in complete tears.

There are three predominant special tests for the diagnosis of subscapularis pathology: belly-press, lift-off, and bear-hug tests. Some physicians also utilize the internal rotation lag sign. All of these tests involve active internal rotation of the shoulder in varying degrees of shoulder flexion. The lift-off test places the dorsum of the hand in the lumbar region so that the humerus is internally rotated and extended [10]. A positive test occurs when the patient is unable to further internally rotate the humerus, indicted by an inability to lift the hand off the back. The internal rotation lag sign is evaluated with the arm in the same starting position as the lift-off test [30]. However, in this test the arm is held at near maximal internal rotation (hand off of the back), and the patient is asked to maintain this position. A positive test occurs when the arm drifts into external rotation (hand nears the back), with the magnitude measured in degrees.

When the patient is not able to perform either of the above tests due to discomfort, the belly-press test may be used by having the patient press the palm of their hand into their abdomen [9]. The test is considered positive when the elbow drops in a posterior direction, internal rotation is lost, and pressure is exerted by extension of the shoulder and flexion of the wrist. More recently, the bear-hug test has also been described [6]. In this test, the palm of the involved side is placed on the opposite shoulder. The patient is asked to hold this position as the examiner tries to pull the patient's hand from the shoulder. The test is considered positive when the patient is not able to resist the examiner and the hand lifts from the shoulder or when there is weakness as compared to the contralateral (unaffected) side.

All of these tests were compared in an investigation by Yoon et al. who performed preoperative isokinetic testing in over 300 patients undergoing rotator cuff repair [31]. They reported that for detecting any tear of the subscapularis, the belly press was the most sensitive (28%), while the lift off was the most specific (100%). For differentiating a full-thickness tear from a partial tear, the most sensitive test was the belly-press test (57%), while the most specific was the lift-off test (97%). Furthermore, a positive lift-off test best correlated with loss of internal rotation strength.

## 25.5 Imaging

Plain radiographs are the first imaging modality performed when evaluating a patient with shoulder pain, including suspected rotator cuff pathology. A typical shoulder series includes a combination of anterior-posterior views in both internal and external rotation, axillary, outlet, and 30° caudal tilt views. Those with subscapularis pathology, particularly chronic tears, may demonstrate lesser tuberosity cortical irregularities and cysts although the sensitivity and specificity of this marker is variable [32].

Magnetic resonance imaging (MRI) of the shoulder remains the gold standard imaging modality for diagnosis of subscapularis pathology. MRI, however, has proved less reliable in the detection of subscapularis tears as compared to tears of the other rotator cuff tendons. Adams et al., in a study examining the MRIs of 120 patients prior to shoulder arthroscopy for rotator cuff repair, found a specificity of 100% but a sensitivity of only 36% in the detection of subscapularis tears by MRI [33]. Another investigation by a separate group supported these findings, reporting an overall sensitivity of 38% for detection of a subscapularis tear by either standard MRI or MR arthrography [34]. Other investigations, however, have reported higher sensitivity values in the range of 70–80% [35, 36]. As with other tendon tears, the larger the size of the subscapularis tear, the more likely MRI evaluation will demonstrate the pathology [36, 37].

There are also many reports on the use of ultrasound for confirming the diagnosis of a subscapularis tear [38–40]. In one investigation which used ultrasound for detection of rotator cuff tears, there was 100% sensitivity and 85% specificity for all rotator cuff tendons, with seven out of eight subscapularis tears being correctly identified preoperatively [40]. Another investigation on the same topic, however, reported a sensitivity of 40% and specificity of 93% [39]. This study broke out partial- and full-thickness tears of the subscapularis, with decreased sensitivity and specificity for partial-thickness and smaller tears. One drawback to the use of ultrasound is that results and accuracy can be operator dependent. For this reason, most clinicians still rely on MRI to confirm their clinical exam findings when planning surgical intervention.

## 25.6 Management of Subscapularis Tears

Nonoperative treatment is undertaken for small, degenerative (nontraumatic) tears of the subscapularis in the older or less physically active individuals. Physical therapy may be utilized, with rehabilitation protocols focusing on rotator cuff and scapular strengthening exercises. Corticosteroid injections and anti-inflammatory medication may also be utilized.

Operative treatment is pursued for all acute subscapularis tears, smaller tears that have failed conservative treatment, larger degenerative tears, as well as all tears visualized arthroscopically, whether they were identified on preoperative MRI or not. While open repair is an option, it is almost always possible to achieve adequate mobilization and secure fixation of the tendon through arthroscopic techniques. The author uses the beach-chair position with an arm holder for all subscapularis and rotator cuff repairs, although the lateral decubitus position is also an option. After a standard posterior viewing portal and anterior working portal are established, a diagnostic arthroscopy is performed.

Evaluation of the subscapularis insertion and less tuberosity can be difficult, but a few techniques can help to improve visualization. Internal rotation of the arm as well as a posteriorly directed force on the humerus (posterior lever push [41]) can bring the tuberosity into view (Fig. 25.1a, b). A 70° arthroscope should be available should increase visualization of the footprint be needed. Lastly, since swelling can impede visualization and working space in the anterior aspect of the shoulder, it is recommended that subscapularis repair be performed first prior to other interventions.

Given the close anatomic relationship of the biceps tendon and pulley to the subscapularis, there is often concomitant pathology. Arai et al. reported that of all biceps tendon lesions, 76% were associated with a subscapularis tear, and all unstable biceps tendons also had subscapularis

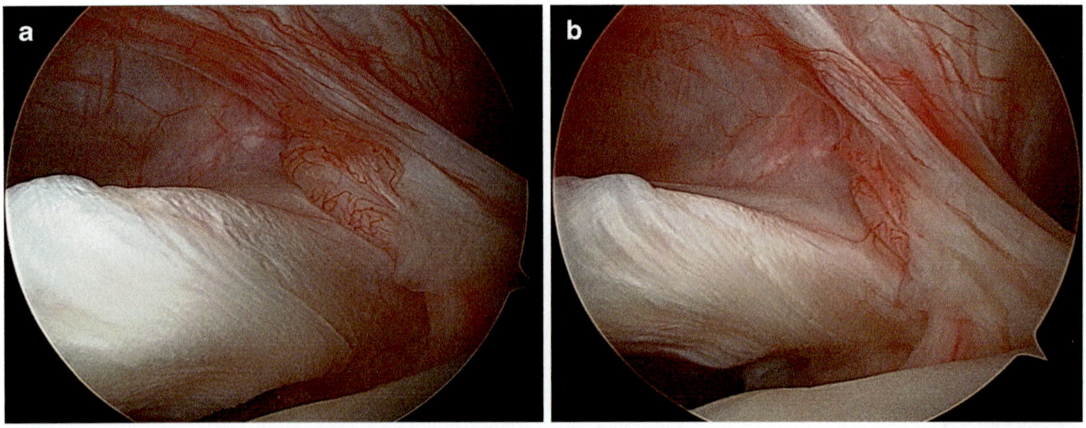


**Fig. 25.1** (**a**, **b**) Arthroscopic images from the posterior viewing portal demonstrating an upper border tear of the subscapularis (**a**) before and (**b**) after a posterior lever push. The posteriorly directed force on the humerus allows the subscapularis tendon to lift away from the lesser tuberosity, revealing the true extent of the pathology

tears [5]. Another investigation found that a subscapularis tear was significantly associated with biceps tendon lesions [12]. Because of this, and particularly in older patients with degenerative tears, a biceps tenodesis or tenotomy is often performed, especially in light of evidence that tenodesis for tenotomy was associated with improved subjective and objective results in a cohort of patients undergoing subscapularis repair [42].

Once the extent and anatomy of the subscapularis tear has been identified, the surgical construct can be determined. A distinction is made between partial-thickness tears (Fig. 25.2a), small full-thickness tears (Fig. 25.2b), and large full-thickness tears with retraction (Fig. 25.2c). A similar but slightly more detailed classification system which divides the subscapularis insertion on the lesser tuberosity into four distinct facets has been proposed [7]. In general, the author utilizes a single-anchor construct for partial-thickness tears, while a double-row construct is used for small and large full-thickness tears. In the author's experience, and in agreement with previously published literature [43], most chronic and retracted subscapularis tears can be repaired arthroscopically given appropriate mobilization techniques. Denard et al. have also shown that medialization of the lesser tuberosity footprint by as much as 7 mm does not result in negative clinical consequences [44].

Following assessment of the tear pattern and mobility, an additional anterosuperolateral working portal is created off the edge of the

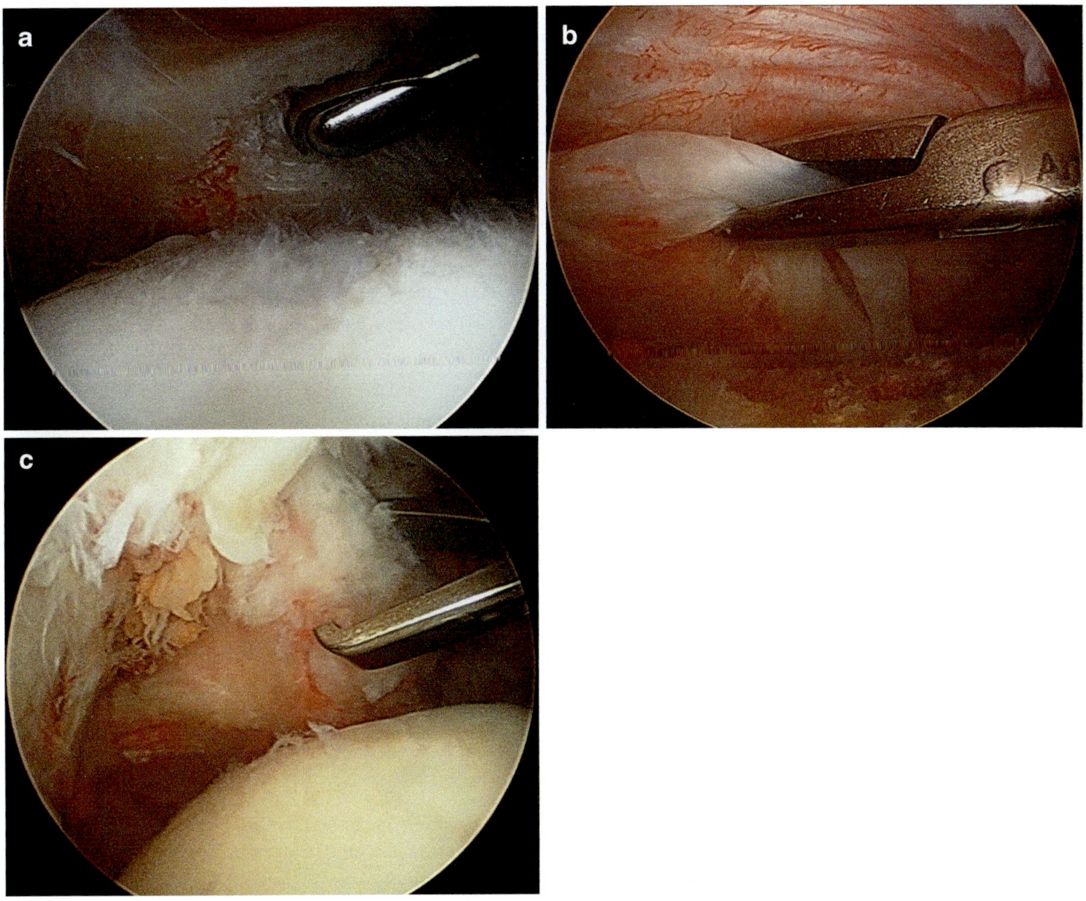


**Fig. 25.2** (**a**–**c**) Arthroscopic images from the posterior portal of three different left shoulders demonstrating (**a**) partial-thickness, (**b**) small full-thickness, and (**c**) large and retracted full-thickness tears of the subscapularis

anterolateral acromion using outside-in technique. The portal should allow an approximately 10° angle of approach to the lesser tuberosity and be mostly aligned with the subscapularis tendon. The exception to this has been in the setting of isolated partial-thickness tears where a coracoplasty is not required, and a single-anchor repair is planned. In this circumstance, the author does not create additional anterosuperolateral portal so as to remove the possibility of damage to the anterior aspect of the supraspinatus tendon. For these cases, a larger cannula may be exchanged for the initial smaller cannula placed anteriorly. After preparation of the footprint, a free suture is passed in mattress fashion through the superolateral border of the tendon using a suture-passing device (Fig. 25.3a). The two suture limbs (exiting the anterior aspect of the tendon) are then placed through the eyelet of a knotless suture anchor and secured to the superolateral aspect of the lesser tuberosity footprint (Figs. 25.3b, c).

For full-thickness tears, mobilization of the tendon is required, and the additional anterosuperolateral portal is created. Working through this portal, the coracoid tip is identified, paying careful attention to the presence of nearby neurovascular structures, and a window in the rotator interval can be created to give access to the anterior aspect of the tendon. The tip and posterolateral base of the coracoid is skeletonized, proving for and giving access to anterior and superior releases. The need for coracoplasty can be determined at this time. Posterior releases can be achieved using a blunt elevator inserted between the subscapularis and anterior glenoid neck. In chronic and retracted tears, the "comma sign," a convergence of the superior glenohumeral ligament and coracohumeral ligament, can aid in identification of the superolateral aspect of the torn tendon (Fig. 25.4) [45]. This tissue can hold a traction stitch to aid in releases and mobilization of the tendon and should be preserved in the final repair.

The author's preferred construct for a full-thickness tear is a double-row knotless repair (Fig. 25.5). Ide et al. reported on a group of patients undergoing subscapularis repairs using either a single-row or double-row technique [46]. While they found that the clinical outcomes for these 61 patients were comparable, subscapularis function and abduction strength were improved in the double-row group, and there was a trend toward a lower failure rate in this same group. For smaller full-thickness tears, a single anchor is placed at the medial aspect of the exposed footprint. For larger tears where more of the footprint is exposed, an inferior and a superior anchor are placed. The anterior portal may need to be adjusted, or a new anterior portal can be created using outside-in technique to allow for appropriate angle for anchor placement. With the use of a grasper or traction stitch through the anterosuperolateral

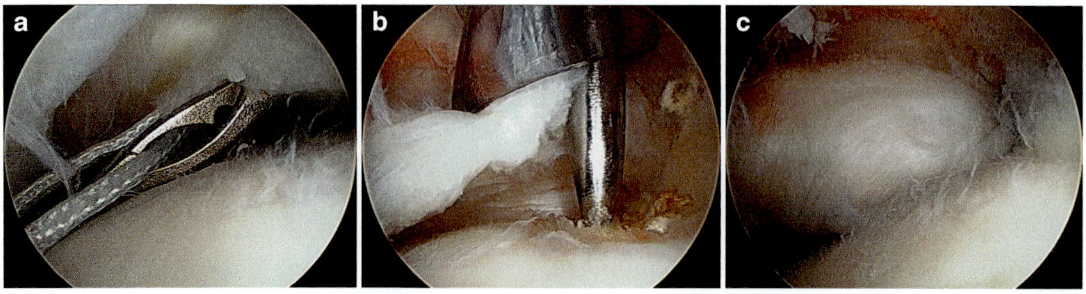


**Fig. 25.3** (**a**–**c**) Arthroscopic images as viewed from the posterior portal demonstrating the steps for repair of a partial-thickness upper border subscapularis tear utilizing single anterior working portal. In this series (**a**) the free end of the sutures are passed in mattress fashion through the superolateral border of the tendon using a suture-passing device. The two suture limbs are then placed through the eyelet of a knotless suture anchor, and (**b**) the anchor hole is created. The final construct demonstrates (**c**) secure fixation of the tendon to the superolateral aspect of the lesser tuberosity footprint

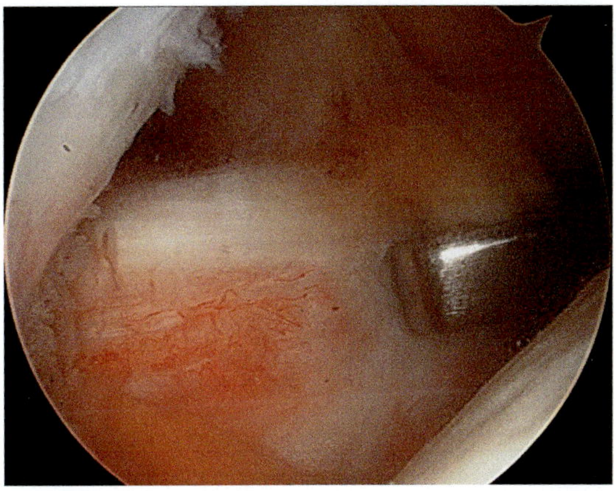

**Fig. 25.4** An arthroscopic image from the posterior viewing portal demonstrating a chronic and retracted subscapularis tear. The grasper is placed through the anterosuperolateral portal and is pulling lateral traction on the tendon, demonstrating the "comma sign," representing the convergence of the superior glenohumeral ligament and coracohumeral ligament attached to the superolateral border of the tendon

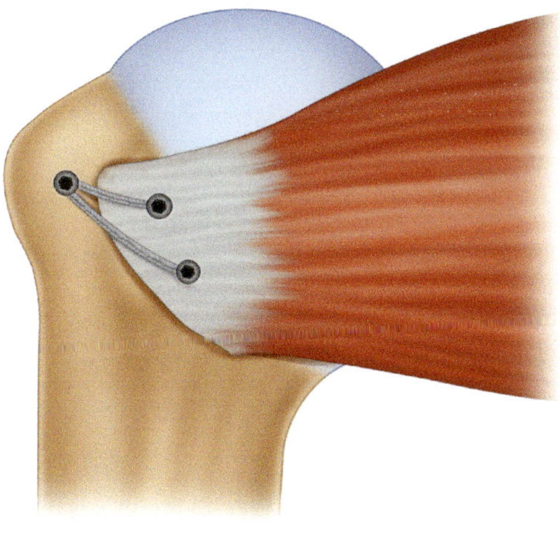

**Fig. 25.5** Schematic drawing of the authors' preferred method for double-row repair of the large, full-thickness subscapularis repair (Adapted from Ide et al. [46])

portal to place tension on the subscapularis, a suture-passing device is utilized to pass each suture limb, from inferior to superior, through the tendon in a mattress configuration. Each limb is then secured with a single knotless anchor to the superolateral aspect of the lesser tuberosity footprint. As mentioned, nearly all subscapularis repairs, even with significant fatty infiltration, are able to be repaired with appropriate releases with or without footprint medialization. In the truly irreparable tears, pectoralis major transfer remains an option [47, 48].

## 25.7 Postoperative Rehabilitation

Postoperatively, patients are placed in a sling for 6 weeks. No weight bearing is allowed during this time. Active motion of the elbow, wrist, and hand is encouraged. In the case of partial-thickness repairs, external rotation is allowed to 30°. For full-thickness tears, external rotation is only allowed to neutral. Forward flexion is limited to 90° and abduction to 60°. At 6 weeks, passive stretching is allowed as well as progression to active range of motion. Strengthening is deferred until 3 months postoperatively.

## 25.8 Results

Burkhart et al. were some of the first to publish preliminary results of arthroscopic subscapularis repair in 2002, reporting 92% good-to-excellent outcomes [49]. This group followed their cohort and reported intermediate-term results which continued to be significantly improved from preoperative status [50]. Numerous other studies have reported similarly good-to-excellent results with arthroscopic subscapularis repair [51–54], and this method has therefore become current standard of care. The exact technique of the repair (single- versus double-row, stitch configuration) is still controversial; however, early reports indicate a trend toward improved outcomes with a double-row technique [46].

**Conclusion**

The subscapularis muscle-tendon unit plays a critical role in the stability and kinematics of shoulder function. Recognition of subscapularis tears has increased with the wide adoption of arthroscopic techniques for the treatment of shoulder pathologies. Both physical exam and advanced imaging modalities can be sensitive for the detection of subscapularis pathology; however, one must maintain a high index of clinical suspicion, particularly for partial-thickness tears, which may not be evident on MRI. Conservative treatment is pursued for small chronic tears in older patients, while operative management is the mainstay of treatment for all other categories. While repair techniques and construct configurations are evolving, good-to-excellent results have been reported for arthroscopic subscapularis repair.

## References


1. Keating JF, Waterworth P, Shaw-Dunn J, Crossan J. The relative strengths of the rotator cuff muscles. A cadaver study. J Bone Joint Surg Br. 1993;75(1):137–40.
2. Bouaicha S, Slankamenac K, Moor BK, Tok S, Andreisek G, Finkenstaedt T. Cross-sectional area of the rotator cuff muscles in MRI – is there evidence for a biomechanical balanced shoulder? PLoS One. 2016;11(6):e0157946.
3. Codman E. Lesions of the supraspinatus tendon and other lesions in or about the subacromial bursa. The Shoulder. Boston: Thomas Todd; 1934. p. 65–7.
4. Warner JJ, Higgins L, Parsons IM, Dowdy P. Diagnosis and treatment of anterosuperior rotator cuff tears. J Shoulder Elbow Surg. 2001;10(1):37–46.
5. Arai R, Sugaya H, Mochizuki T, Nimura A, Moriishi J, Akita K. Subscapularis tendon tear: an anatomic and clinical investigation. Arthroscopy. 2008;24(9):997–1004.
6. Barth JR, Burkhart SS, De Beer JF. The bear-hug test: a new and sensitive test for diagnosing a subscapularis tear. Arthroscopy. 2006;22(10):1076–84.
7. Yoo JC, Rhee YG, Shin SJ, Park YB, McGarry MH, Jun BJ, et al. Subscapularis tendon tear classification based on 3-dimensional anatomic footprint: a cadaveric and prospective clinical observational study. Arthroscopy. 2015;31(1):19–28.
8. Lafosse L, Jost B, Reiland Y, Audebert S, Toussaint B, Gobezie R. Structural integrity and clinical outcomes after arthroscopic repair of isolated subscapularis tears. J Bone Joint Surg Am. 2007;89(6):1184–93.
9. Gerber C, Hersche O, Farron A. Isolated rupture of the subscapularis tendon. J Bone Joint Surg Am. 1996;78(7):1015–23.
10. Gerber C, Krushell RJ. Isolated rupture of the tendon of the subscapularis muscle. clinical features in 16 cases. J Bone Joint Surg Br. 1991;73(3):389–94.
11. Naimark M, Zhang AL, Leon I, Trivellas A, Feeley BT, Ma CB. Clinical, radiographic, and surgical presentation of subscapularis tendon tears: a retrospective analysis of 139 patients. Arthroscopy. 2016;32(5):747–52.
12. Urita A, Funakoshi T, Amano T, Matsui Y, Kawamura D, Kameda Y, et al. Predictive factors of long head of the biceps tendon disorders-the bicipital groove morphology and subscapularis tendon tear. J Shoulder Elbow Surg. 2016;25(3):384–9.
13. Neviaser RJ, Neviaser TJ. Recurrent instability of the shoulder after age 40. J Shoulder Elbow Surg. 1995;4(6):416–8.
14. Neviaser RJ, Neviaser TJ, Neviaser JS. Concurrent rupture of the rotator cuff and anterior dislocation of the shoulder in the older patient. J Bone Joint Surg Am. 1988;70(9):1308–11.
15. Neviaser RJ, Neviaser TJ, Neviaser JS. Anterior dislocation of the shoulder and rotator cuff rupture. Clin Orthop Relat Res. 1993;291:103–6.
16. Elmore KA, Wayne JS. Soft tissue structures resisting anterior instability in a computational glenohumeral joint model. Comput Methods Biomech Biomed Engin. 2013;16(7):781–9.
17. Wirth MA, Rockwood Jr CA. Operative treatment of irreparable rupture of the subscapularis. J Bone Joint Surg Am. 1997;79(5):722–31.
18. Khan KM, Cook JL, Bonar F, Harcourt P, Astrom M. Histopathology of common tendinopathies. Update and implications for clinical management. Sports Med. 1999;27(6):393–408.
19. Fukuda H, Hamada K, Yamanaka K. Pathology and pathogenesis of bursal-side rotator cuff tears viewed from en bloc histologic sections. Clin Orthop Relat Res. 1990;254:75–80.
20. Hashimoto T, Nobuhara K, Hamada T. Pathologic evidence of degeneration as a primary cause of rotator cuff tear. Clin Orthop Relat Res. 2003;415:111–20.
21. Xu Y, Murrell GA. The basic science of tendinopathy. Clin Orthop Relat Res. 2008;466(7):1528–38.
22. Abrams GD, Luria A, Carr RA, Rhodes C, Robinson WH, Sokolove J. Association of synovial inflammation and inflammatory mediators with glenohumeral rotator cuff pathology. J Shoulder Elbow Surg. 2016;25(6):989–97.
23. Balke M, Banerjee M, Greshake O, Hoeher J, Bouillon B, Liem D. The coracohumeral distance in shoulders with traumatic and degenerative subscapularis tendon tears. Am J Sports Med. 2016;44(1):198–201.
24. Hekimoglu B, Aydin H, Kizilgoz V, Tatar IG, Ersan O. Quantitative measurement of humero-acromial, humero-coracoid, and coraco-clavicular intervals for the diagnosis of subacromial and subcoracoid impingement of shoulder joint. Clin Imaging. 2013;37(2):201–10.
25. Li X, Fallon J, Egge N, Curry EJ, Patel K, Owens BD, et al. MRI study of associated shoulder pathology in patients with full-thickness subscapularis tendon tears. Orthopedics. 2013;36(1):e44–50.
26. Richards DP, Burkhart SS, Campbell SE. Relation between narrowed coracohumeral distance and subscapularis tears. Arthroscopy. 2005;21(10):1223–8.

27. Neer 2nd CS. Anterior acromioplasty for the chronic impingement syndrome in the shoulder: a preliminary report. J Bone Joint Surg Am. 1972;54(1):41–50.
28. Bath SS, Bath SS, Tehranzadeh J. Anterosuperior glenoid impingement syndrome. Clin Med Insights Arthritis Musculoskelet Disord. 2012;5:15–8.
29. Longo UG, Berton A, Marinozzi A, Maffulli N, Denaro V. Subscapularis tears. Med Sport Sci. 2012;57:114–21.
30. Hertel R, Ballmer FT, Lombert SM, Gerber C. Lag signs in the diagnosis of rotator cuff rupture. J Shoulder Elbow Surg. 1996;5(4):307–13.
31. Yoon JP, Chung SW, Kim SH, Oh JH. Diagnostic value of four clinical tests for the evaluation of subscapularis integrity. J Shoulder Elbow Surg. 2013;22(9):1186–92.
32. Studler U, Pfirrmann CW, Jost B, Rousson V, Hodler J, Zanetti M. Abnormalities of the lesser tuberosity on radiography and MRI: association with subscapularis tendon lesions. AJR Am J Roentgenol. 2008;191(1):100–6.
33. Adams CR, Schoolfield JD, Burkhart SS. Accuracy of preoperative magnetic resonance imaging in predicting a subscapularis tendon tear based on arthroscopy. Arthroscopy. 2010;26(11):1427–33.
34. Foad A, Wijdicks CA. The accuracy of magnetic resonance imaging and magnetic resonance arthrogram versus arthroscopy in the diagnosis of subscapularis tendon injury. Arthroscopy. 2012;28(5):636–41.
35. Gyftopoulos S, OD J, Shah NP, Goss J, Babb J, Recht MP. Correlation of MRI with arthroscopy for the evaluation of the subscapularis tendon: a musculoskeletal division's experience. Skeletal Radiol. 2013;42(9):1269–75.
36. Malavolta EA, Assuncao JH, Guglielmetti CL, de Souza FF, Gracitelli ME, Bordalo-Rodrigues M, et al. Accuracy of preoperative MRI in the diagnosis of subscapularis tears. Arch Orthop Trauma Surg. 2016;136:1425–30.
37. Smith TO, Daniell H, Geere JA, Toms AP, Hing CB. The diagnostic accuracy of MRI for the detection of partial- and full-thickness rotator cuff tears in adults. Magn Reson Imaging. 2012;30(3):336–46.
38. Iannotti JP, Ciccone J, Buss DD, Visotsky JL, Mascha E, Cotman K, et al. Accuracy of office-based ultrasonography of the shoulder for the diagnosis of rotator cuff tears. J Bone Joint Surg Am. 2005;87(6):1305–11.
39. Narasimhan R, Shamse K, Nash C, Dhingra D, Kennedy S. Prevalence of subscapularis tears and accuracy of shoulder ultrasound in pre-operative diagnosis. Int Orthop. 2016;40(5):975–9.
40. Teefey SA, Hasan SA, Middleton WD, Patel M, Wright RW, Yamaguchi K. Ultrasonography of the rotator cuff. A comparison of ultrasonographic and arthroscopic findings in one hundred consecutive cases. J Bone Joint Surg Am. 2000;82(4):498–504.
41. Burkhart SS, Brady PC. Arthroscopic subscapularis repair: surgical tips and pearls A to Z. Arthroscopy. 2006;22(9):1014–27.
42. Edwards TB, Walch G, Sirveaux F, Mole D, Nove-Josserand L, Boulahia A, et al. Repair of tears of the subscapularis. J Bone Joint Surg Am. 2005;87(4):725–30.
43. Denard PJ, Ladermann A, Burkhart SS. Arthroscopic management of subscapularis tears. Sports Med Arthrosc. 2011;19(4):333–41.
44. Denard PJ, Burkhart SS. Medialization of the subscapularis footprint does not affect functional outcome of arthroscopic repair. Arthroscopy. 2012;28(11):1608–14.
45. Lo IK, Burkhart SS. The comma sign: an arthroscopic guide to the torn subscapularis tendon. Arthroscopy. 2003;19(3):334–7.
46. Ide J, Karasugi T, Okamoto N, Taniwaki T, Oka K, Mizuta H. Functional and structural comparisons of the arthroscopic knotless double-row suture bridge and single-row repair for anterosuperior rotator cuff tears. J Shoulder Elbow Surg. 2015;24(10):1544–54.
47. Jost B, Puskas GJ, Lustenberger A, Gerber C. Outcome of pectoralis major transfer for the treatment of irreparable subscapularis tears. J Bone Joint Surg Am. 2003;85-A(10):1944–51.
48. Nelson GN, Namdari S, Galatz L, Keener JD. Pectoralis major tendon transfer for irreparable subscapularis tears. J Shoulder Elbow Surg. 2014;23(6):909–18.
49. Burkhart SS, Tehrany AM. Arthroscopic subscapularis tendon repair: technique and preliminary results. Arthroscopy. 2002;18(5):454–63.
50. Adams CR, Schoolfield JD, Burkhart SS. The results of arthroscopic subscapularis tendon repairs. Arthroscopy. 2008;24(12):1381–9.
51. Arun GR, Kumar P, Patnaik S, Selvaraj K, Rajan D, Singh A, et al. Outcome of arthroscopic subscapularis tendon repair: are the results improving with improved techniques and equipment?: a retrospective case series. Indian J Orthop. 2016;50(3):297–302.
52. Bennett WF. Arthroscopic repair of anterosuperior (supraspinatus/subscapularis) rotator cuff tears: a prospective cohort with 2- to 4-year follow-up. Classification of biceps subluxation/instability. Arthroscopy. 2003;19(1):21–33.
53. Ide J, Tokiyoshi A, Hirose J, Mizuta H. Arthroscopic repair of traumatic combined rotator cuff tears involving the subscapularis tendon. J Bone Joint Surg Am. 2007;89(11):2378–88.
54. Mall NA, Chahal J, Heard WM, Bach Jr BR, Bush-Joseph CA, Romeo AA, et al. Outcomes of arthroscopic and open surgical repair of isolated subscapularis tendon tears. Arthroscopy. 2012;28(9):1306–14.

# Cartilage Defects

# 26

Julian Mehl and Knut Beitzel

## Contents

**26.1 Etiology** ........ 227

**26.2 Symptoms and Diagnosis** ........ 228

**26.3 Therapy** ........ 229
26.3.1 Bone Marrow Stimulation ........ 229
26.3.2 Autologous Chondrocyte Transplantation ........ 230
26.3.3 Autologous Osteochondral Transplantation ........ 231
26.3.4 Partial Joint Resurfacing (PJR) ........ 234
26.3.5 Shoulder Arthroplasty ........ 234

**26.4 Summary** ........ 235

**References** ........ 235

J. Mehl (✉) • K. Beitzel
Department of Orthopaedic Sports Medicine, Technical University of Munich (TUM), Munich, Germany
e-mail: julian.mehl@tum.de

Articular cartilage shows very limited self-healing capacity, which is why damages to this tissue can lead to significant impairment of the joint function. Despite scientific progress regarding diagnosis and treatment of cartilage defects in recent years, they still represent a challenge to orthopedic clinicians, which is even more applicable for the shoulder in comparison to other joints. Since lesions of the chondral layer are a risk factor for the development of osteoarthritis, early detection and adequate therapy are crucial, especially in young and active patients, to avoid rapid deterioration of the joint function and the need for early arthroplasty.

## 26.1 Etiology

There are various reasons for the development of cartilage defects in the shoulder such as trauma, chronic overuse, chronic instability, osteochondritis dissecans, osteonecrosis, or iatrogenic injuries. Acute trauma like a direct hit to the shoulder leading to a disruption of cartilage from the underlying bone or shoulder luxation with an engaging Hill-Sachs is one of the main causes for focal cartilage defects in the shoulder. But also iatrogenic damages during operation or due to incorrectly inserted anchors can lead to focal defects. In contrast chronic cartilage degeneration of the glenohumeral joint is mostly a result of overuse and is often associated with other

© ISAKOS 2017
A.B. Imhoff, F.H. Savoie III (eds.), *Shoulder Instability Across the Life Span*,
DOI 10.1007/978-3-662-54077-0_26

shoulder joint pathologies like rotator cuff tears. It has been demonstrated that chronic shoulder instability as well plays a crucial role in the etiology of chondral lesions since up to 2/3 of patients needing arthroscopical stabilization of the shoulder show intraoperative articular cartilage lesions [8]. Especially repetitive shoulder dislocations are associated with particularly severe cartilage damages increasing the risk of early osteoarthritis [10]. Anterior shoulder dislocation leads to cartilage damages especially at the posterior-middle humeral head zone, whereas the glenoid is less effected [11].

A separate etiology for cartilage defects is osteonecrosis of the humeral head that can be caused by endogenous, iatrogenous (e.g., chemotherapy), exogenous (e.g., alcohol), or posttraumatic (e.g., humeral head fractures) factors and is usually associated with more extensive lesions of the articular cartilage overlying the necrotic bone.

Because of the very limited self-healing capacity of cartilage tissue, these injuries do not only lead to painful decrease of joint function, but they represent a relevant risk factor for the development of osteoarthritis. Especially the history of shoulder dislocation is associated with an up to 19 times greater risk for arthrosis with higher age at the time of dislocation and longer time between dislocation and operation increasing the risk [3]. So early diagnosis and treatment of both cartilage defects and co-pathologies are necessary to prevent the glenohumeral joint from these consequential damages.

## 26.2 Symptoms and Diagnosis

The main symptoms of cartilage defects in the glenohumeral joint are pain and limited function of the shoulder, which is why several differential diagnoses accompanied by the same symptoms have to be considered. Furthermore, as already mentioned above, cartilage defects of the shoulder often come along with chronic overuse, chronic instability, or with traumatic injuries of other structures in the joint. In these cases solely treatment of the cartilage defect would be wrong. Surgical cartilage repair is only allowed after exclusion of other reasons for pain symptoms or in combination with the treatment of the causal pathology such as chronic instability. Therefore, a careful examination and diagnosis prior to operation are mandatory.

Omarthrosis can often be diagnosed already by means of native radiographs since it shows significant alterations like joint space narrowing, subchondral sclerosis, or osteophytes. Also bigger osteochondral defects of the humeral head or the glenoid can be seen in native x-ray images. However, detection of focal chondral or smaller osteochondral defects in the glenohumeral joint is often quite challenging in comparison to other joints. One of the main reasons for this fact is the lower thickness and the inhomogenous distribution of the chondral layer in the glenohumeral joint. According to a study by Zumstein et al., the mean cartilage thickness is 1.93 mm at the glenoid and 1.74 mm at the humeral head, while the highest thickness was seen in the inferior-anterior parts in the glenoid and in the superior and central parts of the humeral head [14]. Although new MRI sequences like T1ρ mapping seem to be advantageous regarding the detection of cartilage defects in the shoulder [11], evaluation of focal chondral defects with native MRI or even with intravenous contrast medium is often not possible because of the insufficient contrast between the articular cartilage and the surrounding tissues [6]. For sufficient evaluation of the glenohumeral cartilage status, invasive imaging with intra-articular application of contrast medium is necessary, whereas arthro-CT seems to show even better sensitivity compared with arthro-MRI. By means of these images, size and grade of the cartilage defect can be measured preoperatively. Nevertheless the final decision for the definitive treatment can only be made after complete arthroscopical debridement of loose cartilage tissue and intraoperative measurement of the defect's size. On the basis of the arthroscopic findings, several classifications for the grade of chondral lesions have been developed during the past years, whereas the classification according to the International Cartilage Repair Society (ICRS), which was initially developed for the knee joint, is now the international standard for the glenohumeral joint as well (Table 26.1) (Fig. 26.1).

**Table 26.1** ICRS classification

| Grad | |
|---|---|
| 0 | Normal cartilage |
| 1a | Intact surface, fibrillation, and/or cartilage softening |
| 1b | Additional superficial lacerations/fissures |
| 2 | <50% of cartilage thickness affected |
| 3a | >50% of cartilage thickness affected, not involving the calcified layer |
| 3b | >50% of cartilage thickness affected, extend to calcified layer |
| 3c | >50% of cartilage thickness affected, extend to subchondral bone |
| 3d | >50% of cartilage thickness affected, with blistering |
| 4a/b | Complete cartilage defect, extend into subchondral bone |

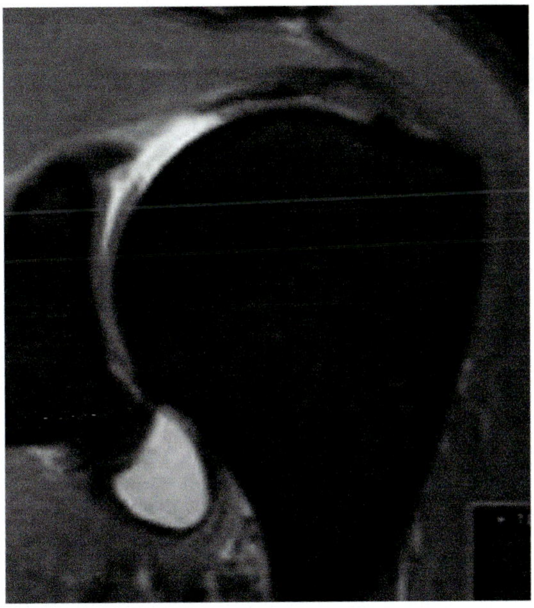

**Fig. 26.1** MRI with intra-articular gadolinium application for better visualization of a chondral lesion at the humerus (ICRS type 4)

## 26.3 Therapy

To date there is only limited evidence regarding diagnosis and therapy of cartilage defects in the shoulder. Because of this lack of high-level studies, it is still a challenge for the clinicians not only to detect focal cartilage defects but above all to draw the correct conclusions from this diagnosis. As cartilage defects of the shoulder are often additional findings with other pathologies, examination has to make sure that the cartilage defect is in fact a relevant reason for the patient's symptoms before planning surgery. In cases of detected comorbidities which do not need immediate surgical treatment, it may be advisable to first treat the shoulder conservatively, e.g., by physical therapy. However, it is important that a conservative treatment attempt must not delay surgical cartilage repair unnecessarily, which is why these patients must be reevaluated in a defined period of time to avoid rapid deterioration.

In general cartilage defects grade 3 or 4 according to ICRS classification associated with symptoms of pain or loss of function are indications for surgical cartilage repair. Nowadays there are several operative treatment options for restoration of articular cartilage in the shoulder, like bone marrow stimulating therapies, autologous osteochondral transplantation (OCT), or autologous chondrocyte transplantation (ACT). The choice of therapy is depending on different factors like size and grade of the defect as well as quality of the subchondral bone. However, due to the lack of clinical trials, the indications for cartilage treatment in the shoulder joint are so far not as clearly defined as for other joints, which is why the indications and contraindications are to a big part based on the data for other joints like the knee (Fig. 26.2).

### 26.3.1 Bone Marrow Stimulation

Bone marrow stimulating therapies like microfracturing are indicated in rather smaller cartilage defects (< 2–3 cm$^2$) with good and healthy subchondral bone. The surgical technique is similar to the treatment of other joints like the knee or ankle and can be performed arthroscopically. Initially a careful debridement of the defect using an arthroscopical shaver or curette is necessary, which must be completed down to the subchondral bone including the calcified layer and into healthy surrounding cartilage. Subsequently the

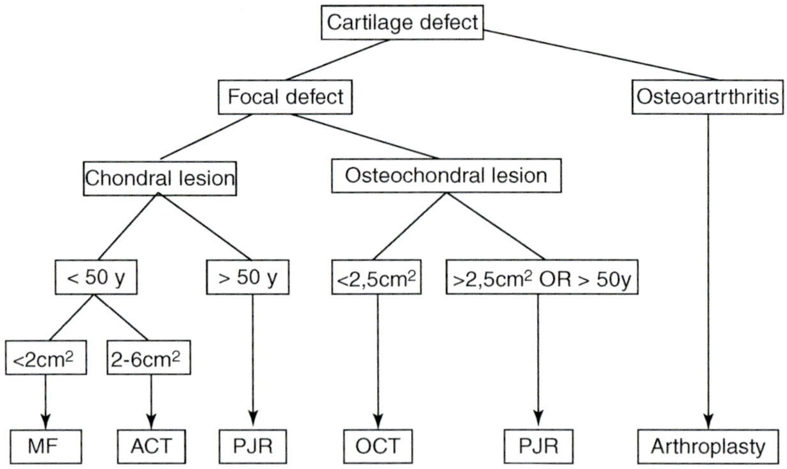


**Fig. 26.2** Flowchart of operative therapy of cartilage defects in the shoulder. *MF* microfracturing, *ACT* autologous chondrocyte transplantation, *PJR* partial joint resurfacing, *OCT* autologous osteochondral transplantation

subchondral surface is perforated with special awls or drills, so blood containing stem cells can escape from the bone marrow and build a clot in the former defect zone, which over time transforms to fibrocartilage tissue [5]. It is crucial that the often sclerotic subchondral bone is completely perforated, which can be ensured by the leakage of grease drops from the underlying bone marrow. Studies have shown that the optimal distance between the perforations is 3 and 4 mm [13]. Microfracturing of the shoulder is a relatively easy and cost-effective therapy with similar good clinical results in comparison to other joints, if the indication is set properly [4]. Furthermore in comparison to other established cartilage regenerative procedures, an additional surgery at the knee for harvesting autologous osteochondral transplants or chondrocytes is not necessary. However, microfracturing is not indicated for bipolar lesions, and it does not seem suitable for larger cartilage defects of more than 3 $cm^2$ and for patients over 40 years of age. Furthermore compared with other locations like the femorotibial joint, microfracturing in the glenohumeral joint can be quite challenging since the surgeon has to avoid an approach, which is too tangential to the defect. While for the humeral head, this problem can be solved by internal or external rotation of the arm; for defects of the glenoid, the arthroscopical portal should be placed more lateral in order to reach the lesion more vertical (Fig. 26.3).

### 26.3.2 Autologous Chondrocyte Transplantation

By now ACT is a standard therapy for the treatment of large (>2$cm^2$) full-thickness chondral lesions with intact subchondral bone in different joints with good clinical outcome. Still clinical experience for the glenohumeral joint is rare, but its application in other joints has shown that ACT is contraindicated in bipolar defects and that previous microfracturing is associated with minor results [9]. In a first operation, chondrocytes are harvested from the posterior-superior zone of the humeral head arthroscopically. Afterward the cells are in vitro cultivated for 4–8 weeks (dependent on the producing company) and then implanted into the defect zone. Also for ACT a careful debridement is necessary prior to implantation; however, in contrast to microfracturing, damage to the subchondral layer and subsequent bleeding from the bone marrow must be avoided as the implanted chondrocytes should not be mixed with stem cells. Especially for defects of the humeral head, matrix-associated ACT (MACT) procedures, where the expanded chondrocytes are imbedded in a three-dimensional collagen bio-scaffold that is fixed in the surrounding cartilage by sutures, have seemed to be advantageous in the past years, as the implanted chondrocytes are distributed more homogeneous in the defect zone on the spherical surface of the humeral

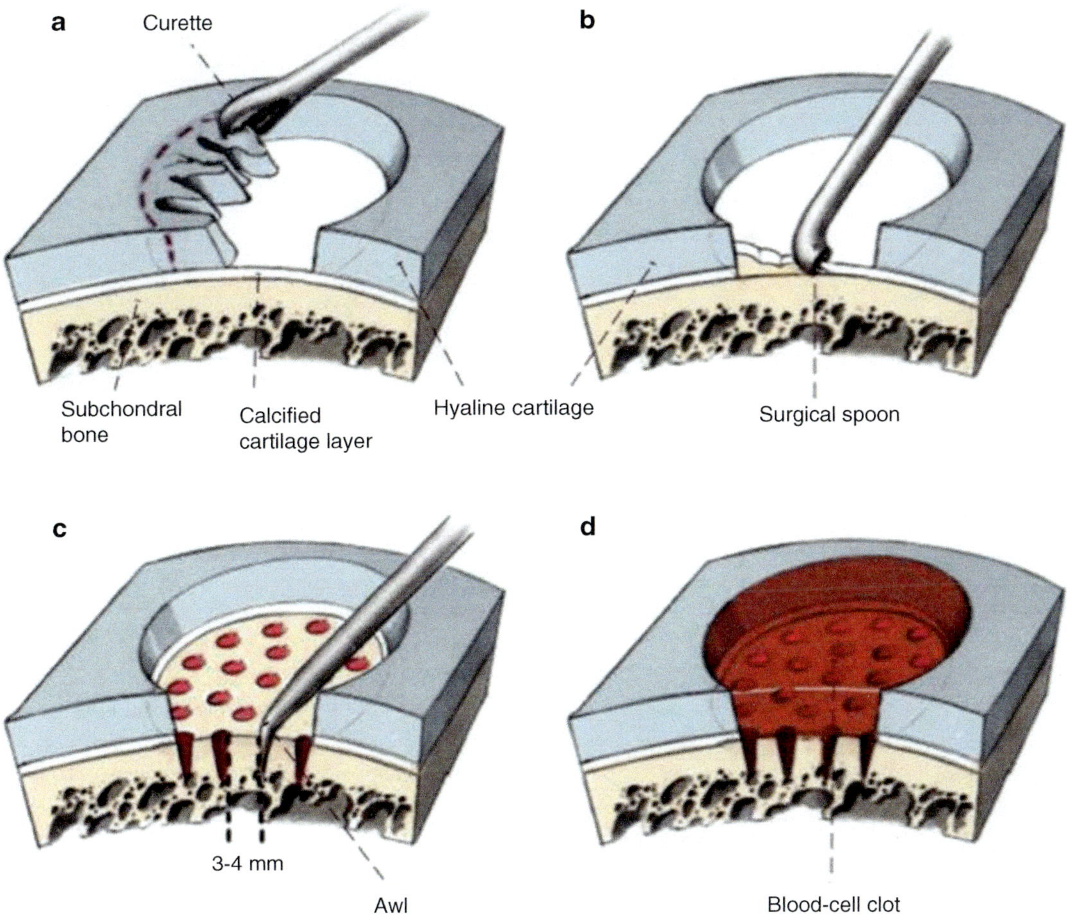


**Fig. 26.3** (**a**–**d**) Schematic representation of the microfracturing technique: (**a**) careful debridement of the defect zone into healthy surrounding cartilage using a curette; (**b**) removal of the calcified layer with a sharp spoon curette; (**c**) perforation of the subchondral bone with the microfracture awl; (**d**) defect filled with blood clot

head [4]. Though this procedure requires an open approach including the detachment of the subscapularis tendon and therefore it causes a more stringent rehabilitation [2]. Following the recent invention of injectable ACT, where the cultivated cells are contained in albumin hyaluronic acid gels, less invasive arthroscopical or arthroscopical-assisted procedures are possible today; however, the arthroscopical technique still requires a high level of experience by the surgeon.

To date there are no clinical high-level studies available regarding the outcome of ACT at the glenohumeral joint in a midterm to long-term perspective. So it is still unclear whether the experience gained from ACT procedures at other joints like the knee can be transferred to the shoulder, especially considering the anatomical differences according to loads, shear forces, and cartilage thickness (Figs. 26.4 and 26.5).

### 26.3.3 Autologous Osteochondral Transplantation

If the defect does not only extend to the cartilage but includes the subchondral bone in terms of an osteochondral lesion, the therapy must also

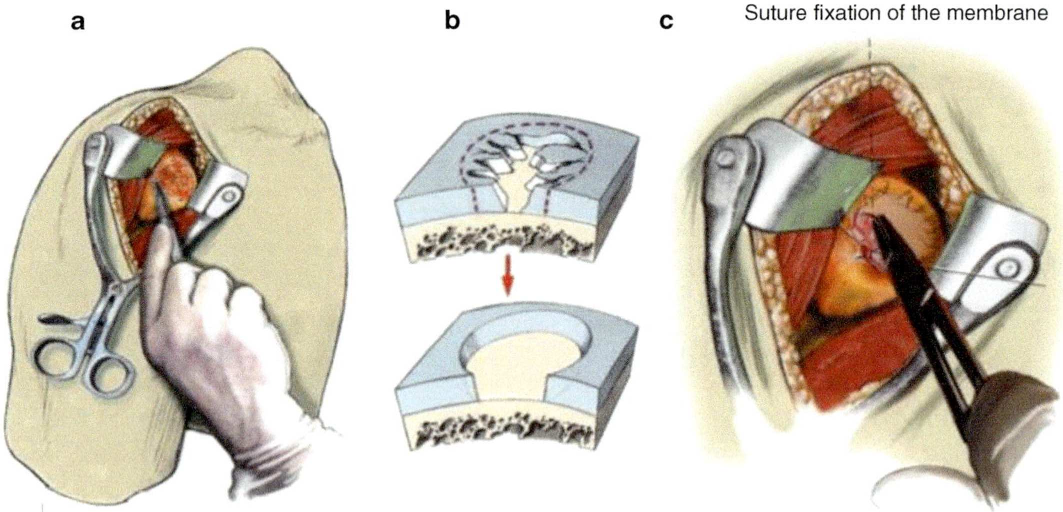


**Fig. 26.4** (**a**–**c**) Schematic representation of MACT at the humeral head: (**a**) open debridement of the whole damaged cartilage; (**b**) creating a stable rim in the surrounding healthy cartilage without damaging the subchondral layer; (**c**) suture fixation of the chondrocyte matrix in the surrounding cartilage

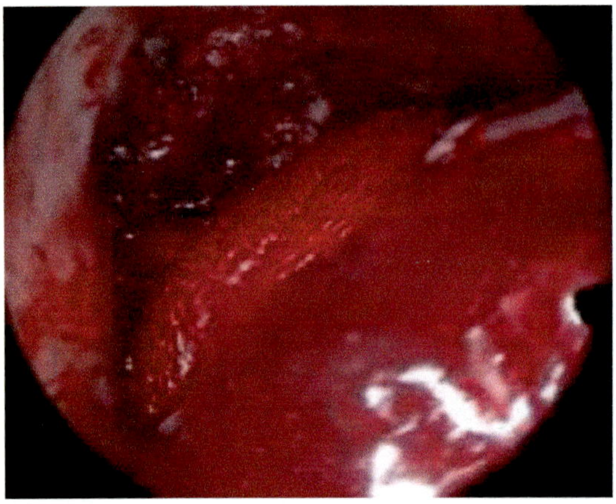

**Fig. 26.5** Arthroscopic view of cartilage defect at the humerus arthroscopically treated with autologous chondrocyte transplantation (Novocart inject)

address both the cartilage and the underlying bone. Autologous osteochondral transplantation is a common and established option for the treatment of these cases, and it is still the only procedure that provides a restoration of chondral defects with hyaline cartilage immediately. After measurement of the defect depth by MRI or CT and measurement of the defect size during arthroscopy, the whole osteochondral defect is punched or cut out. Subsequently an appropriate osteochondral cylinder is harvested from a not weight-bearing area in the knee joint and then brought to the defect site and inserted press fit. Especially for the defects of the humeral head, the dorsal femoral condyle seems to serve as a reasonable donor site because of its spherical shape of the cartilage surface. The operation can be performed via an open or arthroscopical-assisted mini-open approach depending on localization and size of the defect, whereas larger lesions that might even need two cylinders should be performed open.

As for other cartilage regenerative therapy options, there is so far only few evidence for OCT in the shoulder. Case series could show reasonable results with improvement of shoulder function and no relevant donor site morbidity at the knee joint [7, 12]; however, progression of osteoarthritis of the shoulder could not be prevented. In addition to that, the relative invasive procedure of OCT for restoration of chondral defects has to be seen critical in the shoulder, since in many cases it remains unclear, if the patient's symptoms are caused by the cartilage defect or by additional comorbidities (Fig. 26.6).

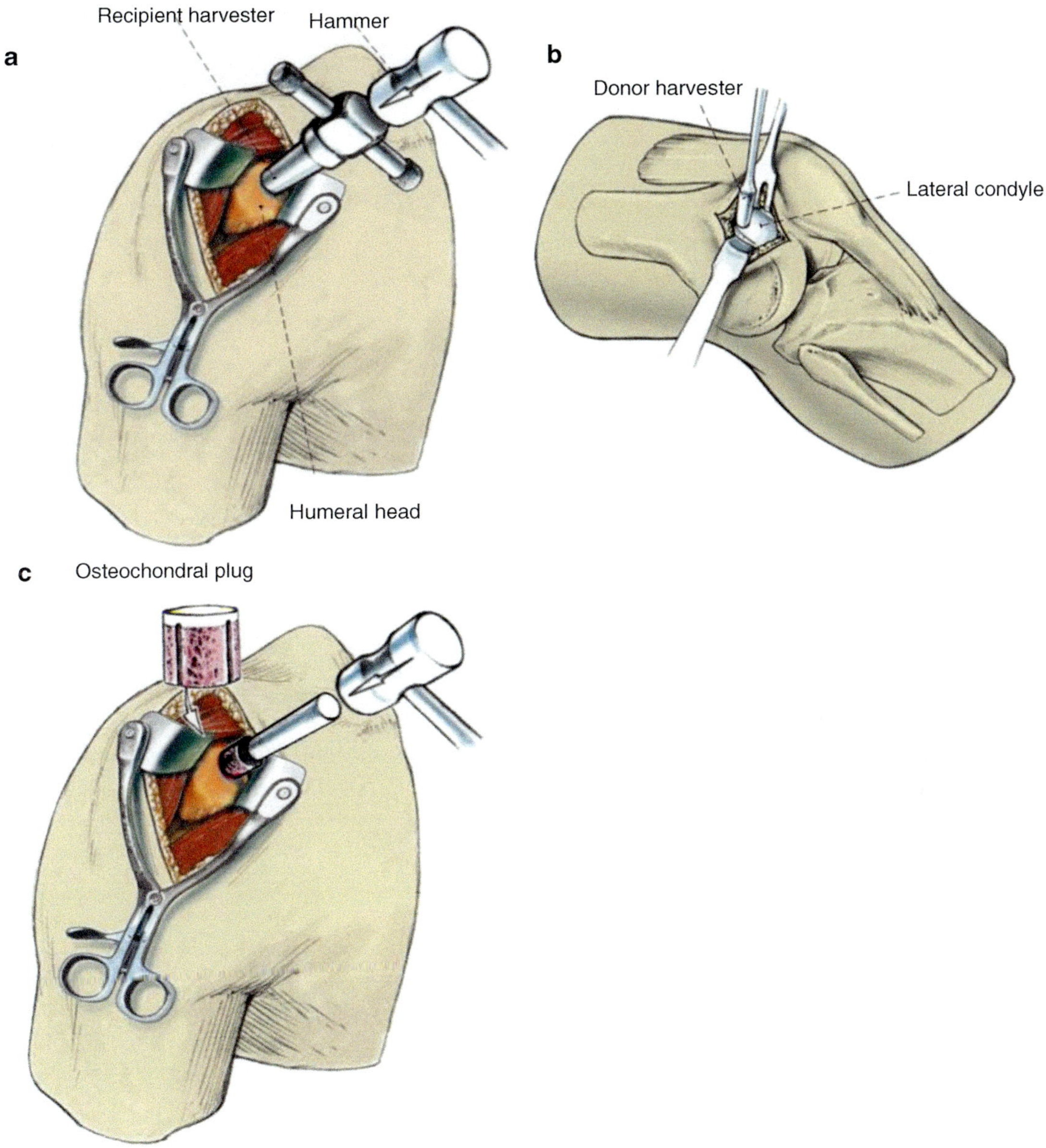


**Fig. 26.6** (**a–c**) Schematic representation of autologous osteochondral transplantation at the humeral head: (**a**) open removal of the osteochondral lesion using a hollow chisel (recipient harvester); (**b**) harvesting the donor cylinder from the proximal lateral trochlea; (**c**) insertion of the donor cylinder into the prepared socket in the humeral head

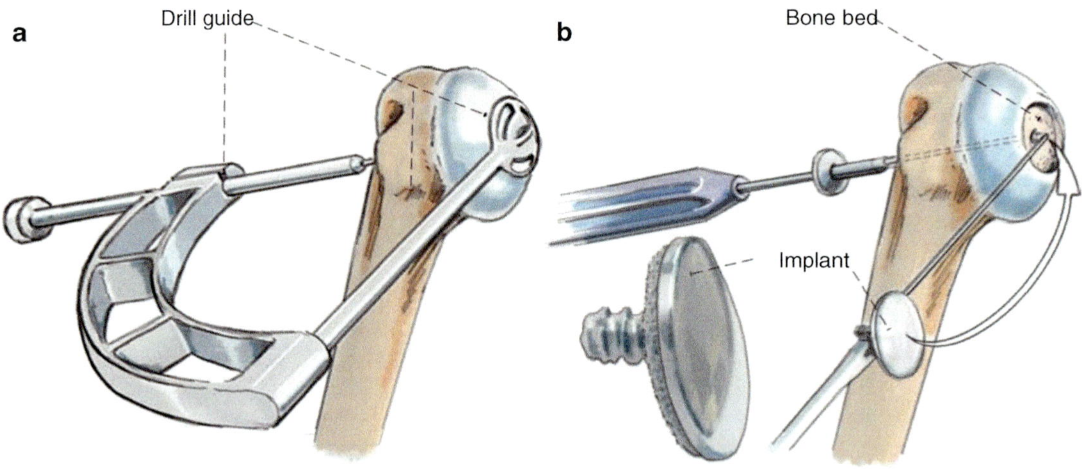


**Fig. 26.7** (**a**, **b**) Schematic representation of arthroscopically assisted partial joint resurfacing at the humeral head (Partial Eclipse™, Arthrex): (**a**) insertion of the drill guide and measuring the defect size to determine the diameter of the implant; (**b**) after reaming of the defect, insertion of the implant via the anterosuperior portal over the seating instrument, centrally placed in the defect

### 26.3.4 Partial Joint Resurfacing (PJR)

In cases of particularly large focal cartilage defects or large osteochondral defects that can occur due to osteonecrosis or after joint dislocation in terms of a large Hill-Sachs lesion, the abovementioned options for restoration of the chondral layer might reach their limits. In these cases replacement of the damaged area by metal implants that are exactly adjusted to the lesion in size and form is a reasonable treatment option, especially for young and active patients. These implants can also be supported by underlying autologous or allogeneic bone in cases with particularly large osteochondral defects.

Meanwhile, in the course of technical progress, this procedure can be performed arthroscopically, which allows the conservation of the subscapularis tendon and therefore a more progressive rehabilitation. According to a recent case series of 11 patients, the arthroscopical technique for partial joint resurfacing at the humeral head can lead to good postoperative short- to midterm results in young and active patients [1] (Figs. 26.7 and 26.8).

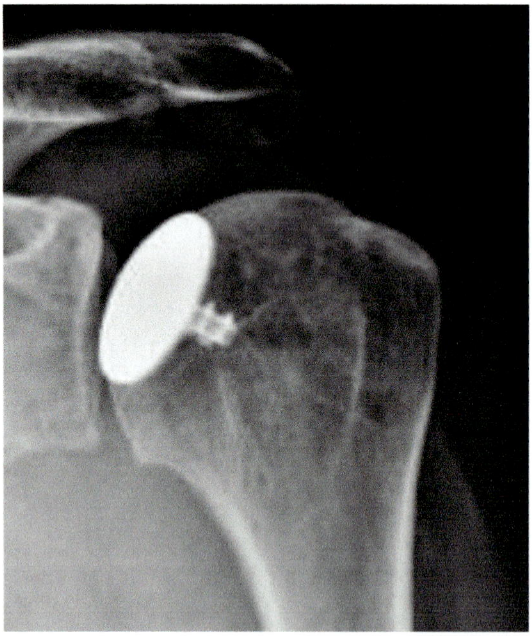

**Fig. 26.8** Postoperative anteroposterior radiograph of a left shoulder after partial joint resurfacing at the humeral head (Partial Eclipse™, Arthrex)

### 26.3.5 Shoulder Arthroplasty

In comparison to focal cartilage defects, the diagnosis of arthrosis does not only differ by more extensive damage to the chondral layer but it is also characterized by chronic inflammation with a tendency to catabolic metabolism. Therefore, it is apparent that cartilage regenerative therapies cannot be successful in these cases, but (partial) joint replacement is the only operative option to restore joint congruency. To date there is a variety of different models of shoulder prosthesis, whose further detailed description is not content of the present chapter.

## 26.4 Summary

Chondral lesions of the shoulder are often associated with glenohumeral instability and can not only cause pain and limited joint function but they represent also a relevant risk factor for the development of osteoarthritis. In comparison to other joints, detection of focal cartilage defects in the shoulder can be challenging, and as these lesions often appear as incidental findings with different comorbidities, the question arises whether they should be restored at all. Due to a lack of clinical trials, it remains also unclear, which cartilage regenerative surgical techniques are most suitable for the shoulder joint, which is why treatment recommendations are to a big part based on the experience from other joints like the knee. The choice of the appropriate treatment option depends on several factors like localization, size, and grade of the chondral defects, as well as on the quality of the subchondral bone. In cases of advanced osteoarthritis, however, the only remaining surgical option is total joint arthroplasty.

## References


1. Anderl W, Kriegleder B, Neumaier M, Laky B, Heuberer P. Arthroscopic partial shoulder resurfacing. Knee Surg Sports Traumatol Arthrosc. 2015;23(5):1563–70. doi:10.1007/s00167-00014-02981-x. Epub 02014 Apr 00122.
2. Buchmann S, Salzmann GM, Glanzmann MC, Wortler K, Vogt S, Imhoff AB. Early clinical and structural results after autologous chondrocyte transplantation at the glenohumeral joint. J Shoulder Elbow Surg. 2012;21(9):1213–21. doi:10.1016/j.jse.2011.1207.1030. Epub 2011 Nov 1212.
3. Cameron ML, Kocher MS, Briggs KK, Horan MP, Hawkins RJ. The prevalence of glenohumeral osteoarthrosis in unstable shoulders. Am J Sports Med. 2003;31(1):53–5.
4. Elser F, Braun S, Dewing CB, Millett PJ. Glenohumeral joint preservation: current options for managing articular cartilage lesions in young, active patients. Arthroscopy. 2010;26(5):685–96. doi:10.1016/j.arthro.2009.1010.1017. Epub 2010 Apr 1018.
5. Frank RM, Van Thiel GS, Slabaugh MA, Romeo AA, Cole BJ, Verma NN. Clinical outcomes after microfracture of the glenohumeral joint. Am J Sports Med. 2010;38(4):772–81.doi:10.1177/0363546509350304. Epub 0363546509352010 Jan 0363546509350321.
6. Hodler J, Loredo RA, Longo C, Trudell D, Yu JS, Resnick D. Assessment of articular cartilage thickness of the humeral head: MR-anatomic correlation in cadavers. AJR Am J Roentgenol. 1995;165(3):615–20.
7. Kircher J, Patzer T, Magosch P, Lichtenberg S, Habermeyer P. Osteochondral autologous transplantation for the treatment of full-thickness cartilage defects of the shoulder: results at nine years. J Bone Joint Surg Br. 2009;91(4):499–503. doi:10.1302/0301-1620X.1391B1304.21838.
8. Krych AJ, Sousa PL, King AH, Morgan JA, May JH, Dahm DL. The effect of cartilage injury after arthroscopic stabilization for shoulder instability. Orthopedics.2015;38(11):e965–9.doi:10.3928/01477447-20151020-01477403.
9. Minas T, Gomoll AH, Rosenberger R, Royce RO, Bryant T. Increased failure rate of autologous chondrocyte implantation after previous treatment with marrow stimulation techniques. Am J Sports Med. 2009;37(5):902–8. doi:10.1177/0363546508330137. Epub 0363546508332009 Mar 0363546508330134.
10. Ruckstuhl H, de Bruin ED, Stussi E, Vanwanseele B (2008) Post-traumatic glenohumeral cartilage lesions: a systematic review. BMC Musculoskelet Disord 9:107. doi:10.1186/1471-2474-1189-1107.
11. Saxena V, D'Aquilla K, Marcoon S, Krishnamoorthy G, Gordon JA, Carey JL, Borthakur A, Kneeland JB, Kelly JDt, Reddy R, Sennett BJ. T1rho magnetic resonance imaging to assess cartilage damage after primary shoulder dislocation. Am J Sports Med. 2016:0363546516655338.
12. Scheibel M, Bartl C, Magosch P, Lichtenberg S, Habermeyer P. Osteochondral autologous transplantation for the treatment of full-thickness articular cartilage defects of the shoulder. J Bone Joint Surg Br. 2004;86(7):991–7.
13. Steadman JR, Rodkey WG, Briggs KK. Microfracture to treat full-thickness chondral defects: surgical technique, rehabilitation, and outcomes. J Knee Surg. 2002;15(3):170–6.
14. Zumstein V, Kraljevic M, Conzen A, Hoechel S, Muller-Gerbl M. Thickness distribution of the glenohumeral joint cartilage: a quantitative study using computed tomography. Surg Radiol Anat. 2014;36(4):327–31. doi:10.1007/s00276-00013-01221-00272. Epub 02013 Oct 00231.

# Part IV

# Instability in the "Older" Patient (Age >50)

# 27 Spectrum of Instability in the Older Patient

A.B. Imhoff, K. Beitzel, and A. Voss

## Content

References ........................................................ 240

Due to demographical changes with a prolonged life experience in the aging active population, the prevalence of anterior traumatic shoulder dislocations has increased [9]. There is an increasing incidence of shoulder dislocations starting with 12.89 (50–59 years)–28.38 (>90 years) per 100.000 person years at risk affecting more women than men, and a recurrence rate in patients older than 60 has been reported to be 11–22% [5, 7, 18]. In this population the active and passive stabilizers are both affected once the shoulder was dislocated [4]. The pathophysiology of anterior shoulder dislocation between a young and active population and the older population is different and is related to changes due to the loss of elasticity in capsulo labral complex as well as degenerative changes to the rotator cuff tendon with distribution of the glenohumeral rhythm [10]. Basically, there are two described mechanisms: The anterior mechanism leads to lesion of the anterior labrum-ligament complex with a sudden eccentric load to the posterior aspect of the rotator cuff. This induces a refectory contracture and over-tensioning of the posterior cuff tendon, which can cause a partial or total rupture of a pre-existing injury of a degenerated infraspinatus and supraspinatus tendon [1, 10]. Additionally, there are also ruptures to the upper part of the subscapularis tendon, commonly seen with a humeral avulsion of the inferior glenohumeral ligament [17]. The posterior mechanism popularized by Craig [3] on the contrary can be explained by a

A.B. Imhoff (✉) • K. Beitzel • A. Voss
Department of Orthopaedic Sports Medicine,
Technical University of Munich, Munich, Germany
e-mail: Imhoff@tum.de

© ISAKOS 2017
A.B. Imhoff, F.H. Savoie III (eds.), *Shoulder Instability Across the Life Span*,
DOI 10.1007/978-3-662-54077-0_27

dislocation with the arm in maximum abduction, flexion, and external rotation. This leads to an impact of the infraspinatus and supraspinatus on superior glenoid rim and subsequently causes a rupture to a degenerative posterior-superior tendon structure. This mechanism can be seen with and without damages to the anterior capsulo-labral complex.

Whereas the young population dislocates because of failure to the anterior capsulo-labral complex (anterior mechanism), the older patient commonly dislocates because of loss of posterior active stabilizing structures, especially the posterior aspect of the rotator cuff (posterior mechanism) [10]. A cadaveric study investigating the influence of rotator cuff muscle activity and stability showed a 50% increase of dislocations in all positions of the glenohumeral joint examined with a 50% decrease of muscle activity [14]. Furthermore, a cuff-deficient model showed that a smaller lesion of the ligamentous-labral complex was needed to cause instability in comparison to an intact shoulder [13]. The frequency of rotator cuff tears after an anterior shoulder dislocation has been reported to be between 7 and 32% and is rising with aging [2, 6, 16]. Additionally, it has been shown that 50% of patients older than 60 years with a primary shoulder dislocation had a rotator cuff tendon tear and even over 70% if they had recurrent dislocations [7].

There is still no consensus about whether a symptomatic degenerative ruff tendon with a lesion to the tendon structure may lead to an abnormal active stabilization and can be seen as the cause of dislocation or if the dislocation itself induces a cuff injury [15, 17]. But a hint for a preexisting rotator cuff lesion can be seen in those patients with shoulder dislocation with a trivial trauma compared to forces needed to dislocate a shoulder in a young population [8, 11, 12]. Therefore, the purpose of the following chapters will focus on treatment of shoulder instability in the older patient, aimed to point out the specifics in regard to a lesion to the anterior capsulo-labral complex as well as a damage to the rotator cuff tendon.

## References


1. Araghi A, Prasarn M, St Clair S, Zuckerman JD. Recurrent anterior glenohumeral instability with onset after forty years of age: the role of the anterior mechanism. Bull Hosp Jt Dis. 2005;62(3–4):99–101.
2. Berbig R, Weishaupt D, Prim J, Shahin O. Primary anterior shoulder dislocation and rotator cuff tears. J Shoulder Elbow Surg. 1999;8(3):220–5.
3. Craig EV. The posterior mechanism of acute anterior shoulder dislocations. Clin Orthop Relat Res. 1984;190:212–6.
4. Gombera MM, Sekiya JK. Rotator cuff tear and glenohumeral instability : a systematic review. Clin Orthop Relat Res. 2014;472(8):2448–56. doi:10.1007/s11999-013-3290-2.
5. Gumina S, Postacchini F. Anterior dislocation of the shoulder in elderly patients. J Bone Joint Surg Br. 1997;79(4):540–3.
6. Imhoff AB, Ansah P, Tischer T, Reiter C, Bartl C, Hench M, Spang JT, Vogt S. Arthroscopic repair of anterior-inferior glenohumeral instability using a portal at the 5:30-o'clock position: analysis of the effects of age, fixation method, and concomitant shoulder injury on surgical outcomes. Am J Sports Med. 2010;38(9):1795–803. doi:10.1177/0363546510370199.
7. Levy O, Pritsch M, Rath E. An operative technique for recurrent shoulder dislocations in older patients. J Shoulder Elbow Surg. 1999;8(5):452–7.
8. Loehr JF, Helmig P, Sojbjerg JO, Jung A. Shoulder instability caused by rotator cuff lesions. An in vitro study. Clin Orthop Relat Res. 1994;304:84–90.
9. Maier M, Geiger EV, Ilius C, Frank J, Marzi I. Midterm results after operatively stabilised shoulder dislocations in elderly patients. Int Orthop. 2009;33(3):719–23. doi:10.1007/s00264-008-0578-z.
10. McLaughlin HL, MacLellan DI. Recurrent anterior dislocation of the shoulder. II. A comparative study. J Trauma. 1967;7(2):191–201.
11. Neer 2nd CS, Craig EV, Fukuda H. Cuff-tear arthropathy. J Bone Joint Surg Am. 1983;65(9):1232–44.
12. Porcellini G, Paladini P, Campi F, Paganelli M. Shoulder instability and related rotator cuff tears: arthroscopic findings and treatment in patients aged 40 to 60 years. Arthroscopy. 2006;22(3):270–6. doi:10.1016/j.arthro.2005.12.015.
13. Pouliart N, Gagey O. Concomitant rotator cuff and capsuloligamentous lesions of the shoulder: a cadaver study. Arthroscopy. 2006;22(7):728–35. doi:10.1016/j.arthro.2006.03.015.
14. Rodosky MW, Harner CD, Fu FH. The role of the long head of the biceps muscle and superior glenoid labrum in anterior stability of the shoulder. Am J Sports Med. 1994;22(1):121–30.

15. Shin SJ, Yun YH, Kim DJ, Yoo JD. Treatment of traumatic anterior shoulder dislocation in patients older than 60 years. Am J Sports Med. 2012;40(4):822–7. doi:10.1177/0363546511434522.
16. Simank HG, Dauer G, Schneider S, Loew M. Incidence of rotator cuff tears in shoulder dislocations and results of therapy in older patients. Arch Orthop Trauma Surg. 2006;126(4):235–40. doi:10.1007/s00402-005-0034-0.
17. Voigt C, Lill H. Shoulder instability and rotator cuff tear. Orthopade. 2009;38(1):70–4. doi:10.1007/s00132-008-1356-8.
18. Zacchilli MA, Owens BD. Epidemiology of shoulder dislocations presenting to emergency departments in the United States. J Bone Joint Surg Am. 2010;92(3):542–9. doi:10.2106/JBJS.I.00450.

# Acute RCT as a Part of Dislocation

# 28

Francesco Franceschi, Edoardo Franceschetti, and Enrique Alberto Salas

## Contents

28.1 **Introduction** ........................ 243

28.2 **Literature Overview Summary: What Is Known** ...................... 243

28.3 **Anatomy** ........................... 244

28.4 **Indication for This Surgery**............ 245

28.5 **Specific Points in Rehabilitation**........ 245

28.6 **Results**............................. 245

**Conclusion** .............................. 246

**References** .............................. 246

F. Franceschi (✉) • E. Franceschetti
Department of Orthopaedic and Trauma Surgery, Campus Bio-Medico University of Rome, Via Alvaro del Portillo, 200, 00128, Trigoria, Rome, Italy
e-mail: f.franceschi@unicampus.it

E.A. Salas
Av Leopoldo Aguerrevere Resd Villa del Este, Universidad Central of Venezuela, Caracas, Venezuela

## 28.1 Introduction

Traumatic anterior dislocation of the shoulder is a relatively common injury in the young, active population. Most of the interest regarding these injuries has focused on recurrence as the primary complication. Recurrence is not typically a problem in the older population; prolonged morbidity secondary to associated rotator cuff injury is more common. In older individuals, the dynamic stabilizers are more likely to fail (rotator cuff), whereas in young individuals, it is more often the static restraints that fail (labrum). Additionally, with increasing age, the incidence of pre-existing, degenerative tears of the rotator cuff is increasing.

When evaluating a patient who cannot abduct the arm after reduction of an anterior dislocation, the physician tends to assume that this inability is caused by an axillary nerve palsy. This assumption frequently results in an unnecessary delay in establishing the correct diagnosis of a ruptured rotator cuff, and the delay can result in a challenging reconstruction.

## 28.2 Literature Overview Summary: What Is Known

The association of a rotator cuff tear and dislocation in the older population is well documented. Ribbans et al. [1] reported a 63% rotator cuff tear

© ISAKOS 2017
A.B. Imhoff, F.H. Savoie III (eds.), *Shoulder Instability Across the Life Span*,
DOI 10.1007/978-3-662-54077-0_28

rate in primary traumatic dislocation in a small number of patients older than 50 years. Hawkins and Mohtadi [2] reported a 90% rotator cuff tear rate in a similar patient population. Toolanen et al. [3] reported a 38% tear rate, and 47% of the patients still complained of shoulder dysfunction at 3 years postinjury. However, 65% of their patients had electromyogram-confirmed axillary nerve or brachial plexus injury, which may have contributed to their poor results. Neviaser et al. [4] reported a 100% rate of rotator cuff tears in patients older than 40 years with a primary traumatic anterior dislocation. However, this was a preselected group of patients, making the true incidence impossible to determine. In their study, most rotator cuff tears were initially misdiagnosed as axillary nerve injuries. They also reported a 30% recurrence rate and emphasized the importance of the rotator cuff to glenohumeral stability. This is consistent with Itoi et al. [5] who used a cadaver model to describe the importance of the rotator cuff muscles and the long head of the biceps, as dynamic stabilizers of the shoulder. Pevny et al. [6] studied 52 patients older than 40 years with a shoulder dislocation. Between these group of patients, 42 showed excellent or good outcomes, and 11 showed fair and poor outcomes. 18 patients out of a total of 52 showed a rotator cuff tear (35%), and only 11 (61%) of these patients obtained an excellent or good outcome. Of the 11 patients with a fair or poor result, seven (64%) had a rotator cuff tear. Of the patients with isolated cuff tears, 84% had an excellent or good result when treated surgically, compared with 50% when treated nonsurgically. These findings indicate that recurrence is not a frequent complication of traumatic anterior shoulder dislocation in this age group (4%). However, prolonged morbidity secondary to rotator cuff tear is more prevalent than in a younger population.

The most important concerns regarding this topic are related to the treatment. The dispute is about the type of treatment, conservative or surgical, open or arthroscopic. And finally on what to repair labral tear, cuff tear or both.

Pevny et al. [6] showed that patients treated surgically had 84% excellent/good results, compared with 50% excellent/good results when treated nonoperatively. In this series, most of the patients had open cuff repairs. Bassett and Coffield [7] also reported better results after surgical cuff repair in terms of functional outcome and pain relief following acute dislocations. In all studies available, the cuff repair was combined with an acromioplasty. Voos et al. [8] showed good clinical outcomes, restoration of motion, and high degree of patient satisfaction in patients treated arthroscopically with rotator cuff and Bankart lesion.

Operation is suggested by many authors, but there is discussion as to which structure should be repaired, only Bankart repair, only rotator cuff repair, or both. The Itoi's results indicate that repair of a Bankart lesion is probably not necessary in older patients [5]. In the elderly, cuff tears are commonly associated with anterior dislocation, and repair of the cuff alone may be sufficient to achieve stability. Voos et al. [8] showed good clinical outcomes, restoration of motion, and high degree of patient satisfaction doing arthroscopic treatment of both labrum lesion and rotator cuff.

Porcellini et al. [9] in a case series stated that patient age and the number of dislocations do not appear to correlate with Bankart or capsular lesions, whereas posterosuperior cuff tears seem to be influenced by the number of dislocations. Although data from this study do not permit to conclude whether repair of the sole cuff tear can achieve shoulder stability nor whether shoulder stabilization alone can resolve the instability, treatment of both lesions should be performed arthroscopically, because the arthroscopic technique allows to treat capsular-labral and cuff lesions in the same procedure.

## 28.3 Anatomy

McLaughlin and MacLellan [10] suggested that anterior dislocation of the shoulder occurs either by disruption of the glenohumeral ligament (anterior mechanism) or by rupture of the rotator cuff (posterior mechanism). They believed that failure of the posterior support was more likely in patients who are older than 40 years, because the tendinous structure usually degenerates and weakens with age. Rupture of the musculotendinous cuff, particularly of the supraspinatus, infraspinatus, and teres minor, can permit anterior dislocation of the humeral head on an intact anterior soft tissue hinge and thus may be termed the posterior mechanism of anterior dislocation [11].

Hsu et al. [12] demonstrated in a cadaveric study that the displacement of the humeral head increases with an increase in tear size with or without translational forces applied and that a rotator interval tear is more crucial than a critical area tear from the viewpoint of instability.

## 28.4 Indication for This Surgery

Treatment regarding primary traumatic dislocation in the older patient is not well defined. Hawkins and Mohtadi [2] recommended physical therapy at 1 week followed by an arthrogram at 4 weeks if there was no clinical improvement. More recently, Sonnabend [13] recommended immobilization for 3 weeks followed by an arthrogram or ultrasound if pain and weakness were still present. In this kind of patients, 3 weeks of immobilization could be too long. This can lead to stiffness. Based on results present in the literature, the diagnosis of a rotator cuff tear should be approached aggressively at 7–10 days (after reduction) by an MRI or arthrogram if significant pain and weakness are still present. If the MRI is consistent with a rotator cuff tear, we recommend shoulder arthroscopy and arthroscopic or open repair. If the MRI is negative or the patient shows improved pain and weakness at 7–10 days, we recommend proceeding with a rehabilitation program aimed at strengthening the rotator cuff and scapular stabilizers. If after 3 weeks of rehabilitation the patient does not show significant improvement, an MRI should be ordered to evaluate the rotator cuff. Special attention should be directed to the subset with greater tuberosity fracture or axillary nerve involvement. If a rotator cuff tear is documented, prompt surgical repair should be pursued to optimize the long-term functional outcome in these patients.

## 28.5 Specific Points in Rehabilitation

In case of nonoperative management, a supervised rehabilitation program should be performed. The program consists of several steps: (1) pain was released by detonisation exercises combined with oral medication and (2) the flexibility and range of motion were restored by stretching exercises. The three steps involved restoration of strength of the internal and external rotators against resistance using a rubber tube or weights and improvement of the deltoid strength. After approximately 6 weeks, the fourth step consists of aerobic exercises and modification of work and sport activities.

In the case of surgical treatment of both rotator cuff tear and labrum damage, a physical therapy protocol was directed toward protecting the rotator cuff repair.

Rehabilitation protocols are not changed on the basis of the type of labrum repair performed. All patients had their arm placed in a sling and permitted passive range of motion in the scapular plane (maximum 90 ° forward flexion) and pendulum motion during the first 6 postoperative weeks. During weeks 6–12, passive range of motion is increased and active range of motion initiated. At 6 weeks, rotator cuff strengthening with a low-resistance TheraBand (the Hygenic Corporation, Akron, Ohio) was allowed. At 10–12 weeks, light weights are added. From week 12–6 months postoperatively, rotator cuff strengthening and scapular stabilizing exercises were progressed with unlimited return to activity at 6 months postoperatively.

## 28.6 Results

Only a few studies dealing with this subject are available in the literature. Pevny et al. [6] reported 84% of good results after early repair, as against only 50% after conservative treatment, and concluded that early surgical repair and treatment yielded better results than did conservative treatment of cuff tears. Bassett and Coffield [7] also reported better results after surgical cuff repair in terms of functional outcome and pain relief following acute dislocations.

**Conclusion**

Rotator cuff tear associated with anterior shoulder dislocation is well documented, although often the cuff injury is initially misdiagnosed. Brachial plexus injury has also been reported in association with rotator cuff tear in the setting of shoulder dislocation. This group of injuries could be considered the "terrible triad" of the shoulder.

The debate about the treatment of these patients is still open. The surgical treatment showed superior results to that conservative. It is not yet clear whether in these patients (elderly) it is better to treat either the injury or only the rotator cuff tear.

## References

1. Ribbans WJ, Mitchell R, Taylor GJ. Computerised arthrotomography of primary anterior dislocation of the shoulder. J Bone Joint Surg Br. 1990;72(2):181–5.
2. Hawkins RJ, Mohtadi NG. Controversy in anterior shoulder instability. Clin Orthop Relat Res. 1991;272:152–61.
3. Toolanen G et al. Early complications after anterior dislocation of the shoulder in patients over 40 years. An ultrasonographic and electromyographic study. Acta Orthop Scand. 1993;64(5):549–52.
4. Neviaser RJ, Neviaser TJ, Neviaser JS. Anterior dislocation of the shoulder and rotator cuff rupture. Clin Orthop Relat Res. 1993;291:103–6.
5. Itoi E et al. Dynamic anterior stabilisers of the shoulder with the arm in abduction. J Bone Joint Surg Br. 1994;76(5):834–6.
6. Pevny T, Hunter RE, Freeman JR. Primary traumatic anterior shoulder dislocation in patients 40 years of age and older. Arthroscopy. 1998;14(3):289–94.
7. Bassett RW, Cofield RH. Acute tears of the rotator cuff. The timing of surgical repair. Clin Orthop Relat Res. 1983;175:18–24.
8. Voos JE et al. Outcomes of combined arthroscopic rotator cuff and labral repair. Am J Sports Med. 2007;35(7):1174–9.
9. Porcellini G et al. Shoulder instability and related rotator cuff tears: arthroscopic findings and treatment in patients aged 40 to 60 years. Arthroscopy. 2006;22(3):270–6.
10. McLaughlin HL, MacLellan DI. Recurrent anterior dislocation of the shoulder. II. A comparative study. J Trauma. 1967;7(2):191–201.
11. Craig EV. The posterior mechanism of acute anterior shoulder dislocations. Clin Orthop Relat Res. 1984;190:212–6.
12. Hsu HC et al. Influence of rotator cuff tearing on glenohumeral stability. J Shoulder Elbow Surg. 1997;6(5):413–22.
13. Sonnabend DH. Treatment of primary anterior shoulder dislocation in patients older than 40 years of age. Conservative versus operative. Clin Orthop Relat Res. 1994;304:74–7.

# Acute Dislocation Superimposed on Chronic RCT

# 29

Mike H. Baums

## Contents


| | | |
|---|---|---|
| 29.1 | **Introduction** | 247 |
| 29.2 | **Biomechanics** | 248 |
| 29.3 | **Mechanisms of RCT** | 248 |
| 29.4 | **Injury Pattern in the "Older" Patient** | 248 |
| 29.5 | **The Pre-existing Rotator Cuff Tear** | 248 |
| 29.6 | **Concomitant Nerve Injuries** | 249 |
| 29.7 | **Therapy** | 249 |
| **References** | | 249 |


## 29.1 Introduction

Rotator cuff tears (RCT) are a frequent concomitant injury of glenohumeral dislocations. Whereas especially in young patients a persistent instability is the most common challenge [12], the problem in the elderly is the associated cuff pathology leading to functional impairments [3, 8]. The incidence of an associated cuff tear increases with patients' age and number of dislocations [14]: in patients between 51 and 60 years of age, the rate after a primary dislocation was less than 10%, whereas 40% of recurrent dislocations resulted in related RCT [8].

Moreover, there are age-linked differences regarding the extent of a tear [11]. an isolated supraspinatus tendon tear mostly occurs during the early fifties. During the mid-fifties, mostly a combination of supra- and infraspinatus tears can be expected, whereas patients with a mean age of 58 years suffer from complex and massive tears of the supra-, infra-, as well as subscapularis tendon.

## 29.2 Biomechanics

Shoulder muscles are an important stabilizer of the glenohumeral joint by a concavity-compression mechanism enabling a concentric rotation [6]. Especially during the mid-ranges of motion, they act as primary stabilizer of the

M.H. Baums
Department of Orthopaedics, Trauma Surgery and Sports Traumatology, St. Elizabeth Hospital Dorsten, Dorsten, Germany
e-mail: m.baums@kkrn.de

© ISAKOS 2017
A.B. Imhoff, F.H. Savoie III (eds.), *Shoulder Instability Across the Life Span*,
DOI 10.1007/978-3-662-54077-0_29

shoulder joint [5] and can decrease strains on the capsular-ligamentous complex at the end ranges of motion [5]. Different studies showed that rotator cuff activity increases the compressive forces at the glenohumeral joint and decreases the amount of humeral head translation [7, 18]. They postulate that a decrease in rotator cuff muscle forces results in an increase of anterior humeral head displacement. Equally, Pouliart et al. revealed in a cadaveric model that the humeral head might dislocate easily when rotator cuff tears are present [11].

## 29.3 Mechanisms of RCT

The anterior dislocation mechanism results in a lesion of the anterior capsular-ligamentous complex as well as an abrupt eccentric load on the posterior rotator cuff. This often results in partial articular-sided or complete lesions of the supra- and infraspinatus tendon [1, 8, 9] and is postulated to be the "anterior mechanism." Moreover, lesions of the upper two-thirds of the subscapularis tendon may be associated with shoulder dislocations. These humeral-sided lesions mostly occur in combination with an injury of the capsule and a humeral avulsion of the inferior glenohumeral ligament (HAGL lesion).

In contrast, forced abduction, flexion, and external rotation frequently consequence a posterosuperior RCT, mainly in patients suffering from pre-existing weakening or partial lesions of the rotator cuff. This phenomenon is postulated to be the "posterior mechanism" [2].

## 29.4 Injury Pattern in the "Older" Patient

Loew et al. evaluated a decreased frequency of capsulo-labral lesions in patients with increased age [8]. In their prospective overview, only 10% of patients older than 40 had combined lesions (RCT lesion of the capsular-ligamentous complex), but 89% of them were combined lesions after more than one dislocation. Therefore, it seems to be more likely for older patients to suffer from RCT after the first shoulder dislocation than from a combined lesion of the capsular-ligamentous complex. This is contrary to repetitive shoulder dislocations in this patient group where combined lesions are common.

## 29.5 The Pre-existing Rotator Cuff Tear

In almost all cases, it is difficult to determine whether the detected RCT in older patients is a "true" pre-existing asymptomatic tear or a tear that is related to the shoulder dislocation but attributed to previous age-related weakening of the soft tissue resulting in a reduced failure load of the tendon. It is well known, based on ultrasound and MRI evaluation, that in patients in their sixth decade of life, the incidence of an asymptomatic RCT is calculated to be 28–55%, respectively [10, 16].

In contrast, a RCT after a first-time shoulder dislocation increases the risk of a repetitive dislocation by a factor of 30 [15]. Particularly in patients older than 40, the risk to develop a repetitive shoulder dislocation is not determined by the age but by the existence of a RCT [19]. But specifically in the group of older patients, RCT may be a consequence as well as a cause of shoulder dislocation. Nonetheless in most cases, it is difficult to determine this pathology retrospectively.

## 29.6 Concomitant Nerve Injuries

The postulated frequency of concomitant lesions of the N. axillaris is about 7–18% [4]. Nerve recovery can take up to 24 months. Especially in the group of patients in their sixth decade, complete recovery is reported to take 3–12 months, but irreversible lesions are rare [4]. Particularly in patients suffering from a significant global loss of strength after a shoulder dislocation associated with a RCT, one should be aware of an associated lesion of the N. axillaris. In these cases, an electromyographic investigation is recommended [17] what can be useful to serve as a reference examination, helping to identify the nerve injury as well as pointing out a prognosis. In cases with supero-posterior RCT, a lesion of the N. suprascapularis may be detected which can be caused either by traction or compression load [17].

## 29.7 Therapy

No standard therapeutic regimen can be advocated regarding the literature. Conservative treatment is recommended for patients older than 40 after a first dislocation with a well-balanced, asymptomatic partial RCT without recurrent instability [4, 13].

The purpose of the surgical repair is to restore the shoulder function by the repair of RCT and to reestablish the shoulder stability. Principally, RCT should be supposed and detected quickly in "older" patients, because a delay in diagnosis may result in tendon retraction that impairs the outcome. Even in cases with neurological injury, a quick repair is suggested to avoid a massive atrophy and retraction during nerve recovery [17]. In patients with high functional demands under 60 years of age, both capsular-ligamentous complex reconstruction and a repair of RCT should be done [4]. Merely in cases with an associated bursal-sided RCT involving less than 50% of the tendon, an isolated (arthroscopic) Bankart repair should be performed [13].

Habermeyer et al. endorse in cases suffering from a non-repairable posterosuperior RCT with clinical flexion/external rotation deficit to do a transfer of the latissimus dorsi [4]. In cases suffering from a huge functional deficit and non-repairable RCT with an existent arthritis, an inverse prosthesis may be a therapeutic option.

## References


1. Araghi A, Prasarn M, St. Clair S, Zuckerman JD. Recurrent anterior glenohumeral instability with onset after forty years of age. Bull Hosp Joint Dis. 2005;62:99–101.
2. Craig EV. The posterior mechanism of acute anterior shoulder dislocations. Clin Orthop Relat Res. 1984;190:212–6.
3. Gumina S, Postacchini F. Anterior dislocation of the shoulder in elderly patients. J Bone Joint Surg Br. 1997;79:540–3.
4. Habermeyer P, Lichtenberg S, Magosch P. Rotator cuff tear and shoulder instability. Arthroskopie. 2007;20:217–22. [German].
5. Howell SM, Kraft TA. The role of the supraspinatus and infraspinatus muscles in glenohumeral kinematics of anterior shoulder instability. Clin Orthop Relat Res. 1991;263:128–34.
6. Karduna AR, Williams GR, Williams JL, Iannotti JP. Kinematics of the glenohumeral joint: influences of muscle forces, ligamentous constraints, and articular geometry. J Orthop Res. 1996;14(6):986–93.
7. Labriola JE, Lee TQ, Debski RE, McMahon PJ. Stability and instability of the glenohumeral joint: the role of shoulder muscles. J Shoulder Elbow Surg. 2005;14(Suppl 1):32S–8S.
8. Loew M, Thomson M, Rickert M, Simank HG. Injury pattern in shoulder dislocation in the elderly patient. Unfallchirurg. 2001;104:115–8. [German].
9. McLaughin H, MacLellan DI. Recurrent anterior dislocation of the shoulder. A comparative study. J Trauma. 1967;7:191–201.
10. Milgrom C, Schaffler M, Gilbert S, van Holsbeeck M. Rotator-cuff changes in asymptomatic adults: the effect of age, hand dominance and gender. J Bone Joint Surg Br. 1995;77:296–8.
11. Pouliart N, Gagey O. Concomitant rotator cuff and capsuloligamentous lesions of the shoulder. A cadaver study. Arthroscopy. 2006;22:728–35.
12. Porcellini G, Campi F, Pegreffi F, Castagna A, Paladini P. Predisposing factors for recurrent shoulder dislocation after arthroscopic treatment. J Bone Joint Surg Am. 2009;91:2537–42.
13. Porcellini G, Caranzano F, Campi F, Paladini P. Instability and rotator cuff tear. In: Mafulli N, editor. Rotator cuff tear. Basel: Karger; 2012.
14. Porcellini G, Paladini P, Campi F, Paganelli M. Shoulder instability and related rotator cuff tears: arthroscopic findings and treatment in patients aged 40 to 60 years. Arthroscopy. 2006;22:270–6.
15. Robinson CM, Kelly M, Wakefield AE. Redislocation of the shoulder during the first six weeks after a primary anterior dislocation: risk factors and results of treatment. J Bone Joint Surg Am. 2002;84:1552–9.

16. Sher JS, Uribe JW, Posada A, Murphy BJ, Zlatkin MB. Abnormal findings on magnetic resonance images of asymptomatic shoulders. J Bone Joint Surg Am. 1995;77:10–5.
17. Simonich SD, Wright TW. Terrible triad of the shoulder. J Shoulder Elbow Surg. 2003;12:556–68.
18. Wuelker N, Korell M, Thren K. Dynamic glenohumeral joint stability. J Shoulder Elbow Surg. 1998;7:43–52.
19. Walch G, Boileau P. Rotator cuff tears associated with anterior instability. In: Warner JJP, Iannotti JP, Gerber C, editors. Complex and revision problems in shoulder surgery. Philadelphia: Lippincott-Raven; 1997.

# Dislocation Arthropathy of the Shoulder

**30**

María Valencia and Emilio Calvo

## Contents


30.1 **Dislocation Arthropathy of the Shoulder** ... 251
30.1.1 Incidence and Related Factors ... 252
30.1.2 Classification ... 252
30.1.3 Clinical Presentation ... 253
30.1.4 Treatment Options and Results ... 255

**Conclusion** ... 257

**References** ... 257


M. Valencia, MD, PhD • E. Calvo, MD, PhD (✉)
Shoulder and Elbow Reconstructive Surgery Unit, Department of Orthopedic Surgery and Traumatology, Fundación Jiménez Díaz, Universidad Autónoma, Madrid, Spain
e-mail: ECalvo@fjd.es

## 30.1 Dislocation Arthropathy of the Shoulder

Samilson and Prieto developed the concept of the spectrum of degenerative changes that appeared after a single episode of shoulder dislocation in 1983 and named it "dislocation arthropathy" [1]. Open surgery first, and arthroscopic techniques nowadays, have become the gold standard for the treatment of shoulder instability. In this context, it is difficult to attribute degenerative changes only to the recurrent dislocations but also to the potential iatrogenic damage to the cartilage occurring during surgery. However, it is well known that degenerative changes might be seen even after just one isolated dislocation episode [1]. It is usually discovered at the age of 30 and approximately 4 years after the first dislocation episode [2]. The grade is mild in most cases. Clinical presentation and treatment options are varied, depending on age, level of activity, and degree of arthritis present. An arthroscopic approach can provide good results in terms of pain relief and increased range of motion, overall in the group of patients with less severe chondral damage and a restricted external rotation. Shoulder arthroplasty would be the end-stage preferred treatment for those patients with a highly degenerated joint that do not respond to conservative treatment [3].

© ISAKOS 2017
A.B. Imhoff, F.H. Savoie III (eds.), *Shoulder Instability Across the Life Span*,
DOI 10.1007/978-3-662-54077-0_30

### 30.1.1 Incidence and Related Factors

It is difficult to clarify the real incidence of degenerative changes due to shoulder instability. Hovelius et al. included in their series from single dislocations to recurrent shoulder dislocations that required surgical treatment. They found an overall rate of 26% of moderate/severe changes in 26% of the patients, and the mean increase seemed to be 1 unit of percentage/year. For mild changes the incidence of arthropathy raised to 56% [4]. However, when looking at arthroscopic findings, the incidence increases compared to the late arthritic radiographic signs. Calvo et al. in their series of patients undergoing an arthroscopic procedure to treat a shoulder instability problem found that 98.5% of them presented with synovial or chondral lesions. At least half of them (54.75%) showed moderate signs, and 40.6% of them showed mild changes. Only 4.7% presented with severe degeneration [5].

The incidence and degree of arthropathy have been correlated to numerous factors. Posterior dislocation is related to a higher degree of osteoarthritis rather than anterior dislocation [1]. Authors attribute this fact to a more traumatic event causing posterior dislocations. Interestingly, Calvo et al. found a higher incidence of degenerative changes in patients that had sustained an anterior dislocation rather than in those suffering multidirectional instabilities [5]. This finding could be associated to hyperlaxity that seems to have a protective effect and is usually present in this population group. However, Cameron et al. did not find any relation in between direction of dislocation and osteoarthritis [6]. Some authors have also reported the presence of bony defects as a cause of osteoarthritis as well as rotator cuff tears [2].

It appears that age at the first time of dislocation (over 25 years old) can determine the presence of a more severe type of degeneration as well as a traumatic onset [1, 2, 4, 7]. On the other hand, some authors have shown that dislocations suffered at a younger age are responsible for a more severe degenerative disease. Time from injury to evaluation or treatment is clearly a risk factor for osteoarthritis [2, 6], but whether or not the number of previous dislocations is important is still controversial. While some studies have found a significant association of cartilage lesions with the number of preoperative dislocations [2, 5, 7, 8], others failed to demonstrate this association [1, 4]. Alcohol and smoking habits are also correlated to a moderate/severe type of arthritis, whereas sex has no influence on it [4].

Controversy exists on whether previous surgery has an influence on the degree of cartilage degeneration. For example, Hovelius et al. did not find any difference in the rate of moderate/severe changes in between the group of patients that underwent surgery and those that did not [4]. Interestingly, they found that the degree of arthritis was lower in the group of shoulders that became stable after surgery than those that became stable spontaneously. On the other hand, Buscayret et al. found a prevalence of osteoarthritis of 9.5% preoperatively and a prevalence of 19.7% postoperatively, at 6.5 years follow-up, in the group that did not have joint degeneration before the surgery. In general, the incidence of arthritis after operative treatment for anterior shoulder dislocation has ranged from 12 to 62% [7]. Numerous surgical factors have been pointed out as possible arthrogenic causes, including intra-articular hardware, the number of anchors used, laterally overhanging bone block, or excessive anterior tightening [7, 9]. No differences have been found still in between open and arthroscopic techniques and soft tissue/bony procedures [4, 10]. What seems clear is that progression rate of osteoarthritis is higher in those patients with a severe disease rather than those in which only mild changes are present [2].

### 30.1.2 Classification

Traditionally, classifications were based on degenerative changes present in conventional x-ray studies. Samilson and Prieto described in 1983 the most widespread classification for dislocation arthropathy [1]. It is based on the osteophyte size (either in the humeral or the glenoid side) measured in the anteroposterior shoulder x-ray view. There are three degrees: mild

(<3 mm), moderate (3–7 mm), or severe (>7 mm) depending on the size of osteophytes. There are several downsides to this system. Firstly, there is a poor inter- and intra-reliability [11]. Secondly, the size of the osteophyte is only one of the elements of the osteoarthritis disease and depends on each patient's osteoblastic response [11]. Moreover, the dimensions observed can vary depending on the rotation of the arm and the position of the x-ray beam during imaging process [4, 12]. Rosenberg et al. described a new classification based not only on osteophytes but on all radiological signs of osteoarthritis including joint space narrowing, sclerosis, and cysts [13]. In 2006, Ogawa et al. [14] introduced a new classification system based on Samilson and Prieto's classification but improved with CT imaging. Osteoarthritis is described as grade I (early osteoarthritis) when the spur formation was less than 3 mm or the humeral head has a margin making an acute angle associated to the addition of sclerotic bone (even in the absence of osteophyte). Grade II (moderate) is indicated by a spur measuring between 3 and 7 mm, and grade III (severe) is indicated when the spur exceedes 7 mm. Grade IV (definitive) is assigned if narrowing of the glenohumeral joint along with sclerosis is present. To record the extent of osteoarthritic changes accurately, the authors recommend that more than two successive slices show the same finding. The extent of the osteophyte should also be recorded as a percentage of the diameter of the humeral head.

However, when bony and articular changes can be detected in a CT scan imaging or even in simple x-ray images, a late-stage osteoarthritis disease is present. That is why some authors have demonstrated that early cartilage changes might be foreseen by means of new MRIs or direct visualization during arthroscopy.

With the advances of arthroscopy, different classifications of chondral damage have been proposed. In this context, Outerbridge classification has been widely used by authors when collecting data based on arthroscopic findings of all joints, including the shoulder [6]. Grade I is defined as softening of the articular cartilage. Grade II consists of fissuring and blistering of the articular cartilage. Grade III is deep ulceration of articular cartilage without exposed bone. Grade IV is full-thickness cartilage loss with exposed subchondral bone [15]. Cameron et al. considered osteoarthritis when changes type III and IV were present. Calvo et al. have also described a new classification system that permits a macroscopic categorization of early chondral damage by arthroscopy and includes also synovial membrane abnormalities [16]. Following this system, the synovial membrane is graded as 0 (normal) or 1 (fibrous and proliferative appearance). For the humeral head and glenoid cartilage, the severity of macroscopic changes is categorized as 0 (normal), 1 (discoloration, mild surface irregularities, or pitting), 2 (partial thickness erosion or fibrillation), and 3 (full-thickness erosion or osteophytes) (Fig. 30.1). To characterize topographically chondral damage, both the humeral head and glenoid articular surfaces are divided in four regions of interest corresponding to quadrants. A partial score is allocated to each quadrant, and the scores are totaled for each patient, obtaining a value ranging from 0 to 24 points summing the four quadrants corresponding both to the humeral head and the glenoid. A score of 1–8 is deemed mild osteoarthritis, 9–16 as moderate, and 17–24 points as severe osteoarthritis.

### 30.1.3 Clinical Presentation

The presence of radiographic glenohumeral osteoarthritis does not necessarily translate into clinically significant osteoarthritis [17]. Hovelius et al. in their series of 255 patients followed during 25 years reported that no patient had surgery because of arthropathy or any other disorder (except for revision due to recurrent instability); [4]. Of them, only seven patients presented arthropathy that was somehow disabling, mainly because of pain. Most patients often reduce their sporting activity or change their working routine in order to minimize the effect of the symptoms.

In general, symptoms might not differ from those of patients suffering primary osteoarthritis of other origin. They typically complain of

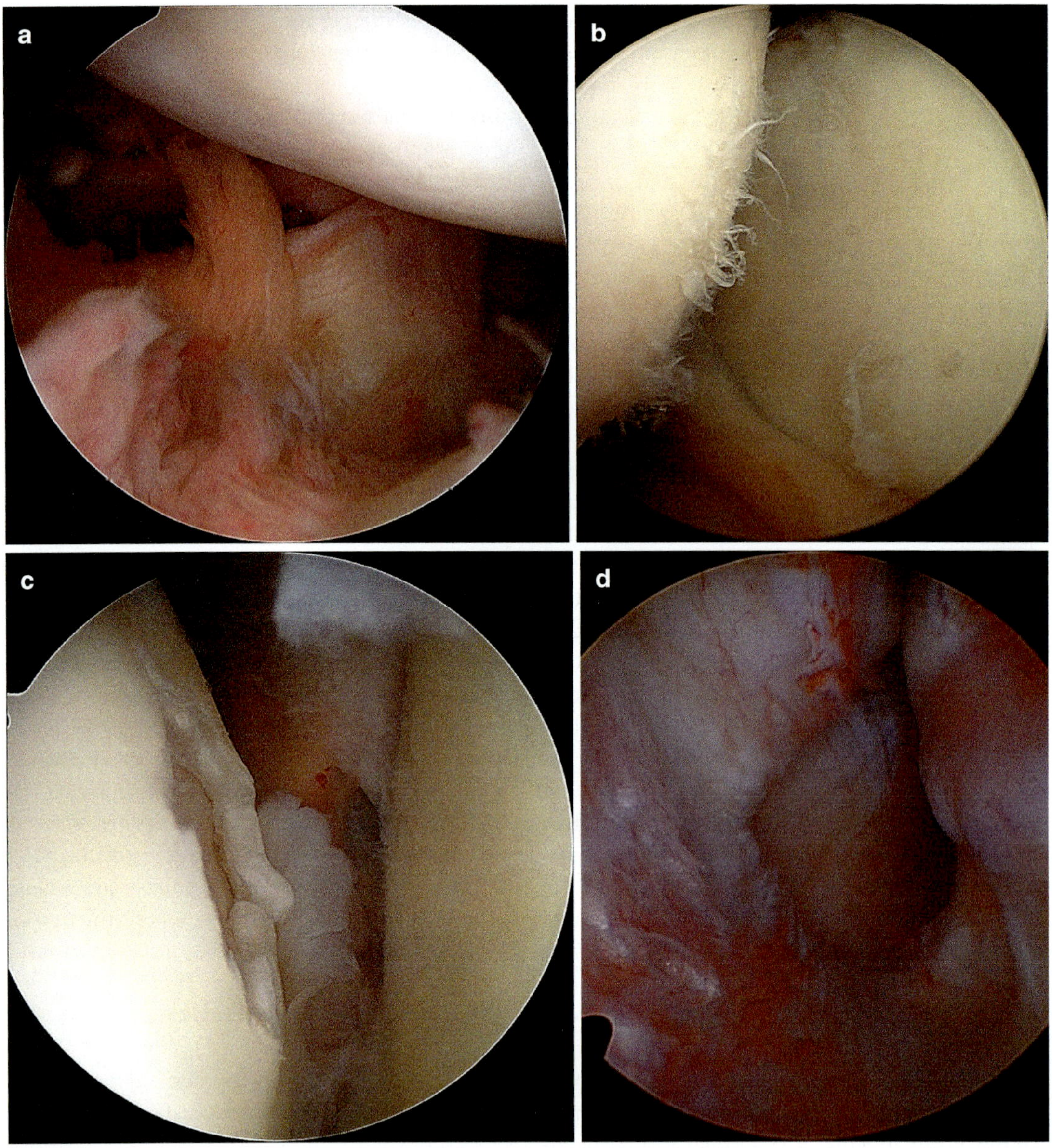


**Fig. 30.1** The spectrum of articular abnormalities that can be found during arthroscopic exam in patients scheduled for shoulder stabilization. (**a**) Synovitis; (**b**) humeral head chondral fibrillation; (**c**) full-thickness ulcer; (**d**) osteophytes located in the inferior margin of humeral head and glenoid

chronic pain with an insidious onset, predominantly in the morning and exacerbated with weather changes. Regarding range of motion, stiffness is frequent. There can be a loss of active and passive external rotation at 90° of abduction and also in neutral position. Whether this is a cause of excessive tightening of anterior structures in previous surgeries or is due to the articular changes that occurred in degenerative disease is still controversial [2]. Audible "clicks" with shoulder motion may indicate bursitis, biceps tendon pathology, osteophytes, or loose bodies. Ellman described a "compression-rotation" test for the arthritic shoulder [18]. The patient is placed in the lateral decubitus position with the affected side up. Then, the humeral head is compressed into the glenoid, and the shoulder is internally and externally rotated. Pain is elicited as the arthritic glenohumeral joint surfaces are compressed together. A subacromial injection can be performed first in order to eliminate subacromial pathology as a source of pain and increase sensibility.

Supraspinatus and infraspinatus fossae should be inspected to look for any rotator cuff atrophies. Shoulder altered kinematics or the presence of a scapular dyskinesia should also be ruled out. A routine physical examination for rotator cuff pathology, acromioclavicular joint osteoarthritis, and shoulder instability is usually recommended. In patients over 40 years old with an instability episode, posterior structures are more likely to fail, secondary to pre-existing rotator cuff weakness [19]. In patients over 60 years old, recurrent instability after an anterior dislocation might be caused by a failure of the posterior rotator cuff [20]. The overall frequency of rotator cuff tears after an anterior dislocation ranges between 7 and 32% and rises with advancing age. In these cases, the patient will present with a limited active forward elevation and abduction. Differential diagnosis should include axillary nerve damage.

### 30.1.4 Treatment Options and Results

Treatment for dislocation arthropathy depends on the presentation and the disability that it causes to the patient. Initial nonoperative measures include anti-inflammatory medications, moderate exercise, physical therapy, and injections. In the cases where a previous surgery was performed, it is mandatory to check if metal hardware is responsible for the symptoms, and sometimes, removing it can avoid progressing symptoms.

Speigl et al. recently published their results of different surgical interventions in the context of glenohumeral osteoarthritis. In this study they compared an arthroscopic approach versus a total shoulder arthroplasty (TSA), and the principal outcome measure was total remaining quality-adjusted life years after each treatment option [21]. They concluded that arthroscopic management was the preferred strategy for patients younger than 47 years, TSA was the preferred strategy for patients older than 66 years, and both treatment options were reasonable for patients aged between 47 and 66.

Arthroscopic management of osteoarthritis would include debridement, removal of loose bodies, synovectomy, osteoplasty, and contracture release [22, 23]. The Comprehensive Arthroscopic Management (CAM) procedure was described by Millett et al. [3]. First, a glenohumeral debridement of degenerative labral tissue and unstable cartilage fragments is performed, and loose bodies are excised. A limited synovectomy can also be performed with the use of the shaver or with the radiofrequency probe, and stable chondral lesions can be treated with microfracture. In the cases where there is a significant inferior osteophyte, it can be excised with a high-speed burr and arthroscopic shaver using a posterosuperior portal for visualization. Internal and external rotation of the arm can help in identifying the spur, and fluoroscopy can be used to ensure adequate bone resection. The capsule release is performed at the end of the procedure as it keeps the axillary nerve out of danger during osteophyte excision and improves visualization of the axillary poach. It can be performed with arthroscopic scissors and a monopolar radiofrequency probe starting from inferior and then complete the anterior and posterior release in a standard fashion. Neurolysis of the axillary nerve can be also performed in patients with posterior or lateral pain, compressive signs detected in the MRI, or direct encroaching seen in the inferior poach during arthroscopy. It is performed from proximal to distal to avoid damage to the nerve branches. Other surgical gestures depending on patient's physical examination can include subacromial decompression, biceps tenotomy or tenodesis, or resection of the acromioclavicular joint.

This procedure provides pain relief, an increase in range of motion, and better functional scores. However, in Millett's series 6 out of 29 patients were dissatisfied with the result and finally underwent TSA at a mean of 1.9 years after the arthroscopic debridement. This group of patients accounted for a lower preoperative ASES score and had less preoperative joint space. A joint space of less than 2 mm increased 7.8 times the risk to progress to an arthroplasty. They also observed that patients with chondral damage grade IV had worse results and those with a more restricted preoperative external rotation were more satisfied with final outcome. The mean survivorship was 95.6% at 1 year, 86.7% at 3 years, and 76.9% at 5 years [24]. Other authors, however, have published worse results with a return to preoperative pain and range of motion levels within 3.8 months after the surgery [22]. Skelley et al. published a rate of unsatisfactory results in 60.6% of their patients, with a TSA conversion rate of 42.4% at an average of 8.8 months after arthroscopy [22].

For isolated unipolar lesions, repair of the chondral defect management with microfractures, cartilage transplantation, osteochondral allografts, or partial resurfacing has been proposed, but to date the results of these procedures are very scant [25, 26] (Fig. 30.2).

With regard to prosthetic options, it is well known that TSA provides pain relief and improves shoulder function [27]. However, there is a risk of component wear and loosening and also a recommendation for activity restriction that is usually a concern for active patients.

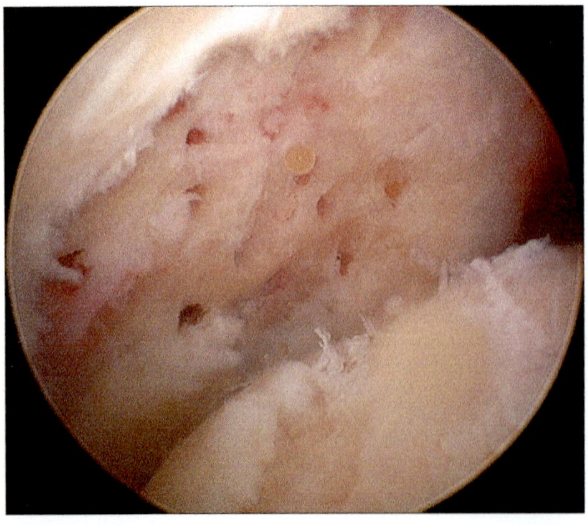

**Fig. 30.2** Full-thickness ulcer involving the vast majority of the glenoid articular surface treated with microfractures

As mentioned before, the symptoms of shoulder arthritis in the context of shoulder instability are mild. This fact often leads the patient to a joint-preserving treatment option even in patients aged over 50 years [4, 28]. Although hemiarthroplasty (HA) could be an intermediate solution, it has been demonstrated that it provides less pain relief and functional improvement than TSA. In younger patients, hemiarthroplasty with biologic glenoid resurfacing as an interposition arthroplasty has been performed using different tissues: fascia lata autograft [29], anterior capsule, lateral meniscus allograft [30], and Achilles tendon allograft [31]. In order to avoid concerns about durability of soft tissue interposition, a concentric glenoid reaming (ream and run) was also proposed [32]. The results of these procedures have been inconsistent (Fig. 30.3).

The results of TSA in patients with dislocation arthropathy are reproducible and satisfactory. Matsoukis et al. reported on the results of TSA in 55 patients with a prior shoulder dislocation [33]. They observed improvements in Constant Score and range of motion, and most of the patients rated the result of their surgery as good or excellent. They did not find differences in between patients with and without previous surgeries for their instability. Negative prognostic factors included older age at the time of the initial dislocation and the presence of a rotator cuff tear. Green and Norris also proved an increase in shoulder function and pain relief [34]. There was a revision rate of 3 out

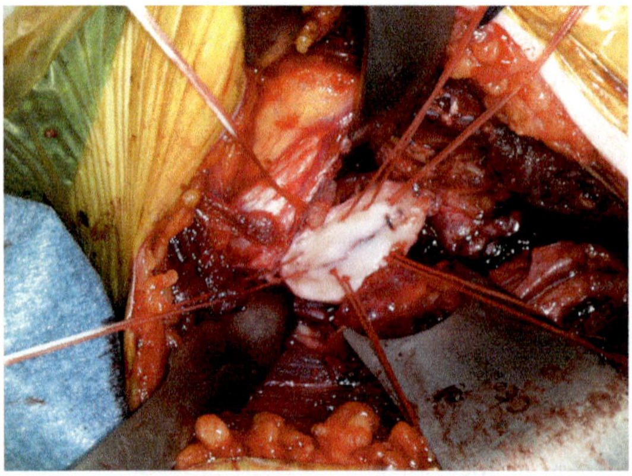

**Fig. 30.3** Biologic resurfacing of the glenoid using a lateral meniscus allograft

of 19. The authors found a more severe arthritis in patients that had previously undergone a nonanatomic procedure and were characterized by a severe internal rotation contracture and subsequent posterior glenoid wear, making the surgery challenging. Sperling et al. reported on 31 cases with a mean age of 46 years consisting of 21 TSA and 10 HA. There was a significant pain relief and increase in abduction and external rotation. However, eight of the TSA and three of the HA required revision surgery [27]. Thus, it is important to mention that results of TSA in this pathology have been proven to be less satisfactory than in primary osteoarthritis [33, 34]. Contracture of the anterior soft tissues and erosion of the posterior glenoid can be related to an increased risk of revision arthroplasty [17, 27].

When a rotator cuff tear is found in combination with osteoarthritis, a reverse shoulder arthroplasty (RSA) should probably be considered. Raiss et al. published their results on 13 patient's series with a mean age of 70 years. They reported good results in terms of Constant Score, forward elevation, and internal rotation. External rotation did not show a significant improvement [35].

**Conclusion**

Osteoarthritis in the context of shoulder instability is frequent and usually presents in a mild grade with moderate symptoms. It can appear after a single episode of shoulder dislocation, but additional surgeries can increase its incidence.

When the symptoms are limiting to the patient, conservative management based on intra-articular injections, physiotherapy, and activity modification should be first advocated. If this fails, even in patients over 50 years, an arthroscopic debridement can provide pain relief and increased range of motion. Total shoulder arthroplasty can also provide satisfactory outcomes in patients with severe degenerative changes, but the results are worse than in primary osteoarthritis. In the cases when a rotator cuff tear is also present, reverse total shoulder arthroplasty is recommended.

## References


1. Samilson RL, Prieto V. Dislocation arthropathy of the shoulder. J Bone Joint Surg Am. 1983;65:456–60.
2. Buscayret F, Edwards TB, Szabo I, Adeleine P, Coudane H, Walch G. Glenohumeral arthrosis in anterior instability before and after surgical treatment: Incidence and contributing factors. Am J Sports Med. 2004;32:1165–72.
3. Millett PJ, Horan MP, Pennock AT, Rios D. Comprehensive arthroscopic management (CAM) procedure: Clinical results of a joint-preserving arthroscopic treatment for young, active patients with advanced shoulder osteoarthritis. Arthroscopy. 2013; 29:440–8.
4. Hovelius L, Saeboe M. Neer award 2008: Arthropathy after primary anterior shoulder dislocation--223 shoulders prospectively followed up for twenty-five years. J Shoulder Elbow Surg. 2009;18(3):339–47.
5. Calvo E, Almaraz M, Gil-Luciano A. Characterization and risk factors for osteoarthritis associated to shoulder instability. 21st Congress of the European Society of Shoulder and Elbow Surgery (ESSSE—SECEC). Brugge. 2008.
6. Cameron ML, Kocher MS, Briggs KK, Horan MP, Hawkins RJ. The prevalence of glenohumeral osteoarthrosis in unstable shoulders. Am J Sports Med. 2003;31(1):53–5.
7. Franceschi F, Papalia R, Del Buono A, Vasta S, Maffulli N, Denaro V. Glenohumeral osteoarthritis after arthroscopic bankart repair for anterior instability. Am J Sports Med. 2011;39:1653–9.
8. Yiannakopoulos CK, Mataragas E, Antonogiannakis E. A comparison of the spectrum of intra-articular lesions in acute and chronic anterior shoulder instability. Arthroscopy. 2007;23;985–90
9. Werner CML, Nyffeler RW, Jacob HAC, Gerber C. The effect of capsular tightening on humeral head translations. J Orthop Res. 2004;22:194–201.
10. Plath JE, Aboalata M, Seppel G, Juretzko J, Waldt S, Vogt S, Imhoff AB. Prevalence of and risk factors for dislocation arthropathy: radiological long-term outcome of arthroscopic Bankart repair in 100 shoulders at an average 13-year follow-up. Am J Sports Med. 2015;43:1084–90.
11. Saito M, Saito S, Ohzono K, Ono K. The osteoblastic response to osteoarthritis of the hip. Its influence on the long-term results of arthroplasty. J Bone Joint Surg Br. 1987;69(5):746–51.
12. Ilg A, Bankes MJ, Emery RJ. The intra- and inter-observer reliability of the samilson and prieto grading system of glenohumeral arthropathy. Knee Surg Sports Traumatol Arthrosc. 2001;9:187–90.
13. Rosenberg BN, Richmond JC, Levine WN. Long-term follow-up of Bankart reconstruction. Incidence of late degenerative glenohumeral arthrosis. Am J Sports Med. 1995;23:538–44.
14. Ogawa K, Yoshida A, Ikegami H. Osteoarthritis in shoulders with traumatic anterior instability:

preoperative survey using radiography and computed tomography. J Shoulder Elbow Surg. 2006;15:23–9.
15. Outerbridge RE, Dunlop JA. The problem of chondromalacia patellae. Clin Orthop Relat Res. 1975;177–96.
16. Calvo E, Palacios I, Delgado E, Ruiz-Cabello J, Hernández P, Sánchez-Pernaute O, et al. High-resolution MRI detects cartilage swelling at the early stages of experimental osteoarthritis. Osteoarthritis Cartilage. 2001;9:463–72.
17. Brophy RH, Marx RG. Osteoarthritis following shoulder instability. Clin Sports Med. 2005;24:47–56.
18. Ellman H, Harris E, Kay SP. Early degenerative joint disease simulating impingement syndrome: Arthroscopic findings. Arthroscopy. 1992;8:482–7.
19. Robinson EC, Thangamani VB, Kuhn MA, Ross G. Arthroscopic findings after traumatic shoulder instability in patients older than 35 years. Orthop J Sports Med. 2015, May;3(5):2325967115584318.
20. Paxton ES, Dodson CC, Lazarus MD. Shoulder instability in older patients. Orthop Clin North Am. 2014;45:377–85.
21. Spiegl UJ, Faucett SC, Horan MP, Warth RJ, Millett PJ. The role of arthroscopy in the management of glenohumeral osteoarthritis: a markov decision model. Arthroscopy. 2014;30:1392–9.
22. Skelley NW, Namdari S, Chamberlain AM, Keener JD, Galatz LM, Yamaguchi K. Arthroscopic debridement and capsular release for the treatment of shoulder osteoarthritis. Arthroscopy. 2015;31:494–500.
23. Pitta M, Davis W, Argintar EH. Arthroscopic management of osteoarthritis. J Am Acad Orthop Surg. 2016;24:74–82.
24. Mitchell JJ, Horan MP, Greenspoon JA, Menge TJ, Tahal DS, Millett PJ. Survivorship and patient-reported outcomes after comprehensive arthroscopic management of glenohumeral osteoarthritis: minimum 5-year follow-up. Am J Sports Med. 2016. pii: 0363546516656372.
25. Scheibel M, Bartl C, Magosch P, Lichtenberg S, Habermeyer P. Osteochondral autologous transplantation for the treatment of full-thickness articular cartilage defects of the shoulder. J Bone Joint Surg Br. 2004;86:991–7.
26. Gobezie R, Lenarz CJ, Wanner JP, Streit JJ. All-arthroscopic biologic total shoulder resurfacing. Arthroscopy. 2011;27:1588–93.
27. Sperling JW, Antuna SA, Sanchez-Sotelo J, Schleck C, Cofield RH. Shoulder arthroplasty for arthritis after instability surgery. J Bone Joint Surg Am. 2002;84:1775–81.
28. Kavaja L, Pajarinen J, Sinisaari I, Savolainen V, Björkenheim JM, Haapamäki V, Paavola M. Arthrosis of glenohumeral joint after arthroscopic bankart repair: a long-term follow-up of 13 years. J Shoulder Elbow Surg. 2012, Mar;21:350–5.
29. Krishnan SG, Nowinski RJ, Harrison D, Burkhead WZ. Humeral hemiarthroplasty with biologic resurfacing of the glenoid for glenohumeral arthritis. J Bone Joint Surg Am. 2007;89:727–34.
30. Lollino N, Pellegrini A, Paladini P, Campi F, Porcellini G. Gleno-Humeral arthritis in young patients: clinical and radiographic analysis of humerus resurfacing prosthesis and meniscus interposition. Musculoskelet Surg. 2011;95:59–63.
31. Sayegh ET, Mascarenhas R, Chalmers PN, Cole BJ, Romeo AA, Verma NN. Surgical treatment options for glenohumeral arthritis in young patients: a systematic review and meta-analysis. Arthroscopy. 2015;31:1156–66.
32. Saltzman MD, Chamberlain AM, Mercer DM, Warme WJ, Bertelsen AL, Matsen FA. Shoulder hemiarthroplasty with concentric glenoid reaming in patients 55 years old or less. J Shoulder Elbow Surg. 2011;20:609–15.
33. Matsoukis J, Tabib W, Guiffault P, Mandelbaum A, Walch G, Némoz C, Edwards TB. Shoulder arthroplasty in patients with a prior anterior shoulder dislocation. Results of a multicenter study. J Bone Joint Surg Am. 2003;85-A:1417–24.
34. Green A, Norris TR. Shoulder arthroplasty for advanced glenohumeral arthritis after anterior instability repair. J Shoulder Elbow Surg. 2001;10:539–45.
35. Raiss P, Zeifang F, Pons-Villanueva J, Smithers CJ, Loew M, Walch G. Reverse arthroplasty for osteoarthritis and rotator cuff deficiency after previous surgery for recurrent anterior shoulder instability. Int Orthop. 2014, Jul;38(7):1407–13.

# Part V

# Miscellaneous Instability Topics in the Various Ages

# Glenoid Fracture

# 31

Jean Michel Hovsepian, Felix Dyrna, and Knut Beitzel

## Contents

31.1 **Introduction** .......... 261
31.2 **Imaging, Classification, and Treatment Algorithm** .......... 262
31.3 **Treatment** .......... 262
31.4 **Acute Fractures (<6 Months)** .......... 263
31.5 **Chronic Fractures and Bone Defects (>6 Months)** .......... 264
31.6 **Summary** .......... 265
**References** .......... 265

J.M. Hovsepian, MD
Department of Orthopaedic Sports Medicine, Technical University of Munich, Munich, Germany

Department of Orthopaedic Surgery, University Hospital of Caracas (HUC), Central University of Venezuela, Caracas, Venezuela
e-mail: jmichelh@gmail.com

F. Dyrna, MD • K. Beitzel, MA, MD (✉)
Department of Orthopaedic Sports Medicine, Technical University of Munich, Munich, Germany

## 31.1 Introduction

Fractures of the scapula rarely occur and account for approximately 0.4–1% of all fractures. About 10% of these fractures include the glenoid, and the same amount is substantially displaced. Within the glenoid fractures, 75–85% are anterior avulsion or rim fractures [1]. A CT analysis of 218 patients showed 21% glenoid rim fractures in patients with single or recurrent dislocations, of which one-half had a detached fragment while the other half had an attached one [2]. Such fractures can result in persisting glenohumeral instability. The average age of the patients is approximately 35 years and seen four times more in men than in women. Two peaks can be found within the age distribution – the first is seen between the age of 20–30 years, mostly because of high energy trauma. The second peak can be found at the age of around 50–60 years due to dislocating trauma [1].

Fractures of the glenoid basically involve two problems. First the physiologic pressure distribution and loading of the glenoid is significantly altered, if the contact area is decreased due to glenoid bone loss. Greis et al. [3] in 2002 showed that a bone loss of 30% results in a decreased contact area of approximately 40% and an increase in pressure of nearly 100% which might be involve in the pathogenesis of osteoarthritis after instability. Second, studies have demonstrated the increased risk of recurrent instability if the bone loss exceeds 20% of the glenoid surface [4, 5].

© ISAKOS 2017
A.B. Imhoff, F.H. Savoie III (eds.), *Shoulder Instability Across the Life Span*, DOI 10.1007/978-3-662-54077-0_31

## 31.2 Imaging, Classification, and Treatment Algorithm

The clinical workup should include a radiological imaging of at least a three-plane X-ray. A true AP, Y-view, and axial (alternative: Velpeau view) are needed to detect and evaluate the fracture. For further assessment, a CT scan with 3D reconstruction (with subtraction of humerus) is the current gold standard. With this, the glenoid surface can exactly be measured and determined. Various techniques could be used, to quantify the glenoid size, fragment size, and bone loss as a percentage area using the inferior perfect circle and the help of a computer software [6–8]. While other techniques use the diameter of the perfect circle to calculate the percentage glenoid bone loss [9, 10], MRI is useful to detect concomitant lesions (e.g., RC tears or LHB lesions) (Fig. 31.1).

Multiple classifications can be used to evaluate fractures of the glenoid. One of the most used is the Ideberg [11] classification that was developed in 1985 from a series of AP and lateral radiographs. It is divided into five groups describing intra-articular glenoid fractures ascending in complexity. Type I are anterior rim fracture differentiating among bony fragments less than 5 mm (Ia) and more than 5 mm (Ib), usually seen in shoulder dislocations. From type II to type V, Ideberg describes higher-grade fractures of the glenoid and the scapula. Nevertheless, prognostic value has not been demonstrated, while therapeutic surgical procedures have been described for each type of fracture. Later on this classification system was modified by Goss et al. [12], adding more subgroups with more details, trying to highlight the mechanism and different patterns that may result looking forward improving the management of these fractures. Moreover, Bigliani [13] in 1998 published a classification more specific for anterior glenoid rim fractures associated with glenohumeral instability, independently of the time frame of the lesion. Type I is a displaced avulsion fracture with attached capsule, type II is a malunited fragment medially displaced to the glenoid rim, and type III is a glenoid rim erosion with bone loss less than 25% (IIIa) or more than 25% (IIIb). Hence, a specific treatment for each kind of lesion is suggested [13]. Recently, in 2009 Scheibel [14] evolves the Bigliani classification, differentiating acute and chronic lesions; isolating lesions between avulsion, solitary, and multifragmented; and adding the types of erosion bone loss used by Sugaya [6].

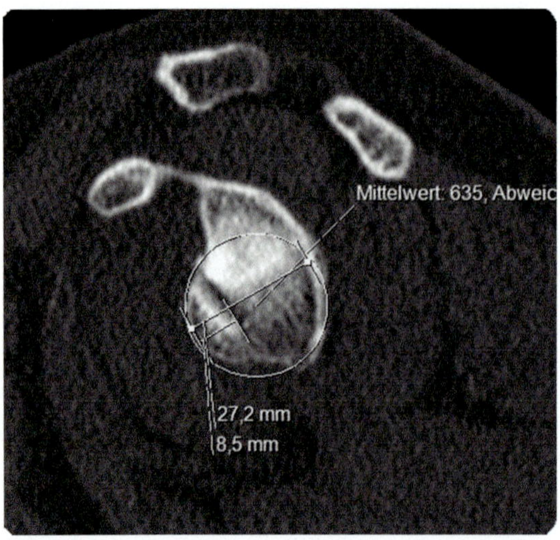


**Fig. 31.1** A CT scan of the glenoid with the "best fit circle" measurement of defect size

## 31.3 Treatment

The optimal treatment of glenoid fractures is dependent on multiple factors and ranges from conservative to surgical and from arthroscopically or open surgery to non-anatomic procedures. The decision is based on multiple variables such as the thorough analysis of the osseous defect size, time from injury, fragment size, and morphology as well as age and demands of the patient.

We suggest a treatment algorithm based primarily on the time since injury (acute < 3 months vs. chronic > 3 months). Porcellini et al. [15] compared the results of 41 acute glenoid fractures to 24 chronic with a mean follow-up of 48 months after suture anchor repair. The Rowe score at final follow-up (acute 59 points vs. chronic 61 points) as well as the percentage of return to sports (78% vs. 40%) was better in the acute group compared to the chronic. Plath et al. [16] also showed advantages for the acutely treated cases, although differences in their study were not significant.

The size of the fragment in correlation to the glenoid size is the second important factor. In addition, the type of fragment (solitary vs. multifragment) has to be considered as well as general factors such as the age and demands of the patient.

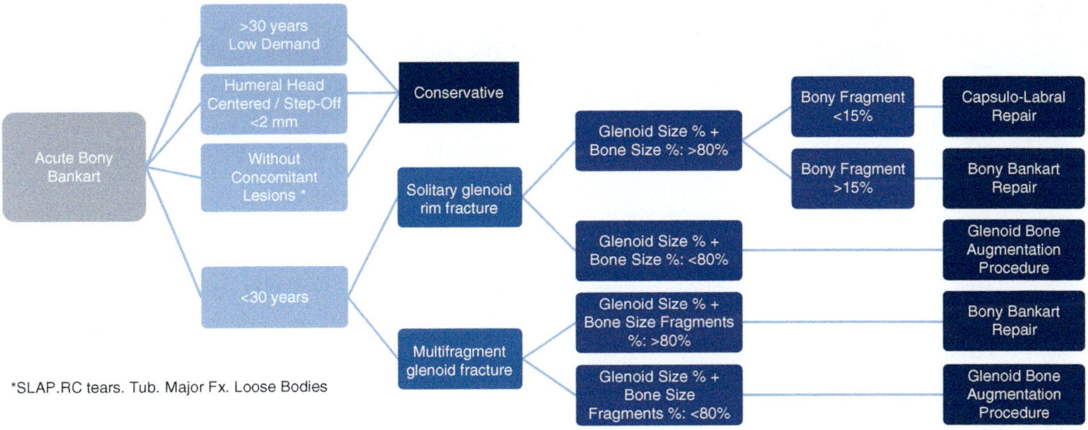


## 31.4 Acute Fractures (<6 Months)

Treatment options for acute fractures highly depend on the size of the fragment and age of the patient. Fragments should be classified to be small rim lesions (<5%), small fragments (<15%), or larger fragments (>15%). This has to be seen in correlation to the glenoid size, which should result in a bony surface of at least 80% after adding together the glenoid surface area with the area of the bony fragment, to permit persisting stability of the glenohumeral joint.

If the fragment is small such as a glenoid rim lesion (<5%), without significant glenoid defect, general risk factors are known from shoulder instability and have to be considered. Salomonsson et al. [17] have shown that in these cases, a solitary fragment smaller than 15% is a positive predictive factor in comparison with labral lesions alone. When a fragment is less than 15%, seems not to increase further the instability process compared to a classic Bankart lesion. Therefore, a patient older than 30 years with no concomitant intra-articular lesions (e.g., SLAP, loose body, etc.) might be treated nonsurgically.

When the patient is younger than 30 years and/or has high athletic demands, an arthroscopic labral repair should be performed to regain stability of the joint because of the overall high reluxation risk of these patients. A recent meta-analysis showed that the luxation rate in the age group between 15–20 and 15–30 is almost 50%; on the contrary with more than 40 years, the recurrence percentage is 11% [18]. The highest odds ratio for presenting recurrent instability was in people with less than 40 years, followed by being male and having hyperlaxity [18].

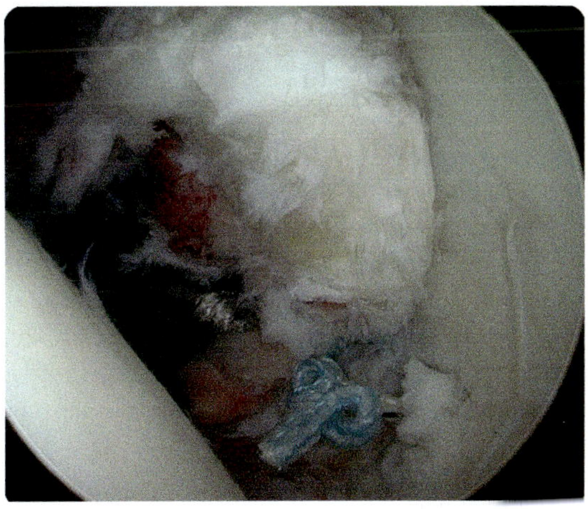

**Fig. 31.2** Arthroscopic view of fragment fixed with suture anchors

Several techniques have been described to achieve this. The fragment can be arthroscopically repositioned and fixed by a suture anchor repair according to the technique described by Sugaya [19]. For this, a suture anchor is positioned inferior and superior to the repositioned fragment (Fig. 31.2).

An alternative fixation for solitary fragments can be achieved by the bony Bankart bridge technique described by Millett et al. [20]. Therefore, a suture anchor is fixed medially to the fragment and then fixed with the second row at the glenoid. Biomechanical studies have shown that both

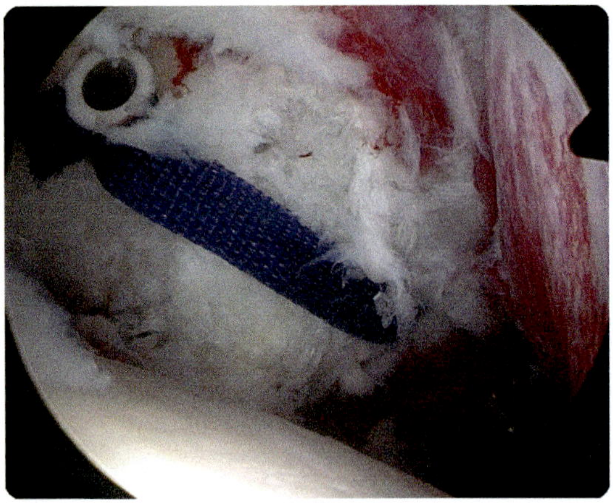

**Fig. 31.3** Arthroscopic view of fragment refixed with a modified "bony Bankart bridge"

techniques have positive results. Although the study from Giles et al. [21], comparing single-point suture anchor vs. double-point, have equivalent failure strengths and load transfers but greater initial fracture fragment stability in favor of the suture-bridge technique. Similarly, Spiegl et al. [22] found improved fracture reduction and superior stability at time zero in the double-row technique (Fig. 31.3).

If a bigger solitary fragment of more than 15% is found, fixation should be intended. However, in cases of a centered joint, a step-off less than 2 mm, no concomitant lesions, and patients with lower demands especially with more than 30 years, a conservative treatment might be successful [23–26]. Gerber et al. [27] demonstrated good clinical results for such conservative treatment in patients with a mean age of 53 years (ratio, 32–73) with concentric reduction of the humeral head after a closed reduction. In the literature the conservative treatment has shown good results following these criteria with 100% of the bony healing [27–30]. Nevertheless, all other cases should be treated surgically. The different methods that have been described to treat bony Bankart, all of them have achieved good clinical results [7, 20, 26, 31–34]. Surgeons can choose between suture fixation, bony Bankart bridge, or screw fixation of the fragment. Arthroscopic and open techniques were proven to achieve positive results. Scheibel et al. [32] published similar scores after open procedures with suture anchors in defects less than 25% and with two cannulated screws in defects larger than 25% of the glenoid surface (mean Constant score, 85.5 points vs. 87.2 points). The second study [35] presented good and excellent clinical results after arthroscopic procedure for large solitary and multifragment lesions with suture anchor, with screws, or with a combined technique (mean Constant score, 84.5 points) without complications; however, 6 patients of 21 presented different grades of osteoarthritis.

Surgeons should keep in mind that, if the addition of the fragment with the glenoid results in a surface area greater than 80%, good prognosis regarding stability can be expected. Otherwise, if the surface area is smaller, the risk for symptomatic instability in an active patient increased significantly. The study from Jian et al. [36] showed in a case series report of 50 patients, where three of four cases with redislocation after arthroscopic fixation of the bony fragment had a reconstructed size of the glenoid less than 80%. Therefore, previous analysis of the fragment must be done before the surgery. Furthermore, poorly reduced fractures will not reconstruct the necessary glenoid surface area. In these cases, surgical techniques like bone grafting from the iliac crest or Latarjet procedures should be aimed at preventing further instability.

## 31.5 Chronic Fractures and Bone Defects (>6 Months)

The indications for chronic cases are symptomatic recurrent instabilities. Again, the surgical technique is primarily based on the size of the fragment as well as the overall bony surface of the glenoid.

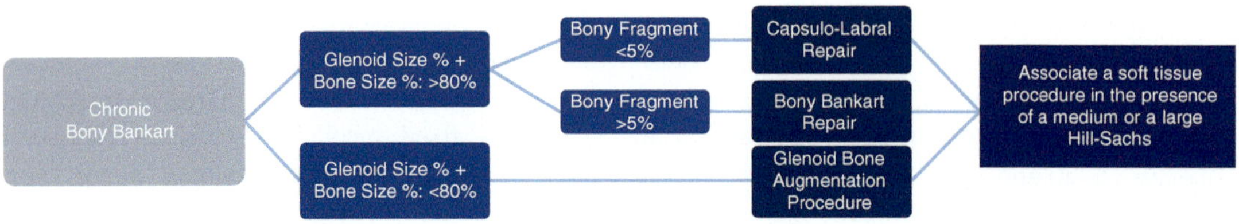

If the glenoid size in combination with the fragment exceeds 80%, smaller bony fragments (<5%) may just be involved in an arthroscopic soft tissue repair with anchors, and this has been shown by Sugaya et al. [8, 19]. Fragments with a bigger size (>5%) may be mobilized and fixated with either soft tissue techniques as described by Sugaya et al. [19] or with a bony Bankart bridge technique according to Millett et al. [20] where they did not find worst outcomes in their reports in chronic patients.

A histologic analysis of chronic bony Bankart fragments has shown that the bony fragment has viability and could be used for repairing the glenoid [37]. Kitayama et al. [8] have published a long follow-up, proving that good functional outcomes could also be obtained in chronic cases. They recommend an extensive labral release, in order to obtain a good fragment reduction in a more superior position. In their postoperative 3D-CT reconstruction, they showed that in all the cases, they restored the normal shape of the glenoid or are slightly hypertrophic – from a mean preoperative glenoid bone loss of 20.4%, they obtained a result of −1.1% with only a mean preoperative fragment size of 4.7%. They suggest that the cause of these results is due to correct restoration the mechanical tension of the inferior glenohumeral ligament, thus improving the healing, formation, and remodeling of the bone. Regardless of this, Park et al. [38] described a cohort where the fragment size decreased from the preoperative measurement 2.2% after a follow-up of 1 year. On the other hand, the nonunion rate in chronic cases is between 10% and 16% but does not influence in the postoperative outcomes scores and instability rates as it does the final size of the glenoid surface after the repair [16, 36, 38]. For this reason, chronic erosions of the glenoid which result in an estimated glenoid size of less than 80% if in combination with a reattached fragment should be treated with either a bone block or Latarjet technique to increase the bone socket or in the case of the Latarjet add additional stabilizing functions [8, 13, 36]. In the presence of a medium or large Hill-Sachs in bony Bankart, the association of a soft tissue procedure may also be beneficial [8]. A glenoid fracture in elderly patients could be a difficult situation to treat. Especially when this population has severe osteopenia and/or multifragment fractures with symptomatic recurrent instability (glenoid size less of 80%). The insertion of an arthroplasty is necessary, usually in combination with bone grafting [39, 40]. In the presence of a really big defect, two surgical steps are needed until the bone graft heals. The type of the prosthesis has to be individualized for every patient.

## 31.6 Summary

After a bony Bankart lesion, the age of the patients and their physical expectations are the first steps for analyzing the therapeutic decision. If the humeral head has a concentric reduction into the glenoid arch preferably visualized with a CT, a conservative management may be preferable if the patients are more than 30 years old. When we are dealing with younger patients, the glenoid surface area in conjunction with the bone defects as percentages should be calculated. When this number is more than 80%, arthroscopic treatment may be performed with fixation of the capsulo-labral complex with the bone defect, if this last one has more than 15% of the surface of the glenoid. Several techniques could be selected as well as different types of fixation (suture anchors and/or screws). Bony Bankart lesions should be treated acutely when the patients manifest recurrent shoulder instability. However, it has been shown that chronic lesions also have good clinical results when they are managed properly.

## References


1. Van Oostveen DPH, Temmerman OPP, Burger BJ, Van Noort A, Robinson M. Glenoid fractures: a review of pathology, classification, treatment and results. Acta Orthop Belg. 2014;80(1):88–98.
2. Griffith JF, Antonio GE, Yung PSH, et al. Prevalence, pattern, and spectrum of glenoid bone loss in anterior shoulder dislocation: CT analysis of 218 patients. Am J Roentgenol. 2008;190(5):1247–54. doi:10.2214/AJR.07.3009.
3. Greis PE, Scuderi MG, Mohr A, Bachus KN, Burks RT. Glenohumeral articular contact areas and pressures following labral and osseous injury to the anteroinferior quadrant of the glenoid. J Shoulder Elbow Surg. 2002;11(5):442–51. doi:10.1067/mse.2002.124526.
4. Itoi E, Lee SB, Berglund LJ, Berge LL, An KN. The effect of a glenoid defect on anteroinferior stability of

the shoulder after Bankart repair: a cadaveric study. J Bone Joint Surg Am. 2000;82(1):35–46. doi:10.1002/sim.5330.
5. Yamamoto N, Itoi E, Abe H, et al. Effect of an anterior glenoid defect on anterior shoulder stability: a cadaveric study. Am J Sports Med. 2009;37(5):949–54. doi:10.1177/0363546508330139.
6. Sugaya H, Moriishi J, Dohi M, Kon Y, Tsuchiya A. Glenoid rim morphology in recurrent anterior glenohumeral instability. J Bone Joint Surg Am. 2003;85-A(5):878–84. doi:10.1053/jars.2000.17715.
7. Sugaya H, Moriishi J, Kanisawa I, Tsuchiya A. Arthroscopic osseous Bankart repair for chronic recurrent traumatic anterior glenohumeral instability. J Bone Joint Surg Ser A. 2005;87(8):1752–60. http://dx.doi.org/10.2106/JBJS.D.02204.
8. Kitayama S, Sugaya H, Takahashi N, et al. Clinical outcome and glenoid morphology after arthroscopic repair of chronic osseous Bankart lesions: A five to eight-year follow-up study. J Bone Joint Surg Am. 2015;97(22):1833–43. doi:10.2106/jbjs.n.01033.
9. Lo IKY, Parten PM, Burkhart SS. The inverted pear glenoid: an indicator of significant glenoid bone loss. Arthrosc – J Arthrosc Relat Surg. 2004;20(2):169–74. doi:10.1016/j.arthro.2003.11.036.
10. Chuang TY, Adams CR, Burkhart SS. Use of preoperative three-dimensional computed tomography to quantify glenoid bone loss in shoulder instability. Arthrosc – J Arthrosc Relat Surg. 2008;24(4):376–82. doi:10.1016/j.arthro.2007.10.008.
11. Ideberg R, Grevsten S, Larsson S. Epidemiology of scapular fractures. Incidence and classification of 338 fractures. Acta Orthop Scand. 1995;66(5):395–7. doi:10.3109/17453679508995571.
12. Goss TP. Fractures of the glenoid cavity: Operative principles and techniques. Tech Orthop. 1993;8(3): 199–204.
13. Bigliani LU, Newton PM, Steinmann SP, Connor PM, McLlveen SJ. Glenoid rim lesions associated with recurrent anterior dislocation of the shoulder. Am J Sports Med. 1998;26(1):41–5.
14. Scheibel M, Kraus N, Gerhardt C, Haas NP. Anteriore glenoidranddefekte der schulter. Orthopade. 2009;38(1):41–53. doi:10.1007/s00132-008-1354-x.
15. Porcellini G, Paladini P, Campi F, Paganelli M. Long-term outcome of acute versus chronic bony Bankart lesions managed arthroscopically. Am J Sports Med. 2007;35(12):2067–72.doi:10.1177/0363546507305011.
16. Plath JE, Feucht MJ, Bangoj R, et al. Arthroscopic suture anchor fixation of bony Bankart lesions: clinical outcome, magnetic resonance imaging results, and return to sports. Arthroscopy. 2015;31(8):1472–81. doi:10.1016/j.arthro.2015.03.005.
17. Salomonsson B, von Heine A, Dahlborn M, et al. Bony Bankart is a positive predictive factor after primary shoulder dislocation. Knee Surg Sports Traumatol Arthrosc. 2010;18(10):1425–31. http://dx.doi.org/10.1007/s00167-009-0998-3
18. Olds M, Ellis R, Donaldson K, Parmar P, Kersten P. Risk factors which predispose first-time traumatic anterior shoulder dislocations to recurrent instability in adults: a systematic review and meta-analysis. Br J Sports Med. 2015;49(14):913–22. doi:10.1136/bjsports-2014-094342.
19. Sugaya H, Kon Y, Tsuchiya A. Arthroscopic repair of glenoid fractures using suture anchors. Arthroscopy. 2005;21(5):635. doi:10.1016/j.arthro.2005.02.006.
20. Millett PJ, Horan MP, Martetschläger F. The "bony Bankart bridge" technique for restoration of anterior shoulder stability. Am J Sports Med. 2013;41(3):608–14. doi:10.1177/0363546512472880.
21. Giles JW, Puskas GJ, Welsh MF, Johnson JA, Athwal GS. Suture anchor fixation of bony Bankart fractures: comparison of single-point with double-point "suture bridge" technique. Am J Sports Med. 2013;41(11): 2624–31. doi:10.1177/0363546513501795.
22. Spiegl U, Smith S, Todd J, Coatney GA, Wijdicks CA, Millett PJ. Biomechanical comparison of arthroscopic single- and double-point repair techniques for acute bony Bankart lesions. Orthop J Sport Med. 2014;2. http://dx.doi.org/10.1177/2325967114S00102.
23. Kim YK, Cho SH, Son WS, Moon SH. Arthroscopic repair of small and medium-sized bony bankart lesions. Am J Sports Med. 2014;42(1):86–94. doi:10.1177/0363546513509062.
24. Königshausen M, Coulibaly M, Nicolas V, Schildhauer TA, Seybold D. Konservative Therapie der antero-inferioren Glenoidrandfraktur (Bankart-Fraktur): Erste Ergebnisse. Obere Extrem. 2013;8(2):96–102. doi:10.1007/s11678-012-0187-8.
25. Kraus N, Gerhardt C, Haas N, Scheibel M. Konservative Therapie anteroinferiorer Glenoidfrakturen. Unfallchirurg. 2010;113(6):469–75. doi:10.1007/s00113-010-1754-3.
26. Osti M, Gohm A, Benedetto KP. Results of open reconstruction of anterior glenoid rim fractures following shoulder dislocation. Arch Orthop Trauma Surg. 2009;129(9):1245–9. doi:10.1007/s00402-009-0828-6.
27. Maquieira GJ, Espinosa N, Gerber C, Eid K. Non-operative treatment of large anterior glenoid rim fractures after traumatic anterior dislocation of the shoulder. J Bone Joint Surg Br. 2007;89(10):1347–51. doi:10.1302/0301-620x.89b10.19273.
28. Kraus N, Gerhardt C, Haas N, Scheibel M. Conservative therapy of antero-inferior glenoid fractures. Unfallchirurg. 2010;113(6):469–75. doi:10.1007/s00113-010-1754-3.
29. Königshausen M, Coulibaly M, Nicolas V, Schildhauer TA, Seybold D. Non-operative treatment of antero-inferior glenoid rim fractures (Bankart fracture): preliminary results. Obere Extrem. 2013;8(2):96–102. doi:10.1007/s11678-012-0187-8.
30. Spiegl UJA, Ryf C, Hepp P, Rillmann P. Evaluation of a treatment algorithm for acute traumatic osseous Bankart lesions resulting from first time dislocation of the shoulder with a two year follow-up. BMC Musculoskelet Disord. 2013;14 http://dx.doi.org/10.1186/1471-2474-14-305
31. Tauber M, Moursy M, Eppel M, Koller H, Resch H. Arthroscopic screw fixation of large anterior glenoid fractures. Knee Surg Sports Traumatol Arthrosc.

2008;16(3):326–32. doi:10.1007/s00167-007-0437-2.
32. Scheibel M, Magosch P, Lichtenberg S, Habermeyer P. Open reconstruction of anterior glenoid rim fractures. Knee Surg Sports Traumatol Arthrosc. 2004;12(6):568–73. doi:10.1007/s00167-004-0495-7.
33. Van Dijkman BA, Schep NWL, Luitse JSK, Ponsen KJ, Kloen P, Goslings JC. Patient related functional outcome of glenoid rim fractures treated with open reduction and internal fixation. Acta Orthop Belg. 2010;76(6):730–4.
34. Maier D, Izadpanah K, Ogon P, et al. Open fixation of acute anterior glenoid rim fractures with bioresorbable pins: analysis of clinical and radiological outcome. Arch Orthop Trauma Surg. 2015;135(7):953–61. doi:10.1007/s00402-015-2242-6.
35. Scheibel M, Hug K, Gerhardt C, Krueger D. Arthroscopic reduction and fixation of large solitary and multifragmented anterior glenoid rim fractures. J Shoulder Elbow Surg. 2016;25(5):781–90. doi:10.1016/j.jse.2015.09.012.
36. Jiang CY, Zhu YM, Liu X, Li FL, Lu Y, Wu G. Do reduction and healing of the bony fragment really matter in arthroscopic bony Bankart reconstruction? A prospective study with clinical and computed tomography evaluations. Am J Sports Med. 2013;41(11):2617–23. doi:10.1177/0363546513499304.
37. Fujii Y, Yoneda M, Wakitani S, Hayashida K. Histologic analysis of bony Bankart lesions in recurrent. 2006:218–23. doi:10.1016/j.jse.2005.06.006.
38. Park JY, Lee SJ, Lhee SH, Lee SH. Follow-up computed tomography arthrographic evaluation of bony bankart lesions after arthroscopic repair. Arthrosc J Arthrosc Relat Surg. 2012;28(4):465–73. doi:10.1016/j.arthro.2011.09.008.
39. Hill JM, Norris TR. Long-term results of total shoulder arthroplasty following bone-grafting of the glenoid. J Bone Joint Surg Am. 2001;83-A(6):877–83. http://jbjs.org/content/83/6/877.abstract
40. Goebel M, Seebauer L. Open operative treatment of acute glenoid fractures following anterior and posterior shoulder dislocation. Oper Orthop Traumatol. 2008;20(3):228–38. doi:10.1007/s00064-008-1305-z.

# Locked Posterior Shoulder Dislocation (LPSD)

# 32

J. Pogorzelski and A.B. Imhoff

## Contents

32.1 **Background** ... 269

32.2 **Physical Examination** ... 270

32.3 **Diagnostics** ... 270

32.4 **Treatment** ... 270
32.4.1 Conservative Treatment ... 272
32.4.2 Operative Treatment ... 272

32.5 **Results** ... 274

**References** ... 274

J. Pogorzelski (✉) • A.B. Imhoff
Department of Orthopaedic Sports Medicine,
Technical University of Munich (TUM),
Munich, Germany
e-mail: jonas.pogorzelski@tum.de

## 32.1 Background

Posterior shoulder dislocation (PSD) is a rare injury associated with trauma and an impression defect of the anterior humeral head ("reverse Hill-Sachs lesion" or "Malgaigne fracture"). When the humeral defect engages into the posterior glenoid rim preventing a spontaneous reduction, it is said to be "locked." The optimal treatment mainly depends on the patient's demands, the size of the humeral head defect, and the time passed since dislocation. Therapy options include non-operative treatment, arthroscopic treatment, or the implantation of a shoulder prosthesis. If diagnosed early, positive outcomes are generally achieved.

When activated involuntary (e.g., during an epileptic seizure or an electric shock), the strong internal rotators of the shoulder overpower the weak external rotators and may result in a locked posterior shoulder dislocation (LPSD). Additionally, high-energy trauma or a fall on the outstretched arm is among the most common causes of LPSD. Diagnosis is often missed or delayed; detailed clinical investigation and radiographic imaging are essential for diagnosing LPSD. The treatment mainly depends on the patient's demands, the size of the humeral impression, as well as the duration of the dislocation.

© ISAKOS 2017
A.B. Imhoff, F.H. Savoie III (eds.), *Shoulder Instability Across the Life Span*,
DOI 10.1007/978-3-662-54077-0_32

## 32.2 Physical Examination

When inspected carefully, an increased anterior prominence of the coracoid process in combination with an increased posterior prominence of the humeral head can be observed. At the same time, the patient often presents with the arm fixed in internal rotation and complains of the loss of active and passive external rotation of the shoulder. There is also restriction of abduction and flexion to between 75° and 100°. A specific test for LPSD published by Rowe/Zarins [9] is the inability to supinate the forearm when the arm is flexed forward due to the locked humeral head.

## 32.3 Diagnostics

A complete radiographic evaluation, including anteroposterior (AP), scapular Y, and axillary lateral views, should be performed as first-line diagnostics when suspecting LPSD. Even though the AP view is regulary seen to be misinterpreted, there exist several radiological signs which are pathognomonic [1, 4]. The "vacant glenoid" sign describes the empty anterior glenoid fossa. The "light bulb" sign is a description of the internally rotated humeral head appearing exceptionally circular on the AP view. The "rim" sign describes more than 6 mm distance between the humeral head and the anterior glenoid rim. Finally, the "through line" sign shows a vertical line caused by the Malgaigne fracture (Fig. 32.1).

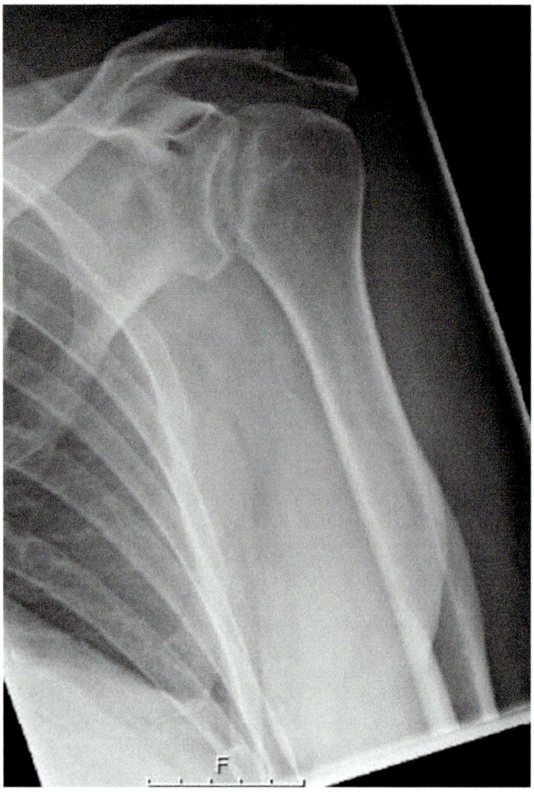

Fig. 32.1 "Through line" sign on an AP radiograph

A computed tomography (CT) scan is essential to determine the size and exact location of the reverse Hill-Sachs defect. Cicak [3] introduced a simple but effective method to determine and classify the size of bony defects of the humeral head in axial sequences of a CT scan (Fig. 32.2). Additionally, further lesions (e.g., of the glenoid) can be excluded.

Magnetic resonance imaging (MRI) are helpful in chronic cases of LPSD to evaluate ligamentous injury or rotator cuff tears. For a primary diagnosis, MRI is generally not recommended.

## 32.4 Treatment

The choice of treatment depends on the size of the humeral defect, the time interval from dislocation to diagnosis, and the patient's demands (Fig. 32.3). In cases where the reverse Hill-Sachs lesion is less than 20% of the articular surface and the duration of the dislocation is less than 3 weeks, closed reduction can be attempted. When the duration of the dislocation is more than 3 weeks, closed reduction is usually impossible and surgery is recommended. In those cases with a Malgaigne fracture of less than 20%, an arthroscopic reduction is considered to be the therapy of choice; further arthroscopic treatment, like tenodesis of the subscapularis tendon in case the reverse Hill-Sachs lesion appears to be engaging (modified McLaughlin procedure, Fig. 32.4), can be performed simultaneously. For Malgaigne fractures >20%, open surgery is usually required

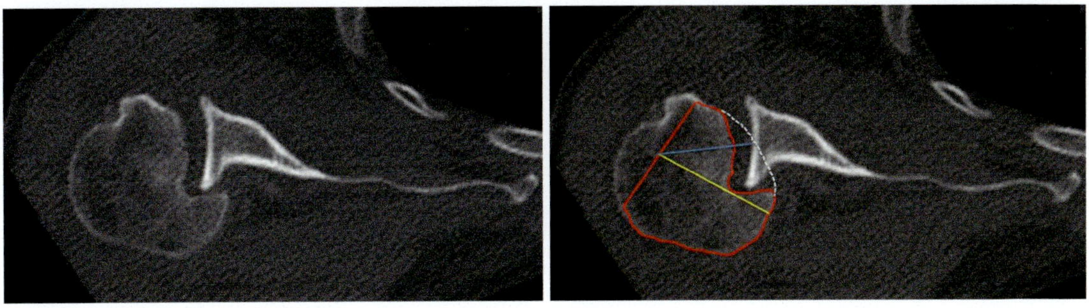

**Fig. 32.2** Determination of the size of the defect of the articular surface of the humeral head in axial sequences of a CT scan. The defect is marked with the white dashed line. According to Cicak it can be estimated by dividing the humeral head into a 25% (*blue line*) zone and a 50% (*yellow line*) zone. In this case the defect is about 30–40% of the articular surface

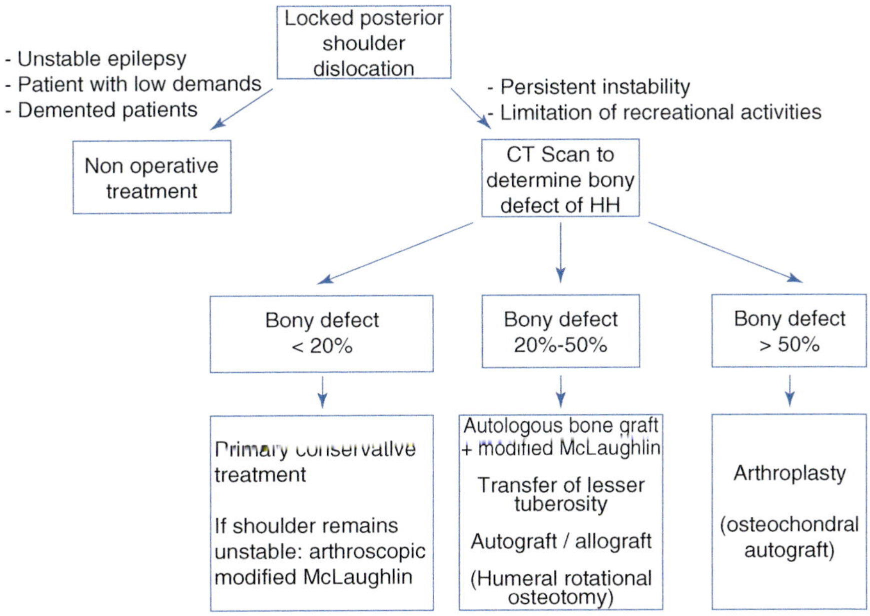


**Fig. 32.3** Treatment algorithm for LPSD

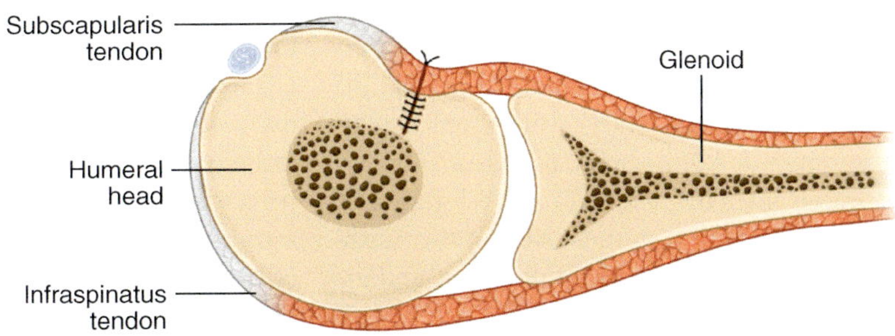


**Fig. 32.4** Modified McLaughlin procedure as described from Krackhardt et al. The subscapularis tendon is attached to the reverse Hill-Sachs lesion and protects the humeral head from engaging at the posterior glenoid rim in internal rotation of the arm

to reduce the dislocation and augment the humeral head through a deltopectoral approach.

### 32.4.1 Conservative Treatment

A locked posterior shoulder dislocation is often well tolerated due to little pain and little limitation of forward elevation allowing the performance of many activities of daily living. For this reason, nonoperative treatment must be considered in certain patients, including those with limited demands, uncontrolled seizures, or inability to comply with postoperative rehabilitation. Moreover, nonoperative management is considered first-line treatment in cases where closed reduction is performed early (within 3 weeks from dislocation), the shoulder appears stable with no further signs of re-dislocation, and the reverse Hill-Sachs lesion covers less than 20% of the articular surface of the humeral head.

In general, conservative treatment consists of immobilization of the shoulder in 10° of abduction and 15° of external rotation in a shoulder orthosis for 6 weeks; passive mobilization up to 60° of abduction and flexion can be performed during this time. Active-assisted mobilization starts 3 weeks after surgery. After 6 weeks, the range of motion is unrestricted, and further physiotherapy is advised to improve sensory-motor stability and scapulothoracic rhythm.

### 32.4.2 Operative Treatment

#### 32.4.2.1 Bony Defect <20% of the Articular Surface of the Humeral Head

As mentioned above, a PLSD with a bony defect of less than 20% can be primarily treated conservatively. If after nonoperative treatment the shoulder remains unstable, arthroscopic treatment is required. Arthroscopic posterior shoulder stabilization involves an anatomic restoration of the posterior labrum, a vertical shift of the posterior capsule, and a tenodesis of the subscapularis tendon into the reverse Hill-Sachs lesion (modified McLaughlin procedure). in cases where the defect of the humeral head engages with the glenoid rim. In general, the tenodesis is performed using suture anchors to secure the subscapularis tendon into the humeral defect (Fig. 32.4).

#### 32.4.2.2 Bony Defect 20–50% of the Articular Surface of the Humeral Head

A common treatment for bony defects of 20–50% is the transfer of the lesser tuberosity with the attached subscapularis tendon into the reverse Hill-Sachs lesion as described by Hughes and Neer [5]. They modified the method of McLaughlin [7] who originally described the transfer of the detached subscapularis tendon secured through drill holes in the humeral head. This modification allowed better bony filling of the defect and better reinsertion of the subscapularis tendon.

In cases of Malgaigne fractures of about 20–40% of the humeral surface, autologous bone grafts (e.g., from the iliac crest) are another reasonable method of reducing the impression fracture and providing a basement for the modified McLaughlin procedure, which should be performed additionally to restore stability (Fig. 32.5).

In reverse Hill-Sachs lesions of 40–50% with the absence of severe shoulder osteoarthritis, reconstruction with an allograft can be considered. Because most fixation techniques require sufficient bone stock in the humeral head, the application of this technique may be limited to younger patients without osteoporosis. In principle, allografts are able to restore the original curvature of the humeral head which is crucial for achieving good outcomes.

Rotational osteotomy of the proximal humerus as treatment for LPSD has also been described in the literature. The increased internal rotation thereby prevents the reverse Hill-Sachs defect engaging with the posterior glenoid rim throughout the entire range of movement. However, as this technique is technically difficult, results in a high percentage of osteoarthritis progression, and has a significant risk of humeral head necrosis, it should only be considered as a salvage procedure in young patients in whom the only other reasonable option would be total shoulder arthroplasty.

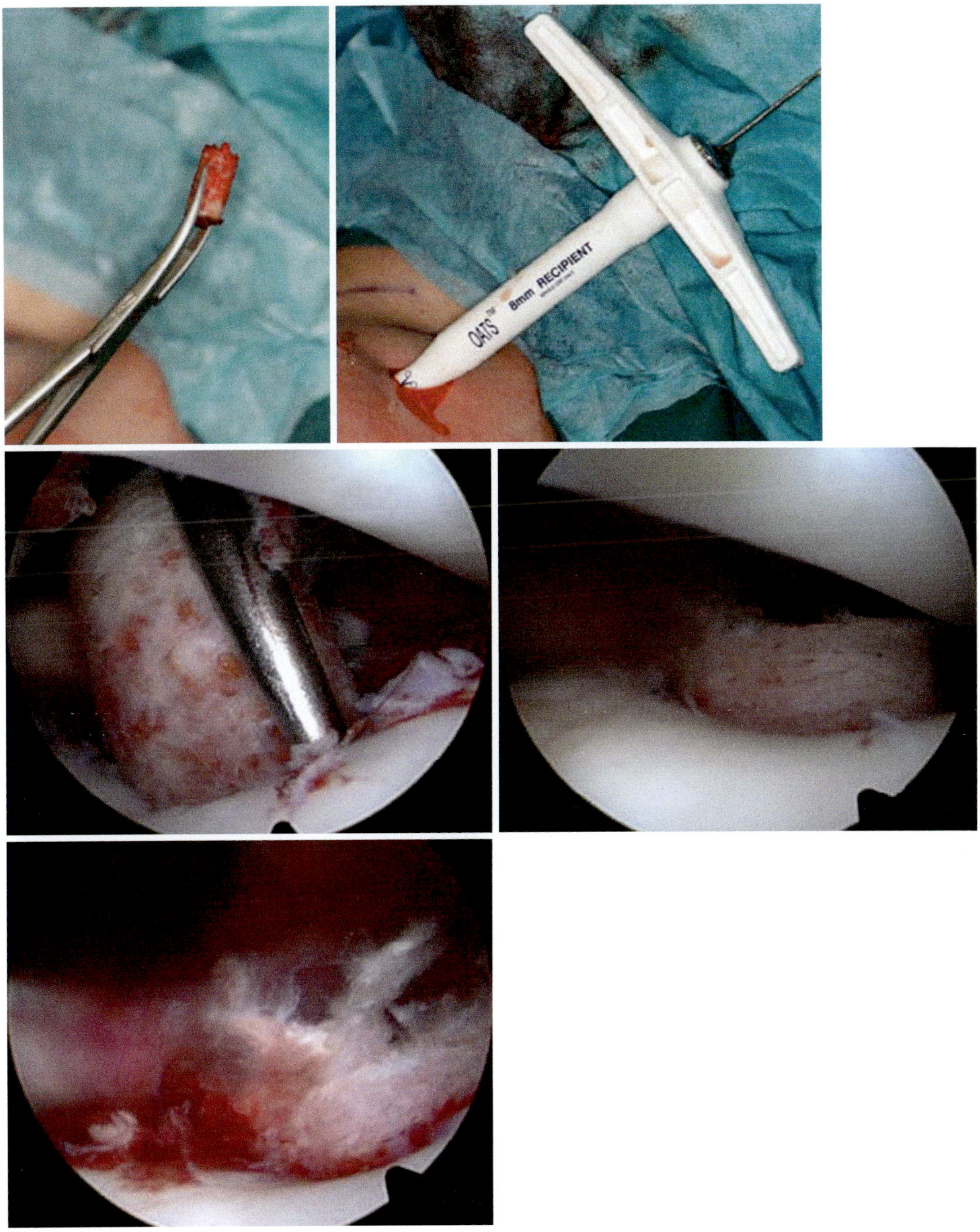


**Fig. 32.5** Autologous bone graft (e.g., from the iliac crest) is used to reduce the impression fracture and provide a basement for the modified McLaughlin procedure, which is performed arthroscopically to restore stability

#### 32.4.2.3 Bony Defect 50% of the Articular Surface of the Humeral Head

In elderly and nonathletic patients with humeral defects of more than 50%, a primary joint replacement is a suitable treatment option. Hemiarthroplasty, total shoulder arthroplasty, and reverse arthroplasty can be used. Hemiarthroplasty is only preferred when the glenoid shows no signs of osteo arthritis, total shoulder arthroplasty is preferred when considerable osteoarthritis exists, and reverse shoulder arthroplasty should be considered in patients with significant rotator cuff pathology.

Another possibility to restore the articular surface is the use of osteochondral autograft. It should only be used in young patients with bilateral acute posterior dislocation and bony defects of more than 50%. After removing the humeral head from one shoulder for implanting a prosthesis, the articular segment of the head can be used as osteochondral autograft and fixed into the reverse Hill-Sachs lesion of the other shoulder.

## 32.5 Results

LPSD is a rare injury; the management may be difficult and diagnosis is often delayed, making treatment even more challenging [8]. There are only a few studies with limited numbers of patients published in literature concerning treatment of LPSD; however, they indicate encouraging results.

Wolke et al. [11] reported on eight patients with acute LPSD who were treated conservatively after successful closed reduction within 14 days after the initial trauma. After 5-year follow-up, they demonstrated good to excellent clinical and radiological long-term results with no cases of recurrent instability. At final follow up, mean forward flexion of all patients included was 169°, mean external rotation 73° and mean internal rotation reached the 11th thoracic vertebra.

Krackhardt et al. [6] reported on 12 patients who were treated with the abovementioned modified McLaughlin procedure. There were no major complications, and there were no reported cases of recurrence of posterior dislocation after short-term follow-up.

Clinical and radiological results of seven patients with locked posterior shoulder dislocation with humeral head defects between 25 and 45% were presented by Banerjee et al. [2] All patients were treated with a lesser tuberosity transfer within 14 days after dislocation. After a mean follow-up of 41 months, all shoulders appeared stable; furthermore, although internal rotation was restricted in all patients, they classified their outcomes as good in one case and excellent in the remaining six cases. The mean Constant score achieved was 92 (range 80–98) with active pain-free abduction of 171°, mean flexion of 176°, and mean external rotation of 54.3°.

Sperling et al. [10] investigated the outcomes of total shoulder arthroplasty after LPSD. Twelve patients were followed up for a minimum of 5 years resulting in one excellent, six satisfactory, and five unsatisfactory results. Three patients underwent revision surgery in the early postoperative period due to recurrent posterior instability or component loosening.

## References


1. Arndt JH, Sears AD. Posterior dislocation of the shoulder. Am J Roentgenol Radium Ther Nucl Med. 1965;94:639–45.
2. Banerjee M, Balke M, Bouillon B, et al. Excellent results of lesser tuberosity transfer in acute locked posterior shoulder dislocation. Knee Surg Sports Traumatol Arthrosc. 2013;21(12):2884–8.
3. Cicak N. Posterior dislocation of the shoulder. J Bone Joint Surg Br. 2004;86(3):324–32.
4. Cisternino SJ, Rogers LF, Stufflebam BC, Kruglik GD. The trough line: a radiographic sign of posterior shoulder dislocation. AJR Am J Roentgenol. 1978;130(5):951–4.
5. Hughes M, Neer 2nd CS. Glenohumeral joint replacement and postoperative rehabilitation. Phys Ther. 1975;55(8):850–8.
6. Krackhardt T, Schewe B, Albrecht D, Weise K. Arthroscopic fixation of the subscapularis tendon in the reverse Hill-Sachs lesion for traumatic unidirectional posterior dislocation of the shoulder. Arthroscopy. 2006;22(2):227.e221–6.

7. Mc LH. Posterior dislocation of the shoulder. J Bone Joint Surg Am. 1952;24 A(3):584–90.
8. Paul J, Buchmann S, Beitzel K, Solovyova O, Imhoff AB. Posterior shoulder dislocation: systematic review and treatment algorithm. Arthroscopy. 2011; 27(11):1562–72.
9. Rowe CR, Zarins B. Chronic unreduced dislocations of the shoulder. J Bone Joint Surg Am. 1982;64(4): 494–505.
10. Sperling JW, Pring M, Antuna SA, Cofield RH. Shoulder arthroplasty for locked posterior dislocation of the shoulder. J Shoulder Elbow Surg. 2004;13(5):522–7.
11. Wolke J, Kruger D, Gerhardt C, Scheibel M. Conservative therapy of acute locked posterior shoulder dislocation: clinical and radiological long-term results. Unfallchirurg. 2014;117(12):1118–24.

# 33

# Chronic Locked Anterior and Posterior Dislocations

Felix H. Savoie and Michael O'Brien

## Contents

33.1 **Introduction** ..... 277
33.2 **Definition** ..... 277
33.3 **Patho-anatomy** ..... 278
33.4 **Clinical Evaluation** ..... 278
33.4.1 History ..... 278
33.4.2 Physical Examination ..... 278
33.5 **Imaging** ..... 279
33.6 **Treatment** ..... 279
33.6.1 Nonoperative Treatment ..... 279
33.6.2 Closed Reduction ..... 279
33.6.3 Surgical Intervention ..... 279
33.7 **Open Reduction and Repair: Anterior Dislocations** ..... 279
33.8 **Anatomic Restoration** ..... 280
33.8.1 Humeral Replacement ..... 281
33.9 **Chronic Posterior Dislocation** ..... 281
33.10 **Post OP Management** ..... 281
33.11 **Results** ..... 281
33.12 **Complications** ..... 282
**Conclusions** ..... 282
**References** ..... 282

F.H. Savoie (✉) • M. O'Brien
Tulane University, New Orleans, LA, USA
e-mail: fsavoie@tulane.edu

## 33.1 Introduction

Dislocation of the glenohumeral joint is a painful injury that requires immediate management. Failure to relocate the joint in a timely fashion usually results in significant destruction of the bone and cartilage of the joint, as well as severe contracture and scar formation in the soft tissues. The incidence of chronic dislocation is unknown, with most reports in the literature citing a limited number of cases. The management of these injuries may vary considerably based on the severity of the destruction.

## 33.2 Definition

There has been controversy over what actually defines a chronic dislocation, with the time frame varying from 24 h to 6 months. In this chapter, we will be addressing the shoulder that has been dislocated for more than 72 h, is irreducible by nonoperative means, and has fixed, severe bone and soft tissue damage that is not amenable to simple repair. In most cases this would mean the shoulder has been dislocated for a period of weeks to months [1, 2, 3, 4].

© ISAKOS 2017
A.B. Imhoff, F.H. Savoie III (eds.), *Shoulder Instability Across the Life Span*,
DOI 10.1007/978-3-662-54077-0_33

## 33.3 Patho-anatomy

In the chronic dislocation, there is much more to consider in the management of this severe injury. In both anterior and posterior dislocations, there is usually a severe bone defect on both the humeral and glenoid side. In anterior dislocations, the defects are usually equal on both sides of the joint and may include up to 1/2 the glenoid and humeral head. Posteriorly, the defect is usually much more severe on the humeral side. The bone of both the humeral head and the glenoid may be severely osteoporotic. The articular cartilage can be absent and thin or may have lost its connection to the subchondral bone and simply slip off the surface of the glenoid when tested. There is usually severe contracture and scar in the associated soft tissues. In posterior dislocations, the subscapularis may be shortened and scarred to the glenoid, while in anterior dislocations, the posterior rotator cuff and capsule will be contracted and fixed to the glenoid in such a way as to prevent the location of the humeral head after anterior soft tissue takedown.

In fixed posterior dislocations, the axillary nerve is at risk at the quadrangular space beneath the teres minor muscle and tendon during release. In the chronic anterior subcoracoid dislocations, the posterior cord of the brachial plexus may be scarred to the displaced humeral head.

## 33.4 Clinical Evaluation

Most patients with chronic dislocation present with only mild pain, but with significant loss of motion. In the early phases, the limitation of motion may be quite severe but will have improved over time due to scapula-thoracic compensation and, unfortunately, increase in the bone defects on the humerus and glenoid.

### 33.4.1 History

In this patient the history is quite an important factor. The initial time the patient noted dysfunction is essential, but interestingly may be quite unclear. Many cases are associated with other issues such as seizures, syncope, and polytrauma. In general chronic posterior dislocation, patients have been previously managed for their shoulder problem by medication or therapy for "stiff shoulder." In the anterior group, about 40% seem to be similarly associated with seizures, but less have had prior treatment.

These patients often have surprisingly little pain. The main complaints are loss of motion and function.

### 33.4.2 Physical Examination

**Inspection** Visualization of the undressed shoulder and comparison to the opposite side remains the hallmark of the physical examination. One will see a prominent acromion on the opposite side of the dislocation as well as significant muscle atrophy. The deltoid muscle is usually quite severely atrophied but can often be stimulated to contract unless there is concomitant posterior cord or axillary nerve injury.

**Palpation** The asymmetry is often easily confirmed by palpating the humeral head in the dislocated position. The posterior dislocation can be felt along the back of the shoulder distal to the acromion. There will also be a palpable defect lateral to a prominent coracoid process.

In the anterior dislocated shoulder, the humeral head will be palpable about the coracoid – indeed in many cases, it will be difficult to determine by palpation what is humeral head and what is coracoid. The acromion will be quite prominent posteriorly with a palpable defect distal to the prominent posterior acromion.

**Motion** In posterior dislocations, the most noticeable limitations are in external rotation. In the adducted position, external rotation will have a hard stop at −10 to 0. Flexion may be surprisingly good, up to 120°. In these patients movement is usually relatively painless.

In chronic anterior dislocations, the movement is more restricted in all planes and is often painful to testing. In attempting to ascertain the amount of passive motion available, the patient will often report neurologic symptoms.

## 33.5 Imaging

**Radiographs** It has been emphasized repeatedly the need for axillary views of the shoulder. Nonetheless, more than half of chronic posterior dislocation, patients will present after having had prior radiographs that were read as "normal" (Ref. Gerber, Sahajpal). It is of critical importance that the axillary and lateral scapular views be performed in all settings. Once the dislocation has become chronic, imaging is a bit more difficult but still helpful. In addition to the regular trauma series, we usually attempt to obtain a Bernageau view, which is most helpful in determining the severity of the bone defects.

**Advanced Imaging** In the younger (age <40) patient with a chronic dislocation, we usually request a CT scan with 3D reconstruction. The CT is most helpful in planning bone restoration, but is limited in its ability to discern significant soft tissue damage. Depending on the etiology, the amount of damage, and the potential surgical interventions, we may do an additional MRI scan. In the older patient, both tests are routinely performed. Shoulder arthroplasty is often considered as a primary surgical treatment option in these patients, and the degree of soft tissue and bone damage are equally important in the decision-making process for replacement surgery.

**Other Studies** In patients with severe atrophy, an EMG-NCS should be considered. The severe disuse of the shoulder is usually the cause of the muscle atrophy, but nerve injuries are frequent. A positive study for injury to the nerves should result in appropriate consultation prior to and during surgery.

## 33.6 Treatment

There are many options available in managing the chronically dislocated shoulder patient. Decision-making needs to consider not only the patho-anatomy but also the patient's pain and functional level and the ability of the surgeon to achieve a successful result. There is a high risk for complications and less than stellar results in the face of the severe damage to the joint.

### 33.6.1 Nonoperative Treatment

Often termed benign neglect, there are several reports in the literature that demonstrate satisfactory results with simply leaving the patient alone. This is usually considered after an extensive discussion with the patient and family. In patients with little to no pain and only relatively minor functional limitations, this may be the best option available. Similarly patients with severe medical problems and uncontrolled seizure disorder or who are unable to participate in the extensive postoperative rehabilitation may be considered for this treatment option.

### 33.6.2 Closed Reduction

There are reports of successful closed reduction of younger patients with relatively recent (less than 4 weeks) posterior dislocations. Although possible in the subacute setting, we feel the risks of increased bone damage and fracture as well as the potential for neurologic stretch injury preclude make this treatment perilous at best.

### 33.6.3 Surgical Intervention

Most of these patients require open reduction, significant soft tissue releases, capsule and tendon repair, and restoration of bone loss. The main factor in the decision-making process is whether to attempt to preserve the native glenohumeral joint or replace the humerus or the entire shoulder joint. This is often based on the status of the articular cartilage as well as the amount of subchondral bone damage on both sides of the joint, with patient age and desired activity playing a role in the preoperative decision-making.

## 33.7 Open Reduction and Repair: Anterior Dislocations

An anterior deltopectoral approach is utilized to expose the rotator cuff and displaced humeral head. The incision should be based on the AC joint and the axialla, as it may be difficult to palpate the coracoid process. It is better to find the deltopectoral interval near the clavicle and track it distally to separate these two muscles. Once the deltopectoral interval has been opened, the displaced humerus can be identified. It is important to then find the coracoid process and the attached conjoined tendon and carefully separate the tendons from the underlying skin. It is often difficult to find this tissue plane, so we often use the biceps to help define the anatomy. We usually find the biceps beneath the pec major tendon and use it to track up to the humeral head to better define the anatomy. There is often a contracture of the upper pectoralis major tendon, which can be released at this time. Identification of the biceps in the rotator interval allows easier definition of the tissue plane between the coracoid process, conjoined tendon, and the displaced humeral head. We try to preserve the coracoid and coracoacromial ligament during this initial dissection to help protect the neurovascular structures. It is quite important to define and preserve as much of the normal structures as possible before beginning the releases necessary to relocate the joint. Once the superior anatomy has been defined, we begin to very carefully dissect along the anterior subscapularis. In these chronic dislocations, the axillary and musculocutaneous nerves are often adhesed to the subscapularis and the brachial plexus – especially the posterior cord – and axillary artery and vein are quite close to the surgical field. In cases in which the anatomy is too distorted, we will do our coracoid osteotomy and then dissect distally to elevate the conjoined tendon off the displaced humerus and subscapularis.

Once the anatomy, especially the location of the plexus and axillary artery and vein are defined, a tenotomy of the subscapularis can be performed. It is often quite shortened, so careful anterior, superior, and posterior releases can be done at this time – the axillary nerve is along the inferior part. The subscapularis is split horizontally at its midpoint and both limbs reflected medially and inferiorly and is used to help protect the neurovascular structures. The humeral head is then visualized and inspected for integrity of the articular cartilage. Gentle distraction may separate it from the underlying glenoid, allowing it to "perch" on the anterior glenoid. At this point the bone loss of the glenoid can be directly evaluated. Rotation of the humeral head can provide the first direct view of the Hill-Sachs lesion, which may be quite large. The posterior capsule and rotator cuff must usually be released off the glenoid to allow the humeral head to be shifted into the center of the glenoid. The glenoid articular cartilage can then be evaluated.

## 33.8 Anatomic Restoration

In young individuals, we usually attempt to reconstruct the native joint. Preoperative planning usually means we have either a fresh osteochondral graft available for the glenoid and humeral head reconstruction, fresh frozen graft for the humeral head with plans to use the coracoid or distal clavicle for the glenoid, or else harvest iliac crest for both. At this point external rotation can expose the HS defect, allowing it to be measured and a graft fashioned to fit the defect. There are multiple options for sizing, including using bone wax or even polymethyl methacrylate. In most cases, we use femoral allograft, finding it to be stouter than the humeral grafts. We recommend using an osteotome or burr to freshen the defect, and then the shaped allograft can be press fit into the defect. Multiple bone options exist, including the coracoid, the distal clavicle, the iliac crest, and fresh osteochondral allograft. Once this has been shaped, tapped into place, and fixated with screws, attention can be directed toward the glenoid.

Anatomic restoration of the glenoid is one of the main keys to successful restoration of stability. The bone loss is usually severe, and in some cases, the coracoid may not be sufficient. This can be determined on the preoperative CT scan and appropriate alternatives considered. In each case, the glenoid is evaluated intraoperatively and the bone graft obtained and stabilized to the residual glenoid. Once adequate bone has been restored to the humeral head and the glenoid, soft tissue reconstruction can begin.

If there is any remaining capsule and labrum, it can be repaired at this time. It has been my experience that is these chronic dislocations the capsule is often nonexistent or too scared to be of much use.

The lower half of the subscapularis is then retrieved from under the conjoined tendon and reattached to the humerus, shifting it superiorly if possible. The upper half is retrieved over the transferred coracoid and its attachment shifted slightly inferiorly to create a T capsular shift on the humerus. The rotator interval is closed to the upper segment and the shoulder tested for motion and stability.

### 33.8.1 Humeral Replacement

In many cases, the humerus is often too damaged to allow anatomic restoration, or the articular cartilage is simply missing. In some cases, it may appear to be in place and viable and a small "push" will separate it from the underlying bone. In these cases, a humeral head replacement should be performed. In this chronic anterior dislocation setting, the soft tissue dissection and glenoid restoration are the same. We place the humerus in 40° of retroversion in order to lessen the risk of recurrent anterior dislocation and often use a smaller humeral head to facilitate motion.

## 33.9 Chronic Posterior Dislocation

In the fixed posterior dislocation, the bone damage is often less severe than in the anterior variant. The glenoid is usually fairly well preserved, and the humeral defect more localized. In many cases, the patient may have reasonable function so one must be careful not to worsen the shoulder.

The initial step once the patient is asleep is to carefully try to reduce the shoulder under fluoroscopic control. Unlike the anterior dislocations, these often can be gently extracted and reduced.

Positioning of the patient is critical as one must be ready for both anterior and posterior approaches. We also like to have the arthroscope available for some intra-articular work if necessary.

The initial approach is the same as anterior, a deltopectoral approach. In these cases, it is best to find the coracoid first and then track the coracoacromial ligament up to the acromion and then follow across the top of the humerus to the back of the shoulder. The bicipital groove can then be located as a guide to the rotator interval. The interval can be split and the glenoid evaluated. The subscapularis should then be carefully tenotomized or removed with a portion of the lessor tuberosity to expose the GH joint more completely. An elevator can then be used to disengage the anterior Hill-Sachs deformity from the glenoid and elevate the humerus, allowing it to reduce.

In many cases of chronic posterior dislocation, the glenoid may not be deficient. In these cases, transfer of the subscapularis into the anterior Hill-Sachs defect ( McLaughlin procedure) with or without using the bone of the lessor tuberosity (Neer modification) may be all that is needed.

In those cases with more damage, a posterior approach to repair the posterior Bankart lesion with or without added bone graft from the iliac crest or distal clavicle may be useful. Alternatively the subscapularis can be transferred, the rotator interval closed, and arthroscopy performed to repair the posterior damage.

Humeral head replacement is utilized similar to the anterior cases. Less retroversion (10–20°) may be utilized to lessen the risk of recurrent instability.

## 33.10 Post OP Management

The patient is placed in a gunslinger brace or pillow sling for 4 weeks to allow the soft tissues to heal. Rehabilitation without stretching and emphasizing correct posture are then performed for 4–6 weeks; if the shoulder remains stable, stretching and strengthening are continued until functions is satisfactory.

## 33.11 Results

The results in general are satisfactory but not excellent. The results of chronic posterior dislocations are discussed in another chapter. In the fixed, chronic anterior dislocation, the results are surprisingly similar between benign neglect, relocations with bone restoration, and humeral replacement. Most reports on benign neglect are relatively older literature and focus more on pain relief. Several reports on open reduction and bone restoration exist, but literature remains limited. Flatow et al. reported on a group of humeral replacements with satisfactory results.

## 33.12 Complications

Motion loss, heterotopic ossification, recurrent dislocation, and brachial plexopathy have all been reported as complications of this procedure.

**Conclusion**

Chronic dislocation of the shoulder remains a difficult problem requiring extraordinary care. In relatively inactive patients, benign neglect may provide satisfactory results. In other cases, bone restoration to both the humeral head and glenoid may be possible, while in other cases replacement surgery may provide better results. Careful assessment of the status of the articular cartilage and the amount of bone damage are necessary to make the correct choice in corrective surgery.

## References

1. Flatlow EL, Miller SR, Neer CS 2nd. Chronic anterior dislocation of the shoulder. J Shoulder Elbow Surg. 1993;2(1):2–10. PMID: 22959291.
2. Gerber C, Hersche O, Farron A. Isolated rupture of the subscapularis tendon. J Bone Joint Surg Am. 1996;78(7):1015–23. PMID: 8698718.
3. Rowe CR, Zarins B. Chronic unreduced dislocations of the shoulder. J Bone Joint Surg Am, 1982;64(4):494–505. PMID: 7068692.
4. Sahajpal DT, Zuckerman JD. Chronic glenohumeral dislocation. J Am Acad Orthop Surg. 2008;16(7):385–98. PMID: 18611996.

# Brachial Plexus Injuries and Rotator Cuff Tears with Dislocations

34

Kevin D. Plancher, Joseph Ajdinovich, and Stephanie C. Petterson

## Contents

| | | |
|---|---|---|
| 34.1 | **Anatomy** | 284 |
| 34.2 | **Examination and Imaging** | 284 |
| 34.3 | **Indication and Technique for Surgery** | 285 |
| 34.3.1 | Release at the Spinoglenoid Notch | 285 |
| 34.3.2 | Release at the Transverse Scapular Ligament | 286 |
| 34.4 | **Specific Points in Rehabilitation** | 287 |
| 34.5 | **Results** | 287 |
| 34.6 | **Complications and Tips to Avoid** | 287 |
| **Conclusion** | | 287 |
| **References** | | 288 |

A myriad of associated shoulder pathologies have been described when considering the entire spectrum of instability leading to untoward functional consequences when underappreciated or unnoticed. One such association, concomitant rotator cuff tear (RCT), is influenced by patient age and history of prior instability or ligamentous laxity with rates as high as 27–100% [1–5]. Nerve injuries associated with shoulder dislocations are often the result of traction of the nerve over the head of the humerus or a result of manipulative reduction of the dislocation [6]. Nerve injuries occur in 19–55% of anterior shoulder dislocations, leading to possible paresis and inability to move the arm [6, 7]. The position of the arm and the time of dislocation dictate where the nerve lesion may occur. A position of internal rotation and abduction causes tension on all nerves and cords, whereas, positions of elbow and wrist extension cause tension on the medial cord and median nerve, and if the elbow is flexed, the medial and posterior cords are placed under tension along with the ulnar and radial nerves [6, 8, 9].

The most common nerve injury in anterior shoulder dislocations is injury to the axillary nerve due to its close proximity to the glenohumeral joint. Typically, associated deficits (e.g., deltoid weakness, sensory disturbance below the shoulder) are transient and resolve within 3–12 months of the initial injury with conservative treatment in 85–100% of cases [6, 7]. Recently, increased

K.D. Plancher (✉) • S.C. Petterson
Department of Orthopaedic Surgery, Albert Einstein College of Medicine, New York, USA
e-mail: kplancher@plancherortho.com

J. Ajdinovich
Orthopaedic Foundation and Plancher Orthopaedics and Sports Medicine, Stamford, CT, USA

© ISAKOS 2017
A.B. Imhoff, F.H. Savoie III (eds.), *Shoulder Instability Across the Life Span*,
DOI 10.1007/978-3-662-54077-0_34

awareness has focused on brachial plexus injuries, specifically, the suprascapular nerve (SSN). Lesions of the SSN are often the result of extreme positions of shoulder abduction and are the most frequent lesions described in the proximal brachial plexus with shoulder dislocation [10]. We believe the association between both RCT and SSN injury in the setting of instability merits a better understanding to guide treatment algorithms and avoid iatrogenic injury.

## 34.1 Anatomy

As the anatomy of the rotator cuff musculature itself has been covered in detail in prior chapters, this chapter will only focus on the role of the rotator cuff in stability and anatomic discussion of the SSN [11, 12].

The SSN is a mixed sensory - sending fibers to both the glenohumeral and acromioclavicular joint - and motor nerve. It arises from the brachial plexus at the level of the superior trunk with contributions from the fifth to sixth cervical roots, with up to 50% of people receiving contributions from C4 as well [13]. The nerve exits the posterior triangle of the neck between the sternocleidomastoid and trapezius muscles and descends on the anterior aspect of the trapezius. It then descends further along the upper border of the scapula alongside the suprascapular artery toward the suprascapular notch. Upon arrival at the notch, the artery and nerve diverge, with the artery coursing above the transverse scapular ligament, while the nerve maintains its course beneath the ligament. Typically, the first motor branch of the nerve to the supraspinatus arises at this point with some minor variations both just proximal and distal to the notch [14]. After passing through the suprascapular notch, the nerve then passes obliquely beneath the supraspinatus muscle, toward the spinoglenoid notch, passing within 20 mm of the glenoid rim [15]. Above the nerve at the level of the spinoglenoid notch lies the inferior transverse scapular, or spinoglenoid, ligament with fibers extending from the lateral aspect of the scapular spine to the posterior aspect of the glenoid and glenohumeral joint capsule. After making the turn around the scapular spine, the nerve gives off three to four motor branches to the infraspinatus muscle belly.

Understanding of the anatomy of the SSN becomes essential when considering the relationship between RCTs and concomitant SSN injuries. Albritton et al. demonstrated that the acuity of the SSN takeoff at its first motor branch at the level of the suprascapular notch increased from 143° in an intact cuff to 98.7° with as little as 1 cm of retraction. As expected, even further levels of retraction, present in chronic tears, lead to even more dramatic angles with the nerve taking a 47° or 35° turn with cuff retraction of 3 cm and 5 cm, respectively [14]. Retraction beyond 2 cm in this cadaveric study provides a possible explanation for the degree of atrophy and fatty changes in the muscle belly with massively retracted tears [16].

One recent multicenter, prospective study attempted to establish a direct correlation between suprascapular neuropathy and fatty infiltration of cuff musculature. Eighty-seven shoulders suspected of suprascapular neuropathy were enrolled and underwent both electromyography/nerve conduction velocity (EMG/NCV) testing and magnetic resonance imaging (MRI). On MRI, cuff musculature was graded according to the Goutallier system, and notation was made regarding the continuity and quality of the tendons. Of the 87 shoulders tested, 32 were found to have objective findings on EMG/NCV consistent with suprascapular neuropathy. A significant association was found between degree of tendon pathology and fatty degeneration (*P* value <0.001), with more severe tendon pathologies correlating with an increasing degree of fatty atrophy. Infraspinatus tendon tears were found to be associated with suprascapular neuropathy ($P = -.01$) [17]. The association seen between infraspinatus tears and suprascapular neuropathy may imply an insult at the level of the spinoglenoid notch, making the spinoglenoid ligament to release a more enticing option in this instance.

## 34.2 Examination and Imaging

Clinical examination, in the setting of instability with suspicion of SSN injury, should assess joint stability, integrity of the cuff musculature, and neurovascular status of the limb, no different than a standard shoulder examination. Findings can be somewhat nebulous when suprascapular neuropathy is expected, especially in the setting of coexisting rotator cuff disease. Periscapular muscle wasting in both the supraspinatus and infraspinatus fossa should prompt consideration for such pathology, though this can also be present in the individual with chronic, massive RTC. Tenderness to palpation might be appreciated either over the suprascapular notch or posterosuperiorly in the region of the spinoglenoid notch. Weakness in external rotation with the arm at the side is often painless, as the sensory portion of the nerve can be unaffected when the pathology originates at the spinoglenoid notch.

The cross-arm adduction test should also be utilized as a means of discerning pathology originating in the area of the spinoglenoid notch. A study published by the senior author demonstrated that the highest pressures measured at the spinoglenoid notch arose in positions of late follow-through or the position of the greatest adduction [18]. Typically patients with positive findings will demonstrate pain in the posterior shoulder in the absence of any findings on plain shoulder imaging, and intra-articular injection of lidocaine into the AC joint can also be used to rule out AC arthralgia.

In the case of uncertain diagnosis without evidence of muscle wasting, diagnostic injections can also be of benefit, as both the suprascapular and spinoglenoid notches can be reached with percutaneous injections in the office setting. The suprascapular notch can be reached via a posterosuperior approach, with an insertion point 3 cm medial to Nevaiser's portal with a trajectory toward the acromion. The spinoglenoid notch can be approached in a direct, posterior fashion, from a point 4 cm medial to the posterolateral corner of the acromion, just inferior to the scapular spine.

EMG/NCV is often of limited use. Due to the dynamic nature of the ligamentous anatomy, positive findings may be lacking despite underlying SSN pathology [19]. EMG/NCV is particularly important in the young patient with an acute massive RCT and/or if symptoms persist beyond 3 weeks [6]. MRI studies will invariably be obtained in the setting of instability with suspicion for rotator cuff pathology and are indispensable for operative planning; however, their utility for further planning in the case of suspected nerve injury is limited and saves the rare occasion of a pre-existing mass lesion in the area of the spinoglenoid or suprascapular notches or unexpected fatty atrophy in the setting of an acute cuff tear. Such findings would be a strong indication for additional decompression of the offending site at the time of the cuff repair/stabilization procedure.

## 34.3 Indication and Technique for Surgery

In the setting of combined instability with RTC and SSN injury, each component of the pathology should be treated according to its own merit. Typically, in the author's practice, instability cases are treated with arthroscopic Bankart repair with a modified inferior capsular shift [20]. Rotator cuff repairs are performed arthroscopically as well, though the exact construct of the repair depends on the anatomy of the tear (e.g., pattern, level of retraction, chronicity, and quality of tissue). Thus, we will largely cover the cases of suspected or documented SSN involvement post dislocation. It is the author's preference to conduct the endoscopic release of the spinoglenoid ligament prior to the commencement of any intra-articular work in the glenohumeral joint.

### 34.3.1 Release at the Spinoglenoid Notch

Endoscopic release of the SSN at the level of the spinoglenoid notch is best approached in a direct, posterior fashion. Intraoperatively, we utilize two primary extra-articular portals placed just inferior to the scapular spine: (1) the viewing portal 8 cm medial to the posterolateral corner of the acromion and (2) a working portal 4 cm from the posterolateral corner of the acromion.

A blunt trocar is first inserted into the viewing portal straight toward the infraspinatus fossa. The soft tissue under the scapular spine is gently swept away as the trocar is progressively directed toward the working portal before passing above the SSN and finally dropping into the spinoglenoid notch. It is important to note that a key step in this process, for visualization, involves the sweeping motion utilized to clear tissue from the curved undersurface of the scapular spine.

The arthroscope is then inserted into the viewing portal in order to first visualize the spinoglenoid ligament as well as the various anatomic landmarks. One must maintain adequate visualization of the spine of the scapula to ensure a successful ligament release and nerve decompression.

Once adequate visualization is obtained, attention is turned to the working portal, through which, after localization with a spinal needle, the blunt trocar is introduced. At this point, the soft tissue can be teased away from the lateral aspect of the SSN, easily localizable at the medal aspect of the spinoglenoid notch. Once this plane is developed, a radiofrequency wand or a small-radius nonaggressive shaver, with suction off, can be used to clear the tissue and specifically isolate the spinoglenoid ligament. Once clearly identified, the ligament may be resected by following along the scapular spine to avoid bleeding. Once released from the spine, the ligament can then be traced to its insertion at the glenohumeral joint to appreciate its anatomy and visually confirm complete resection.

### 34.3.2 Release at the Transverse Scapular Ligament

When releasing the SSN at the TSL, a lateral subacromial portal and an anterolateral portal are utilized in addition to a portal made from outside-in first with an 18-gauge spinal needle 3 cm medial to Nevaiser's portal ensuring that the portal is anterior to the supraspinatus leading edge. The portal is approximately 6–8 cm medial to the anterolateral border of the acromion in between the clavicle and scapular spine. The arthroscope is then introduced into the subacromial space, and a subacromial decompression is completed to allow for adequate visualization. The arthroscope is moved midway to 2/3 of the way posterior along the lateral edge of the acromion or may be placed at the posterolateral corner. The shaver is introduced in a new portal created at the anterolateral edge of the acromion. This portal should be placed as close to the acromion as possible. This entry point will allow for adequate clearance of all soft tissue necessary to complete this operation.

Identification of the various landmarks is completed with the aid of 18-gauge spinal needles. One spinal needle is placed in the center of the AC joint, and a second needle is placed in Nevaiser's portal. The shaver releases the coracoacromial ligament laterally during a subacromial decompression and follows its medial side to the coracoid. Soft tissue is either ablated with a radiofrequency device or removed with a mechanical shaver, but ensuring hemostasis and perfect visualization is maintained throughout the procedure. The leading or anterior edge of the supraspinatus is always maintained in view while proceeding to release the transverse scapular ligament. Upon arriving at the coracoid, the coracoclavicular ligaments are identified first, then laterally the trapezoid, and subsequently the conoid or more medial ligament. The conoid is always more posterior in position, and there is usually an area of fat surrounding this ligament. It is recommended to clear this space with the use of a radiofrequency wand. The spinal needle placed in the AC joint will remind the surgeon of the location of conoid ligament, and the needle in Nevaiser's portal will keep visualization in the correct orientation as the arthroscope is placed more medially as the operation continues. The key to a successful operation is understanding that the most medial border of the conoid ligament is the most lateral attachment of the transverse scapular ligament. If the surgeon stays anterior to the supraspinatus, finding the transverse scapular ligament will not be difficult, but if the arthroscope strays posteriorly, then identification becomes more difficult.

An additional portal is now made upon recognition of the conoid ligament. The 18-gauge spinal needle is introduced 3 cm medial to Nevaiser's portal, and soft tissue is cleared up to this area. Rotation of the arthroscope to look down will identify the artery and/or vein normally lying over the transverse scapular ligament. The outside-in technique allows for a safety factor, and a skin incision is made large enough to introduce the blunt obturator from the arthroscope that will aid in gently pushing away tissue to visualize the transverse scapular ligament and the suprascapular nerve. The blunt obturator will retract the supraspinatus muscle and fat posteriorly which will allow for an excellent view of the transverse scapular ligament, suprascapular artery, and suprascapular nerve. The obturator is then positioned to displace the nerve more medially so that the transverse scapular ligament is isolated. We then make a small incision in the skin and place an arthroscopic scissor in the anatomic position to divide the transverse scapular ligament close to the bone. If the ligament is calcified, we have used a lambotte osteotome in the past through this second small incision. A 3.5 mm burr or small 3.5 mm full-radius shaver may be used safely to smooth any osteophytes that may be encountered. The blunt tip trocar is utilized to assess the mobility and adequate release of the suprascapular nerve.

## 34.4 Specific Points in Rehabilitation

In the author's practice, rehabilitation for isolated release of the SSN involves a week of postoperative sling usage, followed by progressive strengthening, and range of motion. Thus, in cases involving cuff repair and instability, rehabilitation time frames are dictated by the individual surgeon's protocols for cuff repair and stabilization procedures. When rehab is instituted, however, it is important to emphasize early cross-arm stretching, followed later by posterior capsule stretching exercises to prevent recurrence of constriction at the spinoglenoid notch.

## 34.5 Results

As it pertains to isolated SSN release, the author currently has a case series of 13 recreational athletes from age 20 to 56 consisting of 11 males and 2 females. All patients have undergone a pain-free return to sports such as yoga, weightlifting, and martial arts without any incidences of recurrence. No complications have yet to be reported.

## 34.6 Complications and Tips to Avoid

While no complications have yet been noted in the author's series, knowledge of the anatomy at both the suprascapular and spinoglenoid notches remains of paramount importance. Time and care must be taken to adequately expose and identify all surgical landmarks to avoid iatrogenic injury to the SSN and artery. Restoration of the native cuff anatomy will also minimize risk of undue tension on the nerve at both notches. By moving an infraspinatus tendon tear both superiorly and laterally during repair, tension of the SSN at the base of the scapular spine can be minimized. One study demonstrated this effect in patients with massive cuff tears who displayed partial or full recovery of nerve function on EMG/NCV and improvement in pain and function [21]. However, it is important to remember that excessive tendon advancement can cause tension on the SSN at the suprascapular notch [19]; therefore, cuff lateralization greater than 3 cm should be avoided [16].

**Conclusion**

In summary, SSN decompression is a safe and effective way to manage pathology of the SSN at both the suprascapular and spinoglenoid notch. In the setting of instability, RCT, and SSN injury, the author applies an age-based algorithm. Combined arthroscopic Bankart repair, rotator cuff repair, and SSN release is considered in the active patient aged 40–60 years especially when atrophy is observed at either the supraspinatus or infraspinatus fossa. If the patient is greater than 60 years old and presents with a massive, retracted, but repairable cuff tear, he or she will undergo a rotator cuff repair with release of the transverse scapular ligament to avoid iatrogenic tensioning of the nerve at the suprascapular notch. If, however, the tear is deemed irreparable, concerns regarding the tension of the first motor branch of the SSN lead the author to believe that endoscopic release of the spinoglenoid ligament is merited to provide the nerve the greatest chance for recovery.

## References


1. Antonio GE, Griffith JF, Yu AB, Yung PS, Chan KM, Ahuja AT. First-time shoulder dislocation: high prevalence of labral injury and age-related differences revealed by MR arthrography. J Magn Reson Imaging. 2007;26(4):983–91.
2. Simank HG, Dauer G, Schneider S, Loew M. Incidence of rotator cuff tears in shoulder dislocations and results of therapy in older patients. Arch Orthop Trauma Surg. 2006;126(4):235–40.
3. Araghi A, Prasarn M, St Clair S, Zuckerman JD. Recurrent anterior glenohumeral instability with onset after forty years of age: the role of the anterior mechanism. Bull Hosp Joint Dis. 2005;62(3–4):99–101.
4. Atef A, El-Tantawy A, Gad H, Hefeda M. Prevalence of associated injuries after anterior shoulder dislocation: a prospective study. Int Orthop. 2016;40(3):519–24. doi:10.1007/s00264-015-2862-z. Epub 2015 Jul 2.
5. Voigt C, Lill H. Shoulder instability and rotator cuff tear. Orthopade. 2009;38(1):70–4.
6. Visser CPJ, Coene LNJEM, Brand R, Tavy DLG. The incidence of nerve injury in anterior dislocation of the shoulder and its influence on functional recovery. JBJS Br. 1999;81:679–85.
7. Safran MR. Nerve injury about the shoulder in athletes, Part 1: suprascapular nerve and axillary nerve. Am J Sports Med. 2004;32(3):803–19.
8. Coene LNJEM. Axillary nerve lesions and associated injuries. Leiden: Thesis. 1985.
9. Kleinrensink GJ. Influence of posture and motion on peripheral nerve tension. Rotterdam: Thesis. 1997.
10. Coene LN. Mechanisms of brachial plexus lesions. Clin Neurol Neurosurg. 1993;95:24–9. (Zoltan JD. Injury to the SSN associated with anterior dislocation of the shoulder: case report and review of the literature. J Trauma. 1979;19:203–6.
11. Kelkar R, Wang VM, Flatow EL, Newton PM, Ateshian GA, Bigliani LU, Pawluk RJ, Mow VC. Glenohumeral mechanics: a study of articular geometry, contact, and kinematics. JSES. 2001;10(1):73–84.
12. Lee SB, Kim KJ, O'Driscoll SW, Morrey BF, An KN. Dynamic glenohumeral stability provided by the rotator cuff muscles in the mid-range and end-range of motion: a study in cadavers. JBJS Am. 2000;82:849–57.
13. Leung S, Zlotolow DA, Kozin SH, Abzug JM. Surgical anatomy of the supraclavicular brachial plexus. J Bone Joint Surg Am. 2015;97(13):1067–73.
14. Albritton MJ, Graham RD, Richards RS, Basamania CJ. An anatomic study of the effects on the suprascapular nerve due to retraction of the supraspinatus muscle after a rotator cuff tear. JSES. 2003;12(5):497–500.
15. Warner JP, Krushell RJ, Masquelet A, Gerber C. Anatomy and relationships of the suprascapular nerve: anatomical constraints to mobilization of the supraspinatus and infraspinatus muscles in the management of massive rotator-cuff tears. J Bone Joint Surg Am. 1992;74(1):36–45.
16. Greiner A, Golser K, Wambacher M, Kralinger F, Sperner G. The course of the suprascapular nerve in the supraspinatus fossa and its vulnerability in muscle advancement. J Shoulder Elbow Surg. 2003;12(3):256–9.
17. Shi LL, Boykin RE, Lin A, Warner JJ. Association of suprascapular neuropathy with rotator cuff tendon tears and fatty degeneration. J Shoulder Elbow Surg. 2014;23(3):339–46.
18. Luke TA, Rovner AD, Karas SG, Hawkins RJ, Plancher KD. Volumetric change in the shoulder capsule after open inferior capsular shift versus arthroscopic thermal capsular shrinkage: a cadaveric model. J Shoulder Elbow Surg. 2004;13(2):146–9.
19. Collin P et al. Neuropathy of the suprascapular nerve and massive rotator cuff tears: a prospective electromyographic study. J Shoulder Elbow Surg. 2014;23(1):28–34.
20. Plancher KD, Petterson SC. Arthroscopic Bankart repair with suture anchors: tips for success. Oper Tech Sports Med. 2013;21(4):192–200.
21. Costouros JG, Porramatikul M, Lie DT, Warner JJ. Reversal of suprascapular neuropathy following arthroscopic repair of massive supraspinatus rotator cuff tears. Arthroscopy. 2007;23(11):1152–61.

# Part VI

# Complications

# Complications After Instability Surgery

# 35

Andrew J. Sheean and Stephen S. Burkhart

## Contents


| | | |
|---|---|---|
| 35.1 | **Introduction** | 291 |
| 35.2 | **General Complications** | 291 |
| 35.2.1 | Stiffness | 291 |
| 35.2.2 | Infection | 292 |
| 35.3 | **Arthroscopic Stabilization Complications** | 293 |
| 35.3.1 | Nerve Injury | 293 |
| 35.3.2 | Chondrolysis | 293 |
| 35.3.3 | Anchor-Related Complications | 294 |
| 35.3.4 | Recurrent Instability | 294 |
| 35.4 | **Open Stabilization Procedure Complications** | 295 |
| 35.4.1 | Nerve Injury Associated with the Latarjet Procedure | 295 |
| 35.4.2 | Malpositioned Coracoid Graft | 295 |
| **Conclusion** | | 296 |
| **References** | | 296 |



A.J. Sheean, MD
San Antonio Military Medical Center (SAMMC), San Antonio, Texas, USA

S.S. Burkhart, MD (✉)
The San Antonio Orthopaedic Group, Burkhart Research Institute for Orthopaedics (BRIO), San Antonio, Texas, USA
e-mail: ssburkhart@msn.com



© ISAKOS 2017



A.B. Imhoff, F.H. Savoie III (eds.), *Shoulder Instability Across the Life Span*,
DOI 10.1007/978-3-662-54077-0_35


## 35.1 Introduction

Glenohumeral instability is a common condition treated by shoulder surgeons. Given the scope of pathology (generalized ligamentous laxity, deranged capsuloligamentous tissues, osseous abnormalities of the glenoid, and humeral head) implicated in this condition, a variety of open and arthroscopic treatment tactics have been described, and each is associated with unique complications [18, 19, 41, 55, 56]. A thorough history and physical exam, as well as a critical analysis of all available imaging to ascertain the presence of both soft tissue and osseous abnormalities, are crucial when evaluating the patient with glenohumeral instability. Failure to address all of the causes of shoulder instability is perhaps the most widely recognized cause of suboptimal surgical outcomes, and a number of authors have reported on the clinical ramifications of a failure to diagnose and treat all coexisting pathologies [4, 8, 23, 27, 33, 36, 51]. The purpose of this chapter is to provide a synopsis of the relevant literature and a concise update on the complications associated with shoulder stabilization surgery.

## 35.2 General Complications

### 35.2.1 Stiffness

Restriction in external rotation range of motion has been reported following both arthroscopic and open stabilization procedures. Although notably higher rates of stiffness have been observed in the setting of open repairs and revision stabilization surgery, certain arthroscopic procedures can result in significant decreases in external rotation range of motion [26, 29]. In particular, biomechanical data suggest that arthroscopic remplissage commonly results in supraphysiologic shoulder stiffness, and decrements in external rotation can have notable implications on shoulder function [22]. Garcia et al. recently reported that among 50 patients treated with arthroscopic remplissage at a mean follow-up of 60.7 months, 65.5% (19 of 29) of patients reported problems throwing a ball, which was attributable to deficits in external rotation [14]. In the case of an elite, overhead thrower, the surgeon would be wise to carefully balance the goal of treating recurrent instability with the expected decrements in shoulder external rotation associated with remplissage or open stabilization procedures, such as the Latarjet procedure [42]. Conversely, a loss of external rotation would be of less concern for a non-throwing, collision athlete, in whom these decrements would be less likely to impact his ability to return to sport. In this sense, one patient's "complication"—in the case of the overhead thrower, stiffness—is another patient's treatment success, and the surgeon is well served to fully consider these important nuances when determining the optimal surgical tactic.

### 35.2.2 Infection

The incidence of deep infection associated with arthroscopic shoulder stabilization is an exceedingly rare complication as evidenced by a recent review of 9385 arthroscopic procedures, which documented a 0.0016% (15 out of 9385) infection rate [47]. Infection following open stabilization procedures is also relatively uncommon as well. However, higher infection rates ranging from 0.04 to 6% have been reported in association with open procedures [34, 50]. *Propionibacterium acnes*—a gram-positive, non-spore-forming anaerobic bacillus—has become an increasingly recognized pathogen in infections related to both arthroscopic and open shoulder surgery, especially in the setting of a subacute presentation. These infections are seldom associated with draining wounds and/or markedly elevated inflammatory indices. Although more commonly reported in the setting of shoulder arthroplasty, *P. acnes* infections should be considered as a potential cause of insidious, protracted postoperative shoulder pain [24, 39].

Several recent reports based upon large patient registries have identified risk factors for infection and certain steps surgeons can take to mitigate the occurrence of this complication. As is typical throughout orthopedic surgery, obesity is an independent risk factor for infection in shoulder arthroscopy. Using data amassed from the National Surgical Quality Improvement Program database, Sing et al. reviewed 15,589 patients' records that underwent arthroscopic shoulder surgery between 2011 and 2013. Obese patients (6684, 43%) were found to have a significantly higher risk of superficial surgical site infection ($P = 0.015$) when compared to a nonobese cohort [53]. Besides obesity, Werner et al. observed significantly higher rates of infection among 7089 patients that had received an injection within 3 months of arthroscopy (0.7%; odds ratio [OR] 2.2; $P < 0.001$) compared to controls without injection within 3 months of arthroscopy [57]. In order to determine the optimal surgical site preparation method, Saltzman et al. examined the efficacy of various skin preparation solutions on eradicating bacteria from the shoulder. These authors compared culture results obtained before and after shoulders prepared with three randomly selected solutions: ChloraPrep (2% chlorhexidine gluconate and 70% isopropyl alcohol), DuraPrep (0.7% iodophor and 74% isopropyl alcohol), or povidone-iodine scrub and paint (0.75% iodine scrub and 1.0% iodine paint). Positive culture rates for the ChloraPrep group were significantly lower (7%) than either povidone-iodine group (31%) ($P < 0.0001$) or the DuraPrep group (19%) ($P = 0.01$). Of note, there were no significant differences in the ability of any of the tested preparations to eliminate *P. acnes* from the shoulder region [48].

## 35.3 Arthroscopic Stabilization Complications

### 35.3.1 Nerve Injury

Iatrogenic nerve injury related to arthroscopic stabilization procedures is a rare complication, occurring at a rate of 0.3% according to a report published by Owens et al. [43]. Nevertheless, it is imperative that the surgeon possesses a thorough knowledge of the relevant anatomy around the shoulder, particularly with respect to the axillary nerve. Although out of the field of view during shoulder arthroscopy, the axillary nerve is in close proximity to the inferior glenoid, lying within 10–15 mm from the 6 o'clock position on the glenoid [9, 46, 58]. Moreover, Price et al. observed a mean distance of 2.5 mm between the axillary nerve and inferior glenohumeral ligament [46]. With this anatomic relationship in mind, capsular plication stitches should be placed within 10 mm of the 6 o'clock position on the glenoid in order to avoid iatrogenic axillary nerve injury [9]. Additionally, Yoo et al. found that the axillary nerve translated away from the glenoid as the shoulder was moved into 45° of abduction and neutral rotation (Fig. 35.1) [58]. The location of arthroscopic portal placement has also been investigated to determine risk of iatrogenic nerve injury. Meyer et al. scrutinized the proximity of neurovascular structures to 12 commonly used arthroscopic portals and observed that the 5 o'clock portal was consistently found to be in closest proximity (15 mm) to the axillary nerve [38].

### 35.3.2 Chondrolysis

Thermal capsulorrhaphy has been implicated in glenohumeral chondrolysis observed in association with arthroscopic stabilization procedures [32, 44]. Good et al. reported a series of eight patients previously treated with thermal capsulorrhaphy. Six of the eight patients were diagnosed with grade 4 humeral head and glenoid cartilage loss during repeat arthroscopy a mean of 8.2 months following the index procedure [17]. In a cadaveric study investigating the effect of radiofrequency probe use and varying rates of fluid flow on joint fluid temperatures, fluid temperatures were raised above a safe level (defined as below 45 °C based upon basic science data related to temperature-related chondrocyte death) in all testing conditions [28, 54]. Intermittent heating with 100% flow states resulted in the lowest average maximum joint fluid temperature. When the

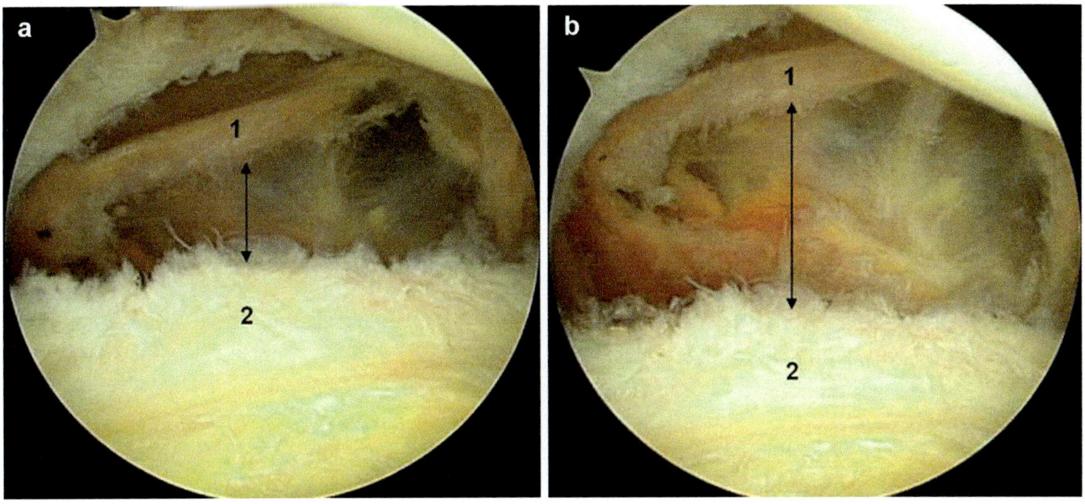


**Fig. 35.1** Arthroscopic view from an anterosuperior portal. (**a**) Demonstration of the relationship between the axillary nerve (*1*) and the inferior margin of the glenoid (*2*). (**b**) The effect of shoulder abduction and external rotation is noted as the distance between axillary nerve and inferior glenoid is increased (Reproduced with permission from Yoo et al. [58])

no-flow state was tested in conjunction with intermittent heating, the average maximum joint fluid temperature was 57.75 °C ± 20.07 °C. Moreover, under these same conditions, joint fluid temperatures required an average of 156 ± 38.64 s to return to a safe level [16]. These data underscore the importance of judicious use of radio-frequency energy in the glenohumeral joint and the importance of adequate fluid egress in order to normalize joint fluid temperatures and avoid chondral injury.

An emerging body of basic science and clinical results has also convincingly shown the negative effects of intra-articular bupivacaine pain pumps. Hansen et al. reported on a series of 12 of 19 patients treated with intra-articular bupivacaine pumps in conjunction with shoulder arthroscopy that developed glenohumeral chondrolysis [21]. Moreover, in several animal models, Chu and associates have demonstrated that local anesthetics as a class may be harmful to chondrocytes, providing further evidence against the use of intra-articular anesthetic pumps as an adjunct for controlling postoperative pain [5, 6, 30].

### 35.3.3 Anchor-Related Complications

Nonmetallic, bioabsorbable suture anchors for arthroscopic stabilization were developed to provide a reliable means of refixation of avulsed capsuloligamentous tissues to the bone while increasing the likelihood of reintegration of autologous tissues as the implants gradually degrade. Recently, several reports have raised concerns regarding the in vivo behavior of poly-L-lactic acid (PLLA) implants. Specifically, substantial rates of intra-articular anchor debris, synovitis, and high-grade chondral damage have been observed in association with PLLA implants [12, 20, 37]. However, the rate of complications from biodegradable anchors is extremely low, and we believe that they are much safer than metallic anchors, which can cause severe articular cartilage damage when they are left "proud" in the shoulder.

Errors in the placement of suture anchors may manifest as recurrent instability or glenoid rim fracture. As higher rates of repair failure have been observed with repairs using less than three anchors, arthroscopic Bankart repair should involve a minimum of three anchors placed below the 3 o'clock position, with the first anchor placed as inferior on the glenoid as possible (between the 5 o'clock and 6 o'clock positions) [3]. Glenoid rim fracture, the so-called postage stamp fracture owing to its serrated appearance, has also been described [2, 13]. In an analysis of four cases of glenoid rim fracture, Fitsch et al. recommended that suture anchors be inserted at varying angles of medial-lateral and superior-inferior inclination so as to avoid narrow bone bridges oriented in a linear fashion. These authors speculated that such an anchor configuration created a zone of weakness that predisposed the anteroinferior glenoid to fracture. The size of the suture anchor may also play a role in the occurrence of glenoid rim fracture, and it is advisable to use the smallest diameter anchor possible.

### 35.3.4 Recurrent Instability

Failure of arthroscopic stabilization techniques resulting in recurrent instability, which has been reported to occur at rates ranging from 4 to 19%, can be attributed to a number of factors, including patient selection, failure to identify and treat associated pathology, and/or poor surgical technique [1, 3, 11, 45]. An accurate assessment of glenoid bone loss is critical prior to undertaking an arthroscopic treatment approach as significant bone loss, commonly recognized as greater than 25% of the inferior glenoid diameter, has been associated with higher rates of recurrence [4, 52]. Additionally, the failure to diagnosis and treat lesions oftentimes found in conjunction with Bankart tears—anterolateral labroligamentous periosteal sleeve avulsion (ALPSA), humeral avulsion of the glenohumeral ligaments (HAGL), Hill-Sachs lesions—jeopardizes the durability of any repair and diminishes the likelihood of a favorable clinical outcome. In particular, an emerging body of literature has validated the role of the engaging ("off-track") Hill-Sachs lesion on clinical outcomes [8]. Shaha et al. evaluated the results of 57 shoulders treated with arthroscopic Bankart repair and observed that 4 out of 49 (8%) patients with "on-track" Hill-Sachs lesions were deemed treatment failures versus 6 out of 8 (75%) patients with "off-track" Hill-Sachs lesions that failed treatment ($P < 0.0001$). Furthermore, these authors determined the positive predictive value for failure of "off-track" to be 75% [51]. Similarly, Locher et al. recently reported on the incidence and association of "off-track" Hill-Sachs lesions in the setting of recurrent instability among 100 patients treated with arthroscopic stabilization. Of the 100 patients, 88 were found to have "on-track" Hill-Sachs lesions and 12 had "off-track" Hill-Sachs lesions. Five patients (6%) with "on-track" Hill-Sachs lesions required revision surgery, while four patients (33%) with "off-track" Hill-Sachs lesions (odds ratio, 8.3, $P = 0.006$) [33].

## 35.4 Open Stabilization Procedure Complications

### 35.4.1 Nerve Injury Associated with the Latarjet Procedure

Neurovascular injuries following open Latarjet procedure have been reported with rates ranging from 1.4 to 10% [19, 50]. Among 47 patients (48 shoulders) treated with open Latarjet procedure, Shah et al. described five nerve palsies (two musculocutaneous nerve, two axillary nerve, one radial nerve), which is a higher rate of previous reports of neurologic complications [50]. Furthermore, Delaney et al. demonstrated that, through the use of intraoperative neuromonitoring, the axillary and musculocutaneous nerves were particularly vulnerable to perturbations in conduction characteristics during glenoid exposure and graft insertion [7]. Thus, it is important to understand the anatomy of the musculocutaneous nerve, which has been described to pierce the coracobrachialis a mean distance of 56 mm from the coracoid with arborization of branches to the coracobrachialis observed as close as 17 mm inferior to the coracoid [10].

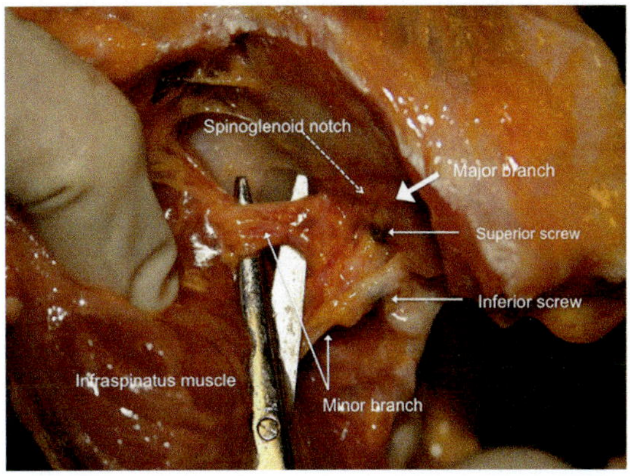


**Fig. 35.2** Demonstration of the close proximity of the suprascapular nerve to the posterior aspect of the superior most screw placed for the Latarjet procedure (Reproduced with permission from Lädermann et al. [31])

Special attention must also be paid to the anatomy of the suprascapular nerve as iatrogenic injuries have been reported [35, 49]. In a cadaveric study to quantify the proximity of the suprascapular nerve to the screw tips used to fix the coracoid graft during the Congruent Arc Latarjet procedure, Lädermann et al. observed that the main trunk of the suprascapular nerve was an average of 4 mm from the posterior exit point of the superior (Fig. 35.2). These authors further observed that the nerve was not in danger as long as the superior screw was oriented less than 10° from the plane of the glenoid [31].

### 35.4.2 Malpositioned Coracoid Graft

The position in which the coracoid graft is fixed to the anterolateral glenoid rim can have deleterious effects on surgical outcomes following the Latarjet procedure. Ghodadra et al. demonstrated that bone grafts fixed 2 mm proud (lateral) relative to the glenoid surface were associated with significant increases in peak anteroinferior contact pressures [15]. These biomechanical observations have been substantiated clinically, with higher rates of arthritis noted by Hovelius et al. among patients with lateral overhang of the bone graft transferred in the traditional Latarjet procedure (43.7% of patients with osteoarthritis versus 3.8% of patients without osteoarthritis, $P < 0.001$) [40]. Conversely, fixation of the graft medial to the glenoid articular surface risks diminishing the stabilizing effect of the bone block and soft tissue sling, thus increasing the likelihood of residual instability [25].

## Conclusion

Complication rates associated with open and arthroscopic shoulder stabilization procedures have historically been low. Nevertheless, suboptimal clinical outcomes have been reported related to recurrent instability, stiffness, infection, iatrogenic nerve injury, and chondrolysis. Higher rates of recurrence should be anticipated in the setting of patients with a history of multiple dislocations and previous stabilization procedures. In order to maximize the likelihood for a favorable outcome, special emphasis must be placed on accurately quantifying glenoid bone loss, assessing for Hill-Sachs lesion engagement, and treating all associated pathology.

## References

1. Balg F, Boileau P. The instability severity index score. A simple pre-operative score to select patients for arthroscopic or open shoulder stabilisation. J Bone Joint Surg Br. 2007;89(11):1470–7.
2. Banerjee S, Weiser L, Connell D, Wallace AL. Glenoid rim fracture in contact athletes with absorbable suture anchor reconstruction. Arthroscopy. 2009;25(5):560–2.
3. Boileau P, Villalba M, Hery JY, Balg F, Ahrens P, Neyton L. Risk factors for recurrence of shoulder instability after arthroscopic Bankart repair. J Bone Joint Surg Am. 2006;88(8):1755–63.
4. Burkhart SS, De Beer JF. Traumatic glenohumeral bone defects and their relationship to failure of arthroscopic Bankart repairs: significance of the inverted-pear glenoid and the humeral engaging Hill-Sachs lesion. Arthroscopy. 2000;16(7):677–94.
5. Chu CR, Coyle CH, Chu CT, et al. In vivo effects of single intra-articular injection of 0.5% bupivacaine on articular cartilage. J Bone Joint Surg Am. 2010;92(3): 599–608.
6. Chu CR, Izzo NJ, Papas NE, Fu FH. In vitro exposure to 0.5% bupivacaine is cytotoxic to bovine articular chondrocytes. Arthroscopy. 2006;22(7):693–9.
7. Delaney RA, Freehill MT, Janfaza DR, Vlassakov KV, Higgins LD, Warner JJ. 2014 Neer Award Paper: neuromonitoring the Latarjet procedure. J Shoulder Elbow Surg. 2014;23(10):1473–80.
8. Di Giacomo G, Itoi E, Burkhart SS. Evolving concept of bipolar bone loss and the Hill-Sachs lesion: from "engaging/non-engaging" lesion to "on-track/off-track" lesion. Arthroscopy. 2014;30(1):90–8.
9. Eakin CL, Dvirnak P, Miller CM, Hawkins RJ. The relationship of the axillary nerve to arthroscopically placed capsulolabral sutures. An anatomic study. Am J Sports Med. 1998;26(4):505–9.
10. Flatow EL, Bigliani LU, April EW. An anatomic study of the musculocutaneous nerve and its relationship to the coracoid process. Clin Orthop Relat Res. 1989;244:166–71.
11. Flinkkila T, Hyvonen P, Ohtonen P, Leppilahti J. Arthroscopic Bankart repair: results and risk factors of recurrence of instability. Knee Surg Sports Traumatol Arthrosc. 2010;18(12):1752–8.
12. Freehill MQ, Harms DJ, Huber SM, Atlihan D, Buss DD. Poly-L-lactic acid tack synovitis after arthroscopic stabilization of the shoulder. Am J Sports Med. 2003;31(5):643–7.
13. Fritsch BA, Arciero RA, Taylor DC. Glenoid rim fracture after anchor repair: a report of 4 cases. Am J Sports Med. 2010;38(8):1682–6.
14. Garcia GH, Wu HH, Liu JN, Huffman GR, Kelly JD. Outcomes of the remplissage procedure and its effects on return to sports: average 5-year follow-up. Am J Sports Med. 2016;44(5):1124–30.
15. Ghodadra N, Gupta A, Romeo AA, et al. Normalization of glenohumeral articular contact pressures after Latarjet or iliac crest bone-grafting. J Bone Joint Surg Am. 2010;92(6):1478–89.
16. Good CR, Shindle MK, Griffith MH, Wanich T, Warren RF. Effect of radiofrequency energy on glenohumeral fluid temperature during shoulder arthroscopy. J Bone Joint Surg Am. 2009;91(2):429–34.
17. Good CR, Shindle MK, Kelly BT, Wanich T, Warren RF. Glenohumeral chondrolysis after shoulder arthroscopy with thermal capsulorrhaphy. Arthroscopy. 2007;23(7): 797.e791–5.
18. Gordins V, Hovelius L, Sandstrom B, Rahme H, Bergstrom U. Risk of arthropathy after the Bristow-Latarjet repair: a radiologic and clinical thirty-three to thirty-five years of follow-up of thirty-one shoulders. J Shoulder Elbow Surg. 2015;24(5):691–9.
19. Griesser MJ, Harris JD, McCoy BW, et al. Complications and re-operations after Bristow-Latarjet shoulder stabilization: a systematic review. J Shoulder Elbow Surg. 2013;22(2):286–92.
20. Haneveld H, Hug K, Diederichs G, Scheibel M, Gerhardt C. Arthroscopic double-row repair of the rotator cuff: a comparison of bio-absorbable and non-resorbable anchors regarding osseous reaction. Knee

Surg Sports Traumatol Arthrosc. 2013;21(7): 1647–54.
21. Hansen BP, Beck CL, Beck EP, Townsley RW. Postarthroscopic glenohumeral chondrolysis. Am J Sports Med. 2007;35(10):1628–34.
22. Hartzler RU, Bui CN, Jeong WK, et al. Remplissage of an off-track Hill-Sachs lesion is necessary to restore biomechanical glenohumeral joint stability in a bipolar bone loss model. Arthroscopy. 2016;32(12): 2466–76.
23. Hawkins RH, Hawkins RJ. Failed anterolateral reconstruction for shoulder instability. J Bone Joint Surg Br. 1985;67(5):709–14.
24. Horneff 3rd JG, Hsu JE, Voleti PB, O'Donnell J, Huffman GR. Propionibacterium acnes infection in shoulder arthroscopy patients with postoperative pain. J Shoulder Elbow Surg. 2015;24(6):838–43.
25. Hovelius L, Sandstrom B, Olofsson A, Svensson O, Rahme H. The effect of capsular repair, bone block healing, and position on the results of the Bristow-Latarjet procedure (study III): long-term follow-up in 319 shoulders. J Shoulder Elbow Surg. 2012;21(5):647–60.
26. Itoi E, Arce G, Bain GI, et al. Shoulder stiffness: current concepts and concerns. Arthroscopy. 2016;32(7): 1402–14.
27. Kang RW, Frank RM, Nho SJ, et al. Complications associated with anterolateral shoulder instability repair. Arthroscopy. 2009;25(8):909–20.
28. Kaplan L, Uribe JW. The acute effects of radiofrequency energy in articular cartilage: an in vitro study. Arthroscopy. 2000;16(1):2–5.
29. Karlsson J, Magnusson L, Ejerhed L, Hultenheim I, Lundin O, Kartus J. Comparison of open and arthroscopic stabilization for recurrent shoulder dislocation in patients with a Bankart lesion. Am J Sports Med. 2001;29(5):538–42.
30. Karpie JC, Chu CR. Lidocaine exhibits dose- and time-dependent cytotoxic effects on bovine articular chondrocytes in vitro. Am J Sports Med. 2007; 35(10):1621–7.
31. Ladermann A, Denard PJ, Burkhart SS. Injury of the suprascapular nerve during latarjet procedure: an anatomic study. Arthroscopy. 2012;28(3):316–21.
32. Levine WN, Clark Jr AM, D'Alessandro DF, Yamaguchi K. Chondrolysis following arthroscopic thermal capsulorrhaphy to treat shoulder instability. A report of two cases. J Bone Joint Surg Am. 2005; 87(3):616–21.
33. Locher J, Wilken F, Beitzel K, et al. Hill-Sachs off-track lesions as risk factor for recurrence of instability after arthroscopic bankart repair. Arthroscopy. 2016;32:1993–9.
34. Mair SD, Hawkins RJ. Open shoulder instability surgery complications. Clin Sports Med. 1999;18(4):719–36.
35. Maquieira GJ, Gerber C, Schneeberger AG. Suprascapular nerve palsy after the Latarjet procedure. J Shoulder Elbow Surg. 2007;16(2):e13–5.
36. McAuliffe TB, Pangayatselvan T, Bayley I. Failed surgery for recurrent anterolateral dislocation of the shoulder. Causes and management. J Bone Joint Surg Br. 1988;70(5):798–801.
37. McCarty 3rd LP, Buss DD, Datta MW, Freehill MQ, Giveans MR. Complications observed following labral or rotator cuff repair with use of poly-L-lactic acid implants. J Bone Joint Surg Am. 2013;95(6): 507–11.
38. Meyer M, Graveleau N, Hardy P, Landreau P. Anatomic risks of shoulder arthroscopy portals: anatomic cadaveric study of 12 portals. Arthroscopy. 2007;23(5):529–36.
39. Millett PJ, Yen YM, Price CS, Horan MP, van der Meijden OA, Elser F. Propionibacterium acnes infection as an occult cause of postoperative shoulder pain: a case series. Clin Orthop Relat Res. 2011;469(10): 2824–30.
40. Mizuno N, Denard PJ, Raiss P, Melis B, Walch G. Long-term results of the Latarjet procedure for anterolateral instability of the shoulder. J Shoulder Elbow Surg. 2014;23(11):1691–9.
41. Moen TC, Rudolph GH, Caswell K, Espinoza C, Burkhead Jr WZ, Krishnan SG. Complications of shoulder arthroscopy. J Am Acad Orthop Surg. 2014;22(7):410–9.
42. Omi R, Hooke AW, Zhao KD, et al. The effect of the remplissage procedure on shoulder range of motion: a cadaveric study. Arthroscopy. 2014;30(2):178–87.
43. Owens BD, Harrast JJ, Hurwitz SR, Thompson TL, Wolf JM. Surgical trends in Bankart repair: an analysis of data from the American Board of Orthopaedic Surgery certification examination. Am J Sports Med. 2011;39(9):1865–9.
44. Petty DH, Jazrawi LM, Estrada LS, Andrews JR. Glenohumeral chondrolysis after shoulder arthroscopy: case reports and review of the literature. Am J Sports Med. 2004;32(2):509–15.
45. Porcellini G, Campi F, Pegreffi F, Castagna A, Paladini P. Predisposing factors for recurrent shoulder dislocation after arthroscopic treatment. J Bone Joint Surg Am. 2009;91(11):2537–42.
46. Price MR, Tillett ED, Acland RD, Nettleton GS. Determining the relationship of the axillary nerve to the shoulder joint capsule from an arthroscopic perspective. J Bone Joint Surg Am. 2004;86-a(10): 2135–42.
47. Randelli P, Castagna A, Cabitza F, Cabitza P, Arrigoni P, Denti M. Infectious and thromboembolic complications of arthroscopic shoulder surgery. J Shoulder Elbow Surg. 2010;19(1):97–101.
48. Saltzman MD, Nuber GW, Gryzlo SM, Marecek GS, Koh JL. Efficacy of surgical preparation solutions in shoulder surgery. J Bone Joint Surg Am. 2009; 91(8):1949–53.
49. Sastre S, Peidro L, Mendez A, Calvo E. Suprascapular nerve palsy after arthroscopic Latarjet procedure: a case report and review of literature. Knee Surg Sports Traumatol Arthrosc. 2016;24(2):601–3.
50. Shah AA, Butler RB, Romanowski J, Goel D, Karadagli D, Warner JJ. Short-term complications of

the Latarjet procedure. J Bone Joint Surg Am. 2012;94(6):495–501.
51. Shaha JCJ, Rowles D, Buttoni C, Shaha S, Tokish J. Clinical validation of the glenoid track concept in anterolateral glenohumeral instability. JBJS Am. 2016;98:1918–23.
52. Shaha JS, Cook JB, Song DJ, et al. Redefining "critical" bone loss in shoulder instability: functional outcomes worsen with "subcritical" bone loss. Am J Sports Med. 2015;43(7):1719–25.
53. Sing DC, Ding DY, Aguilar TU, et al. The effects of patient obesity on early postoperative complications after shoulder arthroscopy. Arthroscopy. 2016;32:2212–7.
54. Voss JR, Lu Y, Edwards RB, Bogdanske JJ, Markel MD. Effects of thermal energy on chondrocyte viability. Am J Vet Res. 2006;67(10):1708–12.
55. Wasserstein D, Dwyer T, Veillette C, et al. Predictors of dislocation and revision after shoulder stabilization in Ontario, Canada, from 2003 to 2008. Am J Sports Med. 2013;41(9):2034–40.
56. Weber SC, Abrams JS, Nottage WM. Complications associated with arthroscopic shoulder surgery. Arthroscopy. 2002;18(2 Suppl 1):88–95.
57. Werner BC, Cancienne JM, Burrus MT, Griffin JW, Gwathmey FW, Brockmeier SF. The timing of elective shoulder surgery after shoulder injection affects postoperative infection risk in Medicare patients. J Shoulder Elbow Surg. 2016;25(3):390–7.
58. Yoo JC, Kim JH, Ahn JH, Lee SH. Arthroscopic perspective of the axillary nerve in relation to the glenoid and arm position: a cadaveric study. Arthroscopy. 2007;23(12):1271–7.

# Index


**A**

Adolescent patients
  arthroscopic repair (*see* Anterior shoulder dislocation)
  Bankart repair (*see* Open Bankart repair)
  dynamic muscular compensation, 4
  humeral physeal/metaphyseal fractures, 3
  hyperlaxity, joint hypermobility, 4
  MDI (*see* Multidirectional instability (MDI))
  posterior dislocation (*see* Posterior shoulder dislocation (PSD))
  recurrence rate
    anatomical-related factors, 3
    bony deficiency, 3–4
    structural age-related factors, 3
  shoulder laxity, acute trauma (*see* Anterior shoulder dislocation)
  skeletal mature and immature patients, 3, 4
  stabilization (*see* Open Bankart repair)
  unidirectional instability, 4
Adson test, 24
Anterior shoulder dislocation
  acute stabilizers, 58
  advantages and disadvantages, 103, 104
  anchor placement, 62
  anterosuperior and anteroinferior portals, 61
  atraumatic MDI
    anatomy, 66
    apprehension and relocation tests, 66
    arthroscopic capsular plication, 70
    Bankart lesion, 67, 70
    bleeding cortical bone, 68
    capsular and labral deficiencies, 66
    clinical evaluation, 66
    complications, 70
    conservative rehabilitation protocol, 69–70
    diagnosis, 66
    examination, 66
    external rotation/stiffness, postoperative loss, 70
    glenoid bone loss, 70
    indications, 67
    insufficient anchors/incorrect anchor placement, 70
    interscalene block, endotracheal anesthesia, 67
    modified 3-portal technique, 67
    open capsular shift, 70
    optimal anchor placement, 67
    radiographic imaging, 66–67
    recurrence rate, 70
    rotator interval closure, 68, 69
    surgical incisions, 68
    suture-passing instrument, 68
  Bankart lesion, 61, 62
  bony defects, glenoid
    arthroscopic bare spot method, 85
    biomechanical studies, 85, 86
    critical defect size, 85–86
    CT methods, 84–85
    Hill-Sachs lesion, 86–87
    location, 83–84
    MRI methods, 85
    prevalence, 83–84
    risk assessment, bipolar lesion, 87–88
    treatment paradigm, 88–89
    WOSI scores, 86
    X-ray methods, 84
  capsular stretching, 62
  complications, 107–108
  description, 104
  dynamic stabilizers, 58
  glenoid decortication, 61, 62
  indications, 104
  lateral decubitus position, 60, 61
  optimal labrum reposition, 62
  optional suture anchors, 106
  portal placement, 61
  posterior knot position, 62
  postoperative hematoma and infection, 107
  progressive bone defects, 58
  scapular neck decortication, 106
  soft tissue damage, 58
  subscapualris tenotomy, 104, 105
  surgical management
    Bankart repair, 59, 63
    lavage, 59–60
    open *vs.* arthroscopic repair, 60
    transglenoid repair, 60
  suture anchors, humeral neck for capsular shift, 106, 107


© ISAKOS 2017
A.B. Imhoff, F.H. Savoie III (eds.), *Shoulder Instability Across the Life Span*,
DOI 10.1007/978-3-662-54077-0

Anterior shoulder dislocation (*cont.*)
traumatic, acute
acquired, 8
active-assisted range of motion exercises, 53
anatomy, 50
anterior-inferior glenoid, labral avulsion, 10
anterior pouch redundancy and hypermobility, 8
AO systems, 7
classic Bankart lesion, 10
classification systems, 7–8
clinical presentation, 51
cryotherapy, 53
dynamic stabilizers, primary, 8, 50
electrical stimulation, 53
inferior glenohumeral ligament, 50
initial postreduction treatment, 52
joint reduction, 52
MDI of (*see* Multidirectional instability (MDI))
muscle relaxation, 51
neurovascular examination, 52
pathophysiology, 50–51
primary surgical repair, 53
radiographs, 51
reduction techniques, 51–52
rehabilitation and physical therapy, 52–53
scapular control and muscle strength, 53
static stabilizers, primary, 8, 50
systemic anti-inflammatory, 53
vertical capsulotomy, 104, 105
Arthroscopic soft tissue repair
anchor-related complications, 294
anterior dislocation
acute stabilizers, 58
anchor placement, 62
anterosuperior and anteroinferior portals, 61
Bankart lesion, 59, 61–63
capsular stretching, 62
dynamic stabilizers, 58
glenoid decortication, 61, 62
lateral decubitus position, 60, 61
lavage, 59–60
open *vs.* arthroscopic repair, 60
optimal labrum reposition, 62
portal placement, 61
posterior knot position, 62
progressive bone defects, 58
soft tissue damage, 58
transglenoid repair, 60
athletic activity, 93
Bankart lesion (Perthes-Bankart lesion) (*see* Bankart repair)
bony fragments, smaller, 265
chondrolysis, 293–294
deep infection, 292
early surgical shoulder stabilization, 94
extended labral injuries
bidirectional instability, 174
complications, 174
diagnostic imaging, 169–170
epidemiology, 169
patient history, 169
physical examination, 170–171
posterior capsule complex, 172
posterior-inferior load shift, 171
progressive rotator cuff strengthening, 174
shuttle suture technique, 173
sport-specific training, 174
surgical technique, 171–173
Hill-Sachs lesion, 94–95
iatrogenic nerve injury, 293
indications, 95
nonmetallic, bioabsorbable suture anchors, 294
open stabilization procedure complications
malpositioned coracoid graft, 295–296
neurovascular injuries, Latarjet procedure, 295
operative evaluation
anesthesia, 96
examination under anesthesia, 96
positioning, 96
preoperative evaluation
history, 95
imaging, 95–96
physical examination, 95
recurrent instability, 294–295
remplissage technique, 96–100
stiffness, 291–292
thermal capsulorrhaphy, 293
Articular cartilage defects
diagnosis, 228, 229
etiology, 227–228
ICRS classification, 228, 229
intra-articular gadolinium application, 228, 229
symptoms, 228
therapy
ACT, 230–231
autologous osteochondral transplantation, 231–233
bone marrow stimulation, 229–230
ICRS classification, 229
PJR, 234
shoulder arthroplasty, 234–235
Athletic young adults. *See also* Overhead athletes (throwers), posterior instability
bone loss (*see* Latarjet procedure, arthroscopic)
coracoid transfer (*see* Open coracoid transfer)
FEDS classification system, 82
HAGL (*see* Humeral avulsion of the glenohumeral ligaments (HAGL))
incidence rate, 81
instability severity index score, 82
modified Bankart repair (*see* Modified open Bankart repair)
neuromuscular factors, 81
PSD (*see* Posterior shoulder dislocation (PSD))
repositioning types, 81
risk factors, 82
soft tissue repair (*see* Arthroscopic soft tissue repair)
Atraumatic multidirectional instability
anatomy, 66
anchor placement, insufficient/incorrect, 70

  apprehension and relocation tests, 66
  Bankart lesion, 70
  capsular and labral deficiencies, 66
  clinical evaluation, 66
  complications, 70
  conservative rehabilitation protocol, 69–70
  diagnosis, 66
  examination, 66
  external rotation/stiffness, postoperative loss, 70
  glenoid bone loss, 70
  indications, 67
  radiographic imaging, 66–67
  recurrence rate, 70
  surgical procedures
    arthroscopic capsular plication, 70
    open capsular shift, 70
  technique
    arthroscopic rotator interval closure, 68
    Bankart repair, 67
    bleeding cortical bone, 68
    interscalene block, endotracheal anesthesia, 67
    modified 3-portal technique, 67
    optimal anchor placement, 67
    rotator interval closure, 68, 69
    surgical incisions, 68
    suture-passing instrument, 68
Autologous chondrocyte transplantation (ACT), 229–231

**B**
Bankart repair
  anatomy, 184
  anterior dislocations, traumatic, 94
  biceps surgery rehabilitation, 206
  cadaver model, 184
  capsule-ligament-labrum complex, 94
  complications, 70
  description, 94
  dynamic stabilizers, 183
  glenohumeral stability, 184
  glenoid bone deficiency, 117
  glenoid track concept, 87
  Hill-Sachs lesion, 86, 88
  incidence, 94
  indications, surgery, 184–185
  inferior capsular shift, 67, 70, 285
  Latarjet procedure, 123
  morbidity, 184
  open/arthroscopic transglenoidal technique, 60
  pathological findings, 184
  postoperative protocol, 61–63
  pre-trauma activity level, 94
  recurrent instability reduction, 59
  and remplissage technique
    ALPSA lesion, 96, 98
    anterolateral superior portal, 96, 97
    SLAP repair, suture anchor, 96, 97
    subscapularis muscle belly, 96, 98
  with suture anchors, 97, 99
  traumatic supraspinatus tears, 183
Belly press test, 24, 38, 219
Biceps tenodesis
  anatomy and examination, 206
  complications, 206
  indications, 206
  neurovascular injury, 204
  open subpectoral, 204
  pain generator, 203
  postoperative stiffness, 206
  proximal *vs.* distal
    complications, 207
    demographic data, 204
    implant costs, 205
    open subpectoral tenodesis, 204
    operative times and perioperative morbidity, 204
    outcome measures, 204, 205
    reoperation rates, 205
  rehabilitation, 206
  SLAP, 198, 199
  subpectoral, 198, 203
  subscapularis repair, 221
Biomechanics, 211, 218, 295
  bony defects, 84, 86
  concavity-compression mechanism, 247
  labral detachment, 194–195
  Latarjet procedure, 122
  RCT, 247
  SLAP tears, 189–190
  and structural capsule modifications, 18
  supraphysiologic shoulder stiffness, 292
  tissue disorders, 17
  unidirectional posterior instability, 166
Bone block procedures. *See* Latarjet procedure, arthroscopic
Bone marrow stimulating therapies, 229–230
Brachial plexus injuries, 130, 138, 244, 246, 283–274. *See also* Suprascapular nerve lesions (SSN)

**C**
Capsulomuscular plication, posterior, 164
Caspari transglenoid capsular shift technique, 22
Chondrolysis, glenohumeral, 293–294, 296
Chronic locked anterior and posterior dislocations
  anatomic restoration, 280–281
  clinical evaluation
    patient history, 278
    physical examination, 278
  closed reduction, 279
  complications, 282
  definition, 277
  deltopectoral approach, 279–280
  humeral head replacement, 281
  imaging, 279
  incidence, 277
  McLaughlin procedure, 281
  nonoperative treatment, 279
  open reduction and repair, 279–280
  pain relief, 281–282
  patho-anatomy, 278

Chronic locked anterior and posterior dislocations (*cont.*)
 patient positioning, 281
 post postoperative management, 281
 rehabilitation, 281
 surgical intervention, 279
Circumduction test, 24, 38, 39
Comprehensive arthroscopic management (CAM) procedure, 255

**D**
Dislocation arthropathy. *See also* Anterior shoulder dislocation; Posterior shoulder dislocation (PSD)
 articular abnormalities, 253, 254
 biologic resurfacing, glenoid, 256
 bony defects, 252
 classification system, 252–253
 clinical presentation, 253–255
 compression-rotation test, 254
 degenerative changes, 251
 glenoid articular surface, microfractures, 256
 hemiarthroplasty, 256
 hyperlaxity, 252
 incidence, 252
 nonoperative measures, 255
 osteoarthritis, 252
 prognostic factors, 256
 supraspinatus and infraspinatus fossae, 255
 surgical interventions, 255
 symptoms, 253–254
 treatment, 255–257

**E**
Ehlers–Danlos syndrome (EDS), 4, 16, 26, 66, 74–75, 95
External rotation test, arm, 24

**F**
Frequency, etiology, direction and severity (FEDS) system
 classification, modified, 11–12
 deficiencies, 9, 11
 definition, 9
 modification to, 11–12
 surgical stabilization, 82

**G**
Genetic approach, unstable shoulder
 acute inflammator, 17
 anterior shoulder dislocations, 16
 biomechanical and structural capsule modifications, 18
 biomechanic tissue disorders, 17
 capsular deformation, 16
 clinical association, 16
 collagen gene expression alterations, 17
 collagen type 1/type 3, 17
 enzymatic cross-linking, 17, 18
 fibrillar collagens, 16
 healing process, damaged ligament/ capsule, 16
 physical activity, 18
 repair process, 17
 transforming growth factor, 17
Glenohumeral internal rotation deficit (GIRD), 37–40, 74
Glenoid fractures
 acute, 263–264
 Bankart lesions, bony, 265
 bone defects, 264–265
 chronic, 264–265
 classification, 262
 fragment size, 262
 histologic analysis, 265
 imaging, 262
 indications, 264
 modified bony Bankart bridge, 264
 physiologic pressure distribution, 261
 prosthesis type, 265
 PSD, 145
 recurrent instability, 261
 Rowe score, 262
 surgical techniques, 264
 suture anchor, 263
 traumatic dislocations, 35
 treatment algorithm, 262

**H**
Healing process, bone, 16, 17, 26, 32, 53, 97, 106, 140, 172, 196, 264, 265
Hill–Sachs lesion
 in ABD group, 87
 abduction and external rotation, 130
 anterior shoulder dislocation, 86–87
 arm abduction, 87
 arthroscopic Latarjet procedure, 128
 Bankart repair, 86, 88
 critical size, 86–87
 debridement, 97, 99
 deltopectoral approach, PSD, 155
 description, 94
 with glenoid track, 86
 incidence, 86
 labrum repair, 94
 open capsular shift, 95
 PJR, 234
 prevalence, 86
 radiographic evaluation, 95
 recurrent dislocation, 94
 severe osteoarthritis, 272
Humeral avulsion of the glenohumeral ligaments (HAGL), 150, 169–170, 248, 294
 anterior, 110
 chronic lesions, 111
 clinical outcomes, 112
 complications, 112
 humeral-based capsuloligamentous damage, 110
 imaging studies, 111
 juxtachondral repair, 112
 knotted/knotless suture anchors, 112

management, 111
open anterior repair, 112
posterior (*see* Posterior humeral avulsion of the glenohumeral ligament (PHAGL))
range of motion, 112
static and dynamic mechanisms, 109
traumatic disorders, 111
traumatic injury, 110
West Point classification system, 110

**J**
Jerk test, 9, 38, 39, 111, 147, 149, 150, 158, 159, 170, 171

**K**
Kim test, 38–39, 149, 150, 158, 159, 170, 171

**L**
Labral repair and capsulorrhaphy, arthroscopic posterior, 165–166
Latarjet procedure, arthroscopic
anterior glenohumeral shoulder stability, 128
*vs.* Bankart repair, 123
biomechanical function, 122
capsulolabral avulsion, 127, 134
clinical outcomes, 133
coracoid transfer, 116
coracoid transfer techniques, 128
Eden-Hybbinette procedure, 119
effects of, 116
glenohumeral joint stability, 116
glenoid defect, 116, 117
Hill–Sachs lesion, 128
intraoperative complications
graft fracture, 138–139
graft positioning, 138
neurovascular injury, 138
long-term studies, 132
neurological complications, 133, 134
nonoperative management, 127
postoperative complications
graft osteolysis, 140
infections, 140
loss of external rotation, 139
nonunion/fibrous union, 139
recurrent glenohumeral instability, 139–140
shoulder arthritis/cartilage damage, 140
risk of osteoarthritis, 134
screw positioning, 133
soft tissue loss, 128
surgical technique
arterial blood pressure, 129
bone block positioning, 129
capsulolabral complex dissection, 130
capsulolabral reattachment, 132
concomitant joint abnormalities, 129
conjoint tendon dissection, 130–131
coracoid preparation and osteotomy, 129
coracoid transfer and fixation, 131–132
extra-articular procedure, 129
general anesthesia, 129
joint evaluation, 130
posterior soft spot portal, visualization, 129
single-shot interscalene regional block, 129
soft tissue stabilization, 129
subscapularis preparation and split, 131
Leffort's test, 24
Locked posterior shoulder dislocation (LPSD)
arthroscopic treatment, 269
autologous bone graft, 272, 273
conservative treatment, 272
diagnostics, 270
high-energy trauma, 269
management, 274
modified McLaughlin procedure, 272, 274
non-operative treatment, 269
operative treatment, 272–273
osteochondral autograft, 274
physical examination, 270
shoulder prosthesis implantation, 269
Long head of the biceps tendon (LHBT)
anatomic structures, 212
arthroscopic findings, 212–215
Bennett's classification, 214
bicipital groove, 211
Coma Sign, 214
coraco-humeral ligament, 211
decision-making criteria, 211, 214
humeral head depressor, 189
preoperative assessment, 212
Ramp Test, 213, 214
residual pain, 211
subscapularis, 211
superior gleno-humeral ligament, 211
supraspinatus, 211
transverse ligament, 211
treatment, 196

**M**
Maffet–Morgan modification, SLAP, 191, 193
Marfan's syndrome, 4, 66, 74–75, 95
Matrix-associated autologous chondrocyte transplantation, 230, 232
McLaughlin technique, bone stability restoration, 37, 43, 154–156, 184, 271–273, 281
Middle age patients
Bankart repair, 183–185
biceps injuries (*see* Biceps tenodesis)
cartilage defects (*see* Articular cartilage defects)
elastic characteristics, 179
incidence rate, 179
LHBT (*see* Long head of the biceps tendon (LHBT))
nerve lesions, 180
RCT, 183–185
SLAP (*see* Superior labrum anterior-posterior (SLAP))
soft tissue repair, 180
subscapularis tears (*see* Subscapularis tears)

Modified open Bankart repair. *See also* Open Bankart repair
advantages and disadvantages, 103, 104
complications, 107–108
description, 104
indications, 104
optional suture anchors, 106
postoperative hematoma and infection, 107
scapualr neck decortication, 106
subscapualris tenotomy, 104, 105
subscapularis reattachment, 106
suture anchors, humeral neck for capsular shift, 106, 107
vertical capsulotomy, 104, 105
Multidirectional instability (MDI)
absorbable/nonabsorbable sutures, 28
anterior capsular laxity, 29
arthroscopic capsular shift, 22
atraumatic
anatomy, 66
apprehension and relocation tests, 66
arthroscopic capsular plication, 70
arthroscopic rotator interval closure, 68
Bankart lesion, 67, 70
bleeding cortical bone, 68
capsular and labral deficiencies, 66
clinical evaluation, 66
complications, 70
conservative rehabilitation protocol, 69–70
diagnosis, 66
examination, 66
external rotation/stiffness, postoperative loss, 70
glenoid bone loss, 70
indications, 67
insufficient anchors/incorrect anchor placement, 70
interscalene block, endotracheal anesthesia, 67
modified 3-portal technique, 67
open capsular shift, 70
optimal anchor placement, 67
radiographic imaging, 66–67
recurrence rate, 70
rotator interval closure, 68, 69
surgical incisions, 68
suture-passing instrument, 68
chondrolysis, 33
circumduction maneuver, 24
complications, 32–33
crochet hook, 29
description, 22
imaging modalities, 24–25
laser-assisted technique, 22
lax capsule, treatment, 28–31
management techniques
contraindications, 26
indications, 25
nonoperative technique, 25
modified arthroscopic capsular shift, 22
operative arthroscopic techniques
anterior capsule, 27–28
diagnostic capability, 27
exposure/setup, 26–27
inferior capsule/axillary pouch, 27–28
instruments/equipment/implants, 27
patho-anatomy, 26
posterior capsule, 27–28
procedure, 27–28
surgical anatomy, 26
pancapsular plication suture technique, 22
patient history, 23
physical examination, 23–24
postoperative regimen, 32
posture control and stability, 23
preoperative rehabilitation, 23
radiographic findings, 24–25
rotator cuff strength, 24
scapular instability, 23
sliding locking knot, 31
subscapularis tendon, 31
suture hook, 29
suture plication technique, 29
symptomatic laxity, 22
synovial rasp, 29
torn labrum, 31
wound closure, 32

**O**

O'Brien's active compression test, 38, 39, 194, 212
Older patient instability
acute RCT (*see* Rotator cuff tears (RCT))
dislocation arthropathy (*see* Dislocation arthropathy)
pathophysiology, 239
posterior active stabilizing structures, 240
rotator cuff muscle activity and stability, 240
Omarthrosis, 228
Open Bankart repair. *See also* Modified open Bankart repair
anatomy, 74
arthroscopic evaluation, 75, 76
complications, 76–77
imaging, 75
indications, 75
in overhead athlete, 76
physical therapy, 74
profound loss of motion, 74
range of motion, 74
recurrence rates, 73, 77
rehabilitation, 76
shoulder scoring systems, 73–74
unidirectional anterior instability, 77
Open capsulomuscular repair, 164
Open coracoid transfer
allograft reconstruction, glenoid bone loss, 119
arthritis, risk factors, 124
bone graft procedures, 119
Bristow-Latarjet coracoid transfer, 116, 123
coracoid transposition surgery, 117
description, 115
diagnostic technique, 117–118
Eden-Hybbinette procedure, 119
fixation, 115

glenoid bone deficiency, 117
glenoid track concept, 118
graft compression, 122–123
horizontal subscapularis splitting technique, 123
ipsilateral distal clavicle resection, 119
Latarjet coracoid transfer, 116
radiographic and arthroscopic method, 118
reabsorption, 124
risk factors, 117
surgical approach
anteroinferior glenoid rim surface, 121
cannulated temporary compression device, 122
coracoid blood supply, 120
deltopectoral approach, 119
interscalene block, 119
microsagittal saw and high-speed burr, 120
self-retaining retractor, 119
subscapularis tendon and muscle, 120
transient nerve injuries, 124
Osteochondral transplantation (OCT), autologous, 230–233
Overhead athletes (throwers), posterior instability
abduction external rotation, 37
anterosuperior migration, humeral head, 37
capsular contracture, 38
GIRD, 37
hyperextension abduction, arm, 38
intra-articular biceps tendon, 38
microtraumatic instability, 189–190
open Bankart repair, 76
pathologic mechanisms, 189
peel-back mechanism, 38
posterior capsular contracture, 37
repetitive microtrauma, 110
repetitive throwing, 37
soft tissue damage, 58
subacromial impingement syndrome, 37

**P**
Partial joint resurfacing (PJR), 234
Posterior humeral avulsion of the glenohumeral ligament (PHAGL), 37, 110
Posterior shoulder dislocation (PSD)
anatomical lesions, 36, 145
anterior-posterior (drawer test), 149
arthroscopic treatment, 42–43
ASES criteria, 44
athletes, unidirectional, 44
bone abnormalities, 145
bone repair procedures, 159
capsular laxity, 147
capsulolabral and posterior glenoid lesions, 147, 158
and chronic locked anterior dislocation, 277–282
classification, 143
clinical evaluation, 38, 143, 149–150
constitutional morphological anomalies, 158
DASH scores, 45
diagnosis, 143
etiology, 36
glenoid chondrolabral and bony version, 146
imaging, 37–38
isolated posterior capsular plication, 166
Jerk Test, 149, 150
Kim lesion, 145, 147, 148
labral flap tear, 147, 148
labrum repair, capsular plication, 166
lesion palpation, 148
LPSD (*see* Locked posterior shoulder dislocation (LPSD))
nonoperative treatment, 38
open procedures, bone deficiency, 43–44
overhead athletes (throwers), 37–38
pathoanatomy, 37
pathogenesis, 144–145
pediatric athletes, 45
physical examination
circumduction test, 37
jerk test, 37
Kim test, 38–39
O'Brien's active compression test, 38
physical therapy, 158, 167
posterior labrum, 37, 38, 147
posterior marginal crack, 147
radiographic examination, 37–38, 150
range of motion, 38
recurrent posterior instability, 144–145
repetitive microtrauma model, 37
rim loading mechanism, 146
rotator interval closure, 166–167
soft tissue repair procedures, 159
surgical treatment
anterior deltopectoral approach, 152–153
arthroscopic/open surgical treatment, 151
bicipital tendon transfer, 151
bone block, 151
capsuloligamentary procedures, 151
deltopectoral approach, Hill-Sachs defect, 155
external rotation deficit, 152
glenoid osteotomy, 151
humeral displacement, 151
humeral impression defect, 155–156
McLaughlin technique, 154
posterior capsular plicature, 151
posterior capsulolabral repair, 151
posterior capsulorrhaphy, 151
posterior iliac bone block, 157
reduction, 152
rotational osteotomy, humerus, 156–157
Scott technique, 151
stabilization, 153
subscapularis tendon transfer, 154
therapeutic strategy, 151, 152
total shoulder arthroplasty, 157–158
therapeutic strategy, 144
traumatic posterior dislocation, 144
tuberosity fractures, 37
Proximal *vs.* distal biceps tenodesis. *See* Biceps tenodesis, proximal *vs.* distal

**R**
Repetitive microtrauma model, posterior instability, 11, 36, 37, 110
Reverse Bankart repair, 37, 151, 153, 158, 164, 165
Reverse shoulder arthroplasty (RSA), 257, 274
Rotator cuff tears (RCT)
  acute, primary traumatic dislocation
    anatomy, 244–245
    cuff repair, 244
    diagnosis, 245
    operation, 244
    physical therapy, 245
    primary traumatic dislocation, 243–244
    rehabilitation protocols, 245
    rotator cuff tear and dislocation, 243
    surgical repair, 245, 246
    treatment, 244
  anatomy, 184
  belly press test, 24
  and brachial plexus injuries (*see* Suprascapular nerve lesions (SSN))
  cadaver model, 184
  chronic dislocation
    anterior dislocation mechanism, 248
    biomechanics, 247–248
    capsulo-labral lesions, older patients, 248
    concavity-compression mechanism, 247
    conservative treatment, 249
    functional impairments, 247
    isolated supraspinatus tendon tear, 247
    nerve injuries, concomitant, 248–249
    pre-existing rotator cuff tear, 248
    therapeutic regimen, 249
  complications, 287
  dynamic stabilizers, 183
  external rotation test, 24
  glenohumeral stability, 184
  indications, surgery, 184–185
  manual scapular retraction, 24
  morbidity, 184
  pathological findings, 184
  patient age, 283
  rehabilitation, 287
  SSN lesions
    anatomy, 284
    clinical examination, 284–285
    cross-arm adduction test, 285
    diagnostic injections, 285
    endoscopic release, spinoglenoid notch, 285–286
    indications, 285
    transverse scapular ligament, 286–287
  supraspinatus isolation test, 24
  supraspinatus stress test, 24
  traumatic supraspinatus tears, 183
  Whipple test, 24
RSA. *See* Reverse shoulder arthroplasty (RSA)

**S**
Scott technique, 151
Snyder classification, SLAP, 187, 190–192
Subacromial impingement syndrome, 37
Subpectoral biceps tenodesis, 198, 203, 207
Subscapularis tears
  anatomy, 221
  belly-press test, 219
  biceps tendon lesions, 221
  chronic and retracted, 221
  clinical presentation, 218–219
  double-row knotless repair, 222, 223
  extrinsic causes of degeneration, 218
  imaging modality, 219–220
  mobilization techniques, 221, 222
  nonoperative treatment, 220
  operative treatment, 220
  pathophysiology, 218
  physical examination, 219
  physical therapy, 220
  postoperative rehabilitation, 223
  preoperative isokinetic testing, 219
  and shoulder stability, 218
  superolateral aspect, 217
Superior labrum anterior-posterior (SLAP)
  activity-related pain, 198
  anatomy
    glenoid cavity, 188
    superior labrum complex vasculature, 188
    variations, labral complex, 188
  anteroinferior labral tear, 187
  biceps fibers, 189
  biceps tenodesis, 198, 199
  biomechanics, 189–190
  cadaveric and arthroscopic studies, 187
  classification
    Bucket handle injury, 191, 192
    lip fibrillation, 191, 192
    Maffet-Morgan modification, 191, 193
    upper lip/biceps glenoid detachment, 191, 192
  clinical history, 194
  management, 199
  mechanism of trauma, 190
  nonoperative treatment, 194
  operative treatment
    anterior shoulder instability, 196
    Bankart lesion, 195
    Bankart reconstruction, 196
    open/arthroscopic biceps tenodesis, 197
    pathoanatomy repair, 195
    superior labral detachment, 194–195
    tenodesis, 196
    trans-rotator cuff portals, 197

patient age, 198
physical exam, 194
postoperative treatment, 197
radiological evaluation, 194
Suprascapular nerve (SSN) lesions
anatomy, 284, 295
clinical examination, 284–285
cross-arm adduction test, 285
diagnostic injections, 285
endoscopic release
spinoglenoid notch, 285–286
transverse scapular ligament, 286–287
graft positioning, 138
indication, 285
treatment algorithms, 284
Supraspinatus isolation test, 24
Supraspinatus stress test, 24
Surgical bone repair procedures
acromial bone block, vascularized deltoid pedicle, 161–162
glenoid osteotomy, 162–163
iliac crest graft, 161
posterior iliac bone block
arthroscopic, 160
by open surgery, 159–160
Surgical soft tissue repair procedures, 88, 103, 144, 159, 164, 180. *See also* Arthroscopic soft tissue repair

**T**
Thermal capsulorrhaphy, 293
Thoracic outlet syndrome, positional/postural, 24
Total shoulder arthroplasty (TSA), 157–158, 255–257, 272, 274

**W**
Whipple test, 24

**Y**
Young patient, shoulder instability. *See* Adolescent shoulder stabilization

Printed by Printforce, the Netherlands